Preface

This concise review of medical pharmacology is designed for medical students, dental students, and others in the health care professions. It is intended primarily to help students prepare for licensing examinations, such as the United States Medical Licensing Examination Step 1 (USMLE) and other similar examinations. This book presents condensed and succinct descriptions of relevant and current Board-driven information pertaining to pharmacology without the usual associated details. It is not meant to be a substitute for the comprehensive presentation of information and difficult concepts found in standard pharmacology texts.

ORGANIZATION

The sixth edition begins with a chapter devoted to the general principles of drug action, followed by chapters concerned with drugs acting on the major body systems. Other chapters discuss autocoids, ergots, anti-inflammatory and immunosuppressive agents, drugs used to treat anemias and disorders of hemostasis, infectious diseases, cancer, and toxicology.

Each chapter includes a presentation of specific drugs with a discussion of their general properties, mechanism of action, pharmacologic effects, therapeutic uses, and adverse effects. A drug list, tables, and figures summarize essential drug information included in all chapters.

Clinically oriented, USMLE-style review questions and answers with explanations follow each chapter to help students assess their understanding of the information. Similarly, a comprehensive examination consisting of USMLE-style questions is included at the end of the book. This examination serves as a self-assessment tool to help students determine their fund of knowledge and diagnose any weaknesses in pharmacology.

Key Features

- Updated with current drug information
- End-of-chapter review tests feature updated USMLE-style questions
- Four-color tables and figures summarize essential information for quick recall
- Updated drug lists for each chapter
- Additional USMLE-style comprehensive examination questions and explanations

Gary C. Rosenfeld, PhD
David S. Loose, PhD

Acknowledgments

The authors acknowledge and thank our colleagues for their support and contributions to this book and our medical students for being our harshest critics.

Our special thanks to the following UT Medical students who reviewed the previous version of this book and offered many helpful suggestions towards this edition: Michael Arriaga, Mark A Barros, Jason S Bluth, John R Burleson, Sean B Bury, Samuel W Carson, Zachary R Compton, Andrew J Coyne, David B Doherty, Brittany L Duyka, Lisa M Evans, Azure G Greeson, Stephen A Herrmann, Hans B Heymann, Ari J Hyman, Jonathon S Jundt, Jacob A Mccoy, Elisabeth W Netherton, Alexander Reskallah, Reem Sabouni, Brittany L Sambrano, Madeleine B Samuelson, David J Savage, Yusra Siddiqui, Sara E Slabisak, Katherine A Smith, Agathe K Streiff, and Annise G Wilson.

BOARD REVIEW SERIES

Pharmacology

SIXTH EDITION

Gary C. Rosenfeld, PhD

Professor
Department of Integrated Biology and Pharmacology and
Graduate School of Biomedical Sciences
Assistant Dean for Education Programs
University of Texas Medical School at Houston
Houston, Texas

David S. Loose, PhD

Associate Professor
Department of Integrated Biology and Pharmacology and
Graduate School of Biomedical Sciences
University of Texas Medical School at Houston
Houston, Texas

Wolters Kluwer | Lippincott Williams & Wilkins
Health

Philadelphia · Baltimore · New York · London
Buenos Aires · Hong Kong · Sydney · Tokyo

Acquisitions Editor: *Sirkka Howes*
Product Manager: *Catherine Noonan*
Marketing Manager: *Joy Fisher-Williams*
Vendor Manager: *Bridgett Dougherty*
Manufacturing Coordinator: *Margie Orzech*
Design Coordinator: *Holly McLaughlin*
Compositor: *Integra Software Services Pvt. Ltd.*

Sixth Edition

351 West Camden Street
Baltimore, MD 21201

Two Commerce Square
2001 Market Street
Philadelphia, PA 19103

Printed in China

9 8 7 6 5 4 3 2 1

Library of Congress Cataloging-in-Publication Data

Rosenfeld, Gary C.
  Pharmacology / Gary C. Rosenfeld, David S. Loose. — 6th ed.
     p. ; cm. — (Board review series)
  Includes index.
  ISBN 978-1-4511-7535-6
  I. Loose, David S. II. Title. III. Series: Board review series.
  [DNLM: 1. Pharmacological Phenomena—Examination Questions. 2. Pharmaceutical Preparations—
Examination Questions. QV 18.2]
  RM301.13
  615'.1076—dc23

                                                                                    2013013307

DISCLAIMER

Care has been taken to confirm the accuracy of the information present and to describe generally accepted practices. However, the authors, editors, and publisher are not responsible for errors or omissions or for any consequences from application of the information in this book and make no warranty, expressed or implied, with respect to the currency, completeness, or accuracy of the contents of the publication. Application of this information in a particular situation remains the professional responsibility of the practitioner; the clinical treatments described and recommended may not be considered absolute and universal recommendations.

The authors, editors, and publisher have exerted every effort to ensure that drug selection and dosage set forth in this text are in accordance with the current recommendations and practice at the time of publication. However, in view of ongoing research, changes in government regulations, and the constant flow of information relating to drug therapy and drug reactions, the reader is urged to check the package insert for each drug for any change in indications and dosage and for added warnings and precautions. This is particularly important when the recommended agent is a new or infrequently employed drug.

Some drugs and medical devices presented in this publication have Food and Drug Administration (FDA) clearance for limited use in restricted research settings. It is the responsibility of the health care provider to ascertain the FDA status of each drug or device planned for use in their clinical practice.

To purchase additional copies of this book, call our customer service department at **(800) 638-3030** or fax orders to **(301) 223-2320**. International customers should call **(301) 223-2300**.

Visit Lippincott Williams & Wilkins on the Internet: http://www.lww.com. Lippincott Williams & Wilkins customer service representatives are available from 8:30 am to 6:00 pm, EST.

BOARD RE

Pharmacology

SIXTH EDITION

Contents

chapter 1

General Principles of Drug Action

I. DOSE–RESPONSE RELATIONSHIPS

A. **Drug effects** are produced by altering the normal functions of cells and tissues in the body via one of the four general mechanisms:
1. *Interaction with receptors,* naturally occurring target macromolecules that mediate the effects of endogenous physiologic substances such as neurotransmitters and hormones.
   a. Figure 1.1 illustrates the four major classes of drug–receptor interactions, using specific examples of endogenous ligands.
      (1) **Ligand-activated ion channels.** Figure 1.1A illustrates acetylcholine interacting with a nicotinic receptor that is a nonspecific Na^+/K^+ transmembrane ion channel. Interaction of a molecule of acetylcholine with each subunit of the channel produces a conformational change that permits the passage of Na^+ and K^+. Other channels that are targets for various drugs include specific Ca^{2+} and K^+ channels.
      (2) **G-protein–coupled receptors** (Fig. 1.1B–D). G-protein–coupled receptors compose the largest class of receptors. All the receptors have seven transmembrane segments, three intracellular loops, and an intracellular carboxy-terminal tail. The biologic activity of the receptors is mediated via interaction with a number of G (GTP binding) proteins.
         (a) **$G\alpha_s$-coupled receptors.** Figure 1.1B illustrates a β-adrenoceptor, which when activated by ligand binding (e.g., epinephrine) exchanges GDP for GTP. This facilitates the migration of $G\alpha_s$ ($G\alpha_{stimulatory}$) and its interaction with adenylyl cyclase (AC). $G\alpha_s$-bound AC catalyzes the production of cyclic AMP (cAMP) from adenosine triphosphate (ATP); cAMP activates protein kinase A, which subsequently acts to phosphorylate and activate a number of effector proteins. The βγ dimer may also activate some effectors. Hydrolysis of the guanosine triphosphate (GTP) bound to the Gα to guanosine diphosphate (GDP) terminates the signal.
         (b) **$G\alpha_i$ ($G_{inhibitory}$)-coupled receptors** (Fig. 1.1C). Ligand binding (e.g., somatostatin) to $G\alpha_i$ ($G\alpha_{inhibitory}$)-coupled receptors similarly exchanges GTP for GDP, but $G\alpha_i$ inhibits AC, leading to reduced cAMP production.
         (c) **G_q (and G_{11})-coupled receptors** (Fig. 1.1D). G_q (and G_{11}) interact with ligand (e.g., serotonin)-activated receptors and increase the activity of phospholipase C (PLC). PLC cleaves the membrane phospholipid phosphatidylinositol 4,5-bisphosphate (PIP_2) to diacylglycerol (DAG) and inositol 1,4,5-triphosphate (IP_3). DAG activates protein kinase C, which can subsequently phosphorylate and activate a number of cellular proteins; IP_3 causes the release of Ca^{2+} from the endoplasmic reticulum into the cytoplasm, where it can activate many cellular processes.
      (3) **Receptor-activated tyrosine kinases** (Fig. 1.1E). Many growth-related signals (e.g., insulin) are mediated via membrane receptors that possess intrinsic tyrosine kinase activity as illustrated for the insulin receptor. Ligand binding

FIGURE 1.1. Four major classes of drug–receptor interactions, with specific examples of endogenous ligands. **A.** Acetylcholine interaction with a nicotinic receptor, a ligand-activated ion channel. **B–D.** G-protein–coupled receptors. **B.** Epinephrine interaction with a $G\alpha_s$-coupled β-adrenoceptor. **C.** Somatostatin interaction with a $G\alpha_i$ ($G_{inhibitory}$)-coupled receptor. **D.** Serotonin interaction with a G_q (and G_{11})-coupled receptor. **E.** Insulin interaction with a receptor-activated tyrosine kinase. **F.** Cortisol interaction with an intracellular nuclear receptor.

causes conformational changes in the receptor; some receptor tyrosine kinases are monomers that dimerize upon ligand binding. The liganded receptors then autophosphorylate tyrosine residues, which recruit cytoplasmic proteins to the plasma membrane where they are also tyrosine phosphorylated and activated.

(4) **Intracellular nuclear receptors** (Fig. 1.1F). Ligands (e.g., cortisol) for nuclear receptors are lipophilic and can diffuse rapidly through the plasma membrane. In the absence of ligand, nuclear receptors are inactive because of their interaction with chaperone proteins such as heat-shock proteins like HSP-90. Binding of ligand promotes structural changes in the receptor that facilitate dissociation of

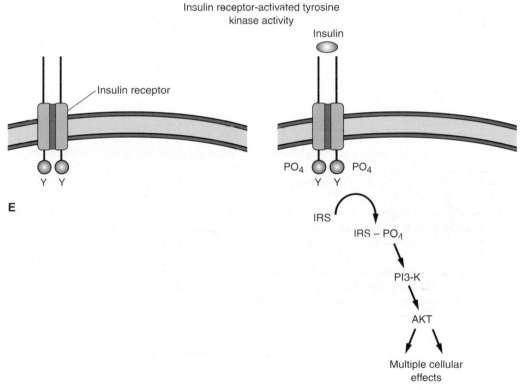

FIGURE 1.1. (*continued*).

chaperones, entry of receptors into the nucleus, hetero- or homodimerization of receptors, and high-affinity interaction with the DNA of target genes. DNA-bound nuclear receptors are able to recruit a diverse number of proteins called coactivators, which subsequently act to increase transcription of the target gene.

2. ***Alteration of the activity of enzymes*** by activation or inhibition of the enzyme's catalytic activity.

3. ***Antimetabolite action*** in which the drug, acting as a nonfunctional analog of a naturally occurring metabolite, interferes with normal metabolism.

4. ***Nonspecific chemical or physical interactions*** such as those caused by antacids, osmotic agents, and chelators.

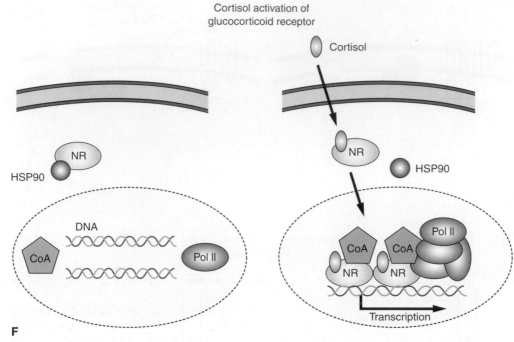

F

FIGURE 1.1. (*continued*).

B. **The graded dose–response curve** expresses an individual's response to increasing doses of a given drug. The magnitude of a pharmacologic response is proportional to the number of receptors with which a drug effectively interacts (Fig. 1.2). The graded dose–response curve includes the following parameters:

1. ***Magnitude of response*** is graded; that is, it continuously increases with the dose up to the maximal capacity of the system, and it is often depicted as a function of the logarithm of the dose administered (to see the relationship over a wide range of doses).

2. ***ED_{50}*** is the dose that produces the half-maximal response; the threshold dose is that which produces the first noticeable effect.

3. ***Intrinsic activity*** is the ability of a drug once bound to activate the receptor.
   a. **Agonists** are drugs capable of binding to, and activating, a receptor.
      (1) **Full agonists** occupy receptors to cause maximal activation; intrinsic activity = 1.

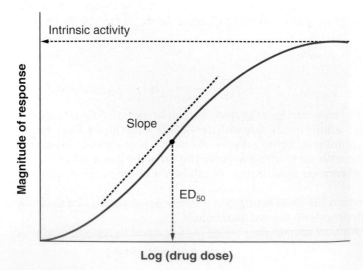

FIGURE 1.2. Graded dose–response curve.

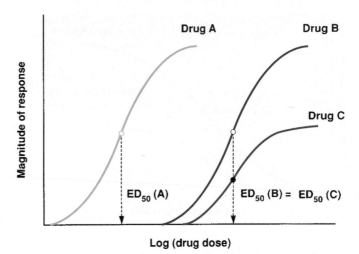

FIGURE 1.3. Graded dose–response curves for two agonists (**A** and **B**) and a partial agonist (**C**).

(2) **Partial agonists** can occupy receptors but cannot elicit a maximal response. Such drugs have an intrinsic activity of <1 (Fig. 1.3; drug C).

  b. **Antagonists** bind to the receptor but do not initiate a response; that is, they block the action of an agonist or endogenous substance that works through the receptor.

    (1) **Competitive antagonists** combine with the same site on the receptor but their binding does not activate the receptor (i.e., their intrinsic activity = 0) so they have no efficacy *per se* but may cause a pharmacological response in some cases by inhibiting the actions of endogenous substances or other drugs. Competitive antagonists may be reversible or irreversible. Reversible, or equilibrium, competitive antagonists are not covalently bound, shift the dose–response curve for the agonist to the right, and increase the ED_{50}; that is, more agonist is required to elicit a response in the presence of the antagonist (Fig. 1.4). Because higher doses of agonist can overcome the inhibition, the maximal response can still be obtained.

    (2) **Noncompetitive antagonists** bind to the receptor at a site other than the agonist-binding site (Fig. 1.5) and either prevent the agonist from binding correctly or prevent it from activating the receptor. Consequently, the effective amount of receptor is reduced. Receptors unoccupied by antagonist retain the same affinity for agonist, and the ED_{50} is unchanged.

  4. *Potency of a drug* is the relative measure of the amount of a drug required to produce a specified level of response (e.g., 50%) compared with other drugs that produce the same effect via the same receptor mechanism. The potency of a drug is determined by the **affinity** of a drug for its receptor and the amount of administered drug that reaches the

FIGURE 1.4. Graded dose–response curves illustrating the effects of competitive antagonists.

FIGURE 1.5. Graded dose–response curves illustrating the effects of non-competitive antagonists.

receptor site. The relative potency of a drug can be demonstrated by comparing the ED_{50} values of two full agonists; the drug with the lower ED_{50} is more potent. (For example, in Fig. 1.3, drug A is more potent than drug B.)

5. *The efficacy of a drug* is the ability of a drug to elicit the pharmacologic response. Efficacy may be affected by such factors as the number of drug–receptor complexes formed, the ability of the drug to activate the receptor once it is bound (i.e., the drug's intrinsic activity), and the status of the target organ or cell.

6. *Slope* is measured at the mid-portion of the dose–response curve. The slope varies for different drugs and different responses. Steep dose–response curves indicate that a small change in dose produces a large change in response.

7. *Variability* reflects the differences between individuals in response to a given drug.

8. *Therapeutic index (TI)* relates the desired therapeutic effect to undesired toxicity; it is determined using data provided by the quantal dose–response curve. The TI is defined as TD_{50}/ED_{50} (i.e., the ratio of the dose that produces a toxic effect in half of the population to the dose that produces the desired effect in half of the population). Note that the TI should be used with caution in instances when the quantal dose–response curves for the desired and toxic effects are not parallel.

C. **The quantal dose–response curve** (Fig. 1.6A and B) relates the dosage of a drug to the frequency with which a designated response will occur within a population. The response may be an "all-or-none" phenomenon (e.g., individuals either do or do not fall asleep after receiving a sedative) or some predetermined intensity of effect. The quantal dose–response curve is obtained via transformation of the data used for a frequency distribution plot to reflect the cumulative frequency of a response. In the context of the quantal dose–response curve, ED_{50} indicates the dose of a drug that produces the response in half of the population. (Note that this differs from the meaning of ED_{50} in a graded dose–response curve.) For example, in Figure 1.6B, the ED_{50} would be 1. The TD_{50} for a drug would be determined from the midpoint of a similar curve indicating the cumulative percent of the population showing a toxic response to a drug.

II. DRUG ABSORPTION

Drug absorption is the movement of a drug from its site of administration into the bloodstream. In many cases, a drug must be transported across one or more biologic membranes to reach the bloodstream.

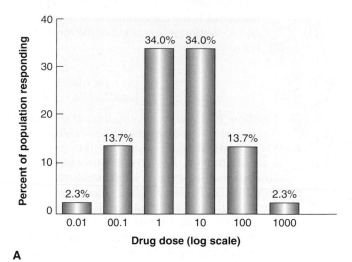

FIGURE 1.6. **A.** Frequency distribution plot. Number of individuals (as percentage of the population) who require the indicated drug dose to exhibit an identical response. As illustrated, 2.3% of the population require 0.01 units to exhibit the response, 13.7% require 0.1 units, and so on. **B.** Quantal dose–response curve. The cumulative number of individuals (as a percentage of the population) who will respond if the indicated dose of drug is administered to the entire population.

A. Drug transport across membranes

1. **Diffusion of unionized drugs** is the most common and most important mode of traversing biologic membranes; drugs diffuse passively down their concentration gradient. Diffusion can be influenced significantly by the lipid-water **partition coefficient** of the drug, which is the ratio of solubility in an organic solvent to solubility in an aqueous solution. In general, absorption increases as lipid solubility (partition coefficient) increases. Other factors that can also influence diffusion include the concentration gradient of the drug across the cell membrane and the surface area of the cell membrane.

2. **Diffusion of drugs that are weak electrolytes**

   a. Only the **unionized** form of a drug can diffuse to any significant degree across biologic membranes.

   b. The degree of ionization of a weak acid or base is determined by the pK of the drug and pH of its environment according to the **Henderson-Hasselbalch equation.**

      (1) For a weak acid, A,

$$HA \rightleftarrows H^+ + A^-,$$
$$pH = pK + \log[A^-]/[HA], \text{ and}$$
$$\log[A^-]/[HA] = pH - pK$$

where HA is the concentration of the protonated, or unionized, form of the acid and A^- is the concentration of the ionized, or unprotonated, form.

(2) For a weak base, B,

$$BH^+ \rightleftarrows H^+ + B,$$
$$pH = pK + \log[B]/[BH^+], \text{ and}$$
$$\log[B]/[BH^+] = pH - pK$$

where BH^+ is the concentration of the protonated form of the base and B is the concentration of the unprotonated form.

c. When the pK of a drug equals the pH of the surroundings, 50% ionization occurs; that is, equal numbers of ionized and unionized species are present. A lower pK reflects a stronger acid; a higher pK corresponds to a stronger base.

d. Drugs with different pK values will diffuse across membranes at different rates.

e. The pH of the biologic fluid in which the drug is dissolved affects the degree of ionization and, therefore, the rate of drug transport.

f. **Ion trapping** occurs when a drug that is a weak acid or weak base moves between fluid compartments with different pHs, for example, when a drug given orally is absorbed from the stomach contents (with a pH of 1 to 2) to plasma with a pH of 7.4. The drug will tend to accumulate in the fluid compartment in which it is most highly ionized, i.e., **weak acids will tend to accumulate in the fluid with the higher pH and weak bases in the fluid with the lower pH**.

3. *Active transport* is an energy-dependent process that can move drugs against a concentration gradient, as in **protein-mediated transport systems.** Active transport occurs in only one direction and is saturable. It is usually the mode of transport for drugs that resemble actively transported endogenous substances such as sugars, amino acids, and nucleosides. Some transport systems may increase drug transport and the entry into cells and increase their effects. Other transport systems cause active efflux of drugs from target cells and decrease their activity, e.g., P-glycoprotein which is also known as ABCB1 (ABC = ATP-binding cassette) or MDR1 (MDR = multi-drug resistance).

4. *Filtration* is the bulk flow of solvent and solute through channels (pores) in the membrane. Filtration is seen with small molecules (usually with a molecular weight <100) that can pass through pores. Some substances of greater molecular weight, such as certain proteins, can be filtered through intercellular channels. Concentration gradients affect the rate of filtration.

5. *Facilitated diffusion* is movement of a substance down a concentration gradient. Facilitated diffusion is carrier-mediated, specific, and saturable; it does not require energy.

B. Routes of administration

1. *Oral administration* is the most convenient, economical, and common route of administration; it is generally safe for most drugs.

   a. Sites of absorption

   (1) Stomach

   (a) Lipid-soluble drugs and **weak acids,** which are normally unionized at the low pH (1 to 2) of gastric contents, may be absorbed directly from the stomach.

   (b) Weak bases and **strong acids** (pK = 2 to 3) are not normally absorbed from this site since they tend to exist as ions that carry either a positive or negative charge, respectively.

   (2) Small intestine

   (a) The small intestine is the **primary site of absorption** of most drugs because of the very large surface area across which drugs, including partially ionized weak acids and bases, may diffuse.

   (b) Acids are normally absorbed more extensively from the small intestine than from the stomach, even though the intestine has a higher pH (approximately 5).

b. The **bioavailability of a drug** is the fraction of drug (administered by any route) that reaches the bloodstream unaltered (bioavailability = 1 for intravenous administration). Bioequivalence refers to the condition in which the plasma concentration versus time profiles of two drug formulations are identical.

   (1) The **first-pass effect** influences drug absorption by metabolism in the liver or by biliary secretion. After absorption from the stomach or small intestine, a drug must pass through the liver before reaching the general circulation and its target site. If the capacity of liver metabolic enzymes to inactivate the drug is great, only limited amounts of active drug will escape the process. Some drugs are metabolized so extensively as a result of hepatic metabolism during the first pass that it precludes their use.

   (2) **Other factors** that may alter absorption from the stomach or small intestine include the following:

   (a) Gastric emptying time and passage of drug to the intestine may be influenced by **gastric contents** and **intestinal motility.** A decreased emptying time generally decreases the rate of absorption because the intestine is the major absorptive site for most orally administered drugs.

   (b) **Gastrointestinal (GI) blood flow** plays an important role in drug absorption by continuously maintaining the concentration gradient across epithelial membranes. The absorption of small, very lipid-soluble molecules is "blood flow limited," whereas highly polar molecules are "blood flow independent."

   (c) **Stomach acid** and inactivating enzymes may destroy certain drugs. Enteric coating prevents breakdown of tablets by the acid pH of the stomach.

   (d) **Interactions** with food, other drugs, and other constituents of the gastric milieu may influence absorption.

   (e) **Inert ingredients** in oral preparations or the special formulation of those preparations may alter absorption.

2. *Parenteral administration* includes three major routes: **intravenous (IV), intramuscular (IM),** and **subcutaneous (SC).** Parenteral administration generally results in more predictable bioavailability than oral administration.

   a. With **IV** administration, the drug is injected directly into the bloodstream (100% bioavailable). It represents the most rapid means of introducing drugs into the body and is particularly useful in the treatment of emergencies when absolute control of drug administration is essential.

   b. After **IM** and **SC** administration, many drugs can enter the capillaries directly through "pores" between endothelial cells. Depot preparations for sustained release may be administered by IM or SC routes, but some preparations may cause irritation and pain.

3. *Other routes of administration*

   a. **Inhalation** results in **rapid absorption** because of the large surface area and rich blood supply of the alveoli. Inhalation is frequently used for gaseous anesthetics, but it is generally not practical. Inhalation may be useful for drugs that act on the airways, such as epinephrine and glucocorticoids, which are used to treat bronchial asthma.

   b. **Sublingual administration** is useful for drugs with **high first-pass metabolism,** such as **nitroglycerin,** since hepatic metabolism is bypassed.

   c. **Intrathecal administration** is useful for drugs that do not readily cross the blood–brain barrier.

   d. **Rectal administration** minimizes first-pass metabolism and may be used to circumvent the nausea and vomiting that sometimes result from oral administration. The use of rectal administration may be limited by inconvenience or patient noncompliance.

   e. **Topical administration** is used widely when a local effect is desired or to **minimize systemic effects,** especially in dermatology and ophthalmology. Preparations must be nonirritating. Note that drugs administered topically may sometimes produce systemic effects.

III. DRUG DISTRIBUTION

Drug distribution is the movement of a drug from the bloodstream to the various tissues of the body.

A. **Distribution of drugs** is the process by which a drug leaves the bloodstream and enters the extracellular fluids and tissues. A drug must diffuse across cellular membranes if its site of action is intracellular. In this case, lipid solubility is important for effective distribution.
   1. *Importance of blood flow*
      a. In most tissues, drugs can leave the circulation readily by diffusion across or between capillary endothelial cells. Thus, the **initial rate of distribution** of a drug **depends heavily on blood flow** to various organs (brain, liver, kidney > muscle, skin > fat, bone).
      b. At **equilibrium,** or **steady state,** the amount of drug in an organ is related to the mass of the organ and its properties, as well as to the properties of the specific drug.
   2. *Volume of distribution (V_d)* is the **volume of total body fluid** into which a drug "appears" to distribute after it reaches equilibrium in the body. Volume of distribution is determined by administering a known dose of drug (expressed in units of mass) intravenously and measuring the initial plasma concentration (expressed in units of mass/volume):

      V_d = amount of drug administered (mg)/initial plasma concentration (mg/L)

      Volume of distribution is expressed in units of volume. In most cases, the "initial" plasma concentration, C_0, is determined by extrapolation from the elimination phase (see VII).
      a. **Standard values** of volumes of fluid compartments in an average 70-kg adult are as follows: plasma = 3 L; extracellular fluid = 12 L; and total body water = 41 L.
      b. **Features** of volume of distribution:
         (1) **V_d values** for most drugs do **not** represent their **actual distribution** in bodily fluids. The use of V_d values is primarily conceptual; that is, drugs that distribute extensively have relatively large V_d values and vice versa.
         (2) A very low V_d value may indicate extensive plasma protein binding of the drug. A very high value may indicate that the drug is extensively bound to tissue sites.
         (3) Among other variables, V_d may be **influenced by age, sex, weight,** and **disease processes** (e.g., edema, ascites).
   3. *Drug redistribution* describes when the relative distribution of a drug in different tissues or fluid compartments of the body changes with time. This is usually seen with highly lipophilic drugs such as **thiopental** that initially enter tissues with high blood flow (e.g., the brain) and then quickly redistribute to tissues with lower blood flow (e.g., skeletal muscle and adipose tissue).
   4. *Barriers to drug distribution*
      a. Blood–brain barrier
         (1) Because of the nature of the blood–brain barrier, **ionized** or **polar drugs distribute poorly to the CNS,** including certain chemotherapeutic agents and toxic compounds, because they must pass through, rather than between, endothelial cells.
         (2) **Inflammation,** such as that resulting from meningitis, may increase the ability of ionized, poorly soluble drugs to cross the blood–brain barrier.
         (3) The blood–brain barrier may not be fully developed at the time of birth.
      b. Placental barrier
         (1) **Lipid-soluble drugs** cross the placental barrier more easily than polar drugs; drugs with a molecular weight of <600 pass the placental barrier better than larger molecules.
         (2) The possibility that drugs administered to the mother may cross the placenta and reach the fetus is always an important consideration in therapy.
         (3) Drug transporters (e.g., the **P-glycoprotein transporter**) transfer drugs out of the fetus.

B. **Binding of drugs by plasma proteins.** Drugs in the plasma may exist in the free form or may be bound to plasma proteins or other blood components, such as red blood cells.

1. *General features of plasma protein binding*

   a. The extent of plasma protein binding is **highly variable** and ranges from virtually 0% to more than 99% bound, depending on the specific drug. Binding is generally reversible.

   b. Only the **free drug is small enough to pass through the spaces between the endothelial cells that form the capillaries;** extensive binding retards the rate at which the drug reaches its site of action and may prolong duration of action.

   c. Some plasma proteins bind many different drugs, whereas other proteins bind only one or a limited number. For example, **serum albumin tends to bind many acidic drugs, whereas** α_1-acid glycoprotein tends to bind many basic drugs.

   d. There are few, if any, documented changes in a drug's effect due to changes in plasma protein binding.

IV. DRUG ELIMINATION AND TERMINATION OF ACTION

A. **Mechanisms of drug elimination and termination of action**

1. In most cases, the action of a drug is terminated by **enzyme-catalyzed conversion** to an inactive (or less active) compound and/or **elimination from the body** via the kidney or other routes.

2. Redistribution of drugs from the site of action may terminate the action of a drug, although this occurs infrequently. For example, the action of the anesthetic **thiopental** is terminated largely by its redistribution from the brain (where it initially accumulates as a result of its high lipid solubility and the high blood flow to that organ) to the more poorly perfused adipose tissue.

B. **Rate of drug elimination from the body**

1. *First-order elimination.* The elimination of most drugs at therapeutic doses is "first-order," where **a constant fraction of drug is eliminated per unit time**; that is, the rate of elimination depends on the concentration of drug in the plasma and is equal to the plasma concentration of the drug multiplied by a **proportionality constant:**

   $$\text{Rate of elimination from body (mass/time)} = \text{Constant} \times [\text{Drug}]_{\text{plasma}}(\text{mass/vol})$$

   Because the rate of elimination is given in units of mass/time and concentration is in units of mass/volume, the units of the constant are volume/time. This constant is referred to as the "clearance" of the drug (see IV C).

2. *Zero-order kinetics.* Infrequently, the rate of elimination of a drug is "zero-order," where **a constant amount of drug is eliminated per unit time.** In this case, the mechanism by which the body eliminates the drug (e.g., metabolism by hepatic enzymes, active secretion in the kidney) is saturated. The rate of drug elimination from the body is thus **constant** and does **not depend on plasma concentration.**

C. **Clearance (CL).** Conceptually, clearance is a measure of the capacity of the body to remove a drug. Mathematically, clearance is the proportionality constant that relates the rate of drug elimination to the plasma concentration of the drug. Thus, drugs with "high" clearance are rapidly removed from the body, and drugs with "low" clearance are removed slowly. As noted in IV B, the units of clearance are volume/time.

1. *Specific organ clearance* is the capacity of an individual organ to eliminate a drug. Specific organ clearance may be due to metabolism (e.g., "hepatic clearance" by the liver) or excretion (e.g., "renal clearance" by elimination in the urine).

   $$\text{Rate of elimination by organ} = \text{CL}_{\text{organ}} \times [\text{Drug}]_{\text{plasma perfusing organ}}$$

or

$$CL_{organ} = \text{Rate of elimination by organ}/[Drug]_{plasma\ perfusing\ organ}$$

2. ***Whole body clearance*** is the capacity of the body to eliminate the drug by all mechanisms. Therefore, whole body clearance is equal to the sum of all of the specific organ clearance mechanisms by which the active drug is eliminated from the body:

$$CL_{whole\ body} = CL_{organ\ 1} + CL_{organ\ 2} + CL_{organ\ N}$$

The term "clearance" generally refers to whole body clearance unless otherwise specified. In this case,

$$\text{Rate of elimination from body} = CL_{whole\ body} \times [Drug]_{plasma}$$

and

$$CL = \text{Rate of elimination from body}/[Drug]_{plasma}$$

3. ***Plasma clearance*** is numerically the same as whole body clearance, but this terminology is sometimes used because clearance may be viewed as the volume of plasma that contains the amount of drug removed per unit time (recall that the units of clearance are volume/time). If not specified, this term refers to the volume of plasma "cleared" of drug by all bodily mechanisms (i.e., whole body clearance). The term may also be applied to clearance by specific organs; for example, renal plasma clearance is the volume of plasma containing the amount of drug eliminated in the urine per unit time.

V. BIOTRANSFORMATION (METABOLISM) OF DRUGS

A. **General properties**
1. Biotransformation is a major mechanism for **drug elimination**; most drugs undergo biotransformation, or metabolism, after they enter the body. Biotransformation, which almost always produces metabolites that are more polar than the parent drug, usually terminates the pharmacologic action of the parent drug and, via excretion, increases removal of the drug from the body. However, other consequences are possible, notably after phase I reactions, including similar or different pharmacologic activity, or toxicologic activity.
2. Many drugs undergo several sequential biotransformation reactions. Biotransformation is catalyzed by **specific enzyme systems,** which may also catalyze the metabolism of endogenous substances such as steroid hormones.
3. The liver is the major site of biotransformation, although specific drugs may undergo biotransformation primarily or extensively in other tissues.
4. Biotransformation of drugs is **variable** and can be affected by many parameters, including **prior administration** of the drug in question or of other drugs; **diet; hormonal status; genetics; disease** (e.g., decreased in cardiac and pulmonary disease); **age** and **developmental status** (the very elderly and very young may be more sensitive to drugs, in part, because of decreased or undeveloped levels of drug-metabolizing enzymes); and **liver function** (in cases of severe liver damage, dosage adjustments may be required for drugs eliminated largely via this route).
5. Possible consequences of biotransformation include the production of **inactive metabolites** (most common), metabolites with increased or decreased potencies, metabolites with qualitatively different pharmacologic actions, toxic metabolites, or active metabolites from inactive prodrugs.
6. **Metabolites carry ionizable groups** and are often **more charged and more polar** than the parent compounds. This increased charge may lead to a more rapid rate of clearance because of possible secretion by acid or base carriers in the kidney; it may also lead to decreased tubular reabsorption.

B. Classification of biotransformation reactions

1. *Phase I (nonsynthetic) reactions* involve enzyme-catalyzed biotransformation of the drug without any conjugations. Phase I reactions include **oxidations, reductions,** and **hydrolysis reactions;** they frequently introduce a functional group (e.g., $-OH$) that serves as the active center for sequential conjugation in a phase II reaction.

2. *Phase II (synthetic) reactions* include **conjugation reactions,** which involve the enzyme-catalyzed combination of a drug (or drug metabolite) with an endogenous substance. Phase II reactions require a functional group—an **active center**—as the site of conjugation with the endogenous substance. Phase II reactions require energy indirectly for the synthesis of "activated carriers," the form of the endogenous substance used in the conjugation reaction (e.g., uridine diphosphate-glucuronate).

C. Enzymes catalyzing phase I biotransformation reactions include cytochrome P-450, aldehyde and alcohol dehydrogenase, deaminases, esterases, amidases, and epoxide hydratases. **Enzymes catalyzing phase II biotransformation reactions** include glucuronyl transferase (glucuronide conjugation), sulfotransferase (sulfate conjugation), transacylases (amino acid conjugation), acetylases, ethylases, methylases, and glutathione transferase. These enzymes are present in numerous tissues; some are present in plasma. Subcellular locations include cytosol, mitochondria, and endoplasmic reticulum. Only those enzymes located in the endoplasmic reticulum are inducible by drugs.

1. *Cytochrome P-450 monooxygenase (mixed function oxidase)*

   a. **General features**

      (1) Cytochrome P-450 monooxygenase plays a central role in drug biotransformation. A large number of families (at least 18 in mammals) of cytochrome P-450 (abbreviated as "CYP") enzymes exist, each member of which catalyzes the biotransformation of a unique spectrum of drugs, with some overlap in the substrate specificities. In humans, over 50 individual P-450s have been identified but only about a dozen are involved in the metabolism of most drugs and xenobiotics. This enzyme system is the one most frequently involved in **phase I reactions.**

      (2) The cytochrome P-450 families are referred to using an arabic numeral (e.g., CYP1, CYP2, etc.). Each family has a number of subfamilies denoted by an upper case letter (e.g., CYP2A, CYP2B, etc.). The individual enzymes within each subfamily are denoted by another arabic numeral (e.g., CYP3A1, CYP3A2, etc.). Three sub-families CYP2C, CYP2D, and CYP3A are responsible for metabolism of the majority of clinically used drugs.

      (3) Cytochrome P-450 catalyzes numerous reactions, including aromatic and aliphatic hydroxylations; dealkylation at nitrogen, sulfur, and oxygen atoms; heteroatom oxidations at nitrogen and sulfur atoms; reductions at nitrogen atoms; and ester and amide hydrolysis.

      (4) The **CYP3A** subfamily is responsible for up to half of the total cytochrome P-450 in the liver. **CYP3A4 is the most abundant hepatic enzyme and is involved in the metabolism of over 50% of clinically important drugs.** Drugs or other agents (e.g., components of grapefruit juice) that inhibit this enzyme or induce its levels may cause untoward effects of numerous drugs based upon their altered metabolism that in turn alters plasma and tissue levels via effects on absorption or elimination.

   b. **Localization.** The **primary location** of cytochrome P-450 is the **liver,** which has the greatest specific enzymatic activity and the highest total activity and very significant levels are also found in the small and large intestine. P-450 activity is also found in many other tissues, including the adrenals, ovaries and testis, and tissues involved in steroidogenesis and steroid metabolism. The enzyme's subcellular location is the **endoplasmic reticulum.** Lipid membrane location facilitates the metabolism of lipid-soluble drugs.

   c. Mechanism of reaction

     (1) In the overall reaction, the drug is oxidized and oxygen is reduced to water. Reducing equivalents are provided by **nicotinamide adenine dinucleotide phosphate (NADPH),** and generation of this cofactor is coupled to **cytochrome P-450 reductase.**

     (2) The overall reaction for aromatic hydroxylation can be described as

$$\text{Drug} + O_2 + \text{NADPH} + H^+ \rightarrow \text{Drug} - \text{OH} + \text{NADP}^+ + H_2O$$

   d. Genetic polymorphism of several clinically important cytochrome P-450s, particularly **CYP2C** and **CYP2D,** is a source of variable metabolism in humans, including differences among racial and ethnic groups. These enzymes have substantially different properties (V_{max} or K_m).

   e. Induction

     (1) Induction is brought about by **drugs** and **endogenous substances,** such as hormones. Any given drug preferentially induces one form of cytochrome P-450 or a particular set of P-450s.

     (2) When caused by drugs, induction is pharmacologically important as a major source of **drug interactions.** A drug may induce its own metabolism (metabolic tolerance) and that of other drugs catalyzed by the induced P-450.

     (3) Induction can be caused by a wide variety of clinically useful drugs (**drug–drug interactions**), such as **quinidine, phenytoin, griseofulvin, phenobarbital, troglitazone, omeprazole, rifampin, carbamazepine,** and **St. John's wort,** and by environmental agents such as **tobacco smoke.**

     (4) Some of the same drugs that induce CYP3A4 can induce the drug efflux transporter P-glycoprotein (e.g., **rifampin, St. John's wort**).

   f. Inhibition

     (1) Competitive or noncompetitive (clinically more likely) inhibition of P-450 enzyme activity can result in the **reduced metabolism** of other drugs or endogenous substrates such as **testosterone.**

     (2) Inhibition can be caused by a number of commonly used drugs, including **cimetidine, fluconazole, fluoxetine,** and **erythromycin or environmental or dietary agents (e.g., grapefruit juice),** and is another major source of **drug–drug interactions.**

     (3) Some of the same drugs that inhibit CYP3A4 can inhibit the drug efflux transporter **P-glycoprotein** (e.g., **amiodarone, clarithromycin, erythromycin, ketoconazole**).

 2. *Glucuronyl transferase*

   a. General features

     (1) Glucuronyl transferase is a set of enzymes with unique but overlapping specificities that are involved in **phase II reactions.**

     (2) It catalyzes the conjugation of glucuronic acid to a variety of active centers, including $-$OH, $-$COOH, $-$SH, and $-$NH$_2$.

   b. Location and induction

     (1) Glucuronyl transferase is located in the **endoplasmic reticulum.**

     (2) It is the only phase II reaction that is **inducible by drugs** and is a possible site of drug interactions.

D. Hepatic extraction of drugs. General extraction by the liver occurs because of the liver's large size (1,500 g) and high blood flow (1 mL/g/min).

 1. The **extraction ratio** is the amount of drug removed in the liver divided by the amount of drug entering the organ; a drug completely extracted by the liver would have an extraction ratio of 1. Highly extracted drugs can have a hepatic clearance approaching 1,500 mL/min.

 2. First-pass effect. Drugs taken orally pass across membranes of the GI tract into the portal vein and through the liver before entering the general circulation.

   a. Bioavailability of orally administered drugs is **decreased** by the fraction of drug removed by the first pass through the liver. For example, a drug with a hepatic extraction ratio of 1 would have 0% bioavailability; a drug such as lidocaine, with an extraction ratio of 0.7, would have 30% bioavailability.

b. In the presence of hepatic disease, drugs with a high first-pass extraction may reach the systemic circulation in higher than normal amounts, and dose adjustment may be required.

VI. EXCRETION OF DRUGS

A. Routes of excretion may include urine, feces (e.g., unabsorbed drugs and drugs secreted in bile), saliva, sweat, tears, milk (with possible transfer to neonates), and lungs (e.g., alcohols and anesthetics). Any route may be important for a given drug, but the kidney is the major site of excretion for most drugs.

1. Some drugs are secreted by liver cells into the bile, pass into the intestine, and are eliminated in the feces (e.g., **rifampin, indomethacin, estradiol**).
2. Drugs may be also be reabsorbed from the intestine (i.e., **undergo enterohepatic circulation**). In this manner, the persistence of a drug in the body may be prolonged.

B. Net renal excretion of drugs

1. **Net renal excretion** of drugs is the result of **three separate processes:** the amount of drug filtered at the glomerulus, plus the amount of drug secreted by active transport mechanisms in the kidney, minus the amount of drug passively reabsorbed throughout the tubule.

   a. Filtration

   (1) Most drugs have low molecular weights and are thus freely filtered from the plasma at the glomerulus.

   (2) Serum protein binding reduces filtration because plasma proteins are too large to be filtered.

   (3) The glomerular filtration rate (GFR) is 30%–40% lower during newborns' first year of life than in adults.

   b. Secretion

   (1) The kidney proximal tubule contains **two transport systems** that may secrete drugs into the ultrafiltrate, one for **organic acids** (organic acid transporters or OATs) and a second for **organic bases** (organic base transporters or OBTs). There are multiple OATs and OBTs with specificities for different organic molecules in the tubule. These systems require energy for active transport against a concentration gradient; they are a site for potential **drug–drug interactions** because drugs may compete with each other for binding to the transporters.

   (2) Plasma protein binding does not normally have a large effect on secretion because the affinity of the transport systems for most drugs is greater than the affinity of plasma-binding proteins.

   c. Reabsorption

   (1) Reabsorption may occur throughout the tubule; some compounds, including endogenous compounds such as glucose, are actively reabsorbed.

   (2) Reabsorption of the unionized form of drugs that are weak acids and bases can occur by simple **passive diffusion,** the rate of which depends on the lipid solubility and pK of the drug and also on the concentration gradient of the drug between the urine and the plasma.

   (3) Reabsorption may be affected by **alterations of urinary pH,** which affects elimination of weak acids or bases by altering their ionization (i.e., **ion trapping**—see II.A.f). For example, alkalinization of the urine will result in a higher proportion of the ionized form of an acidic drug that will decrease its reabsorption and hence increase its elimination.

2. **Renal clearance of drugs**

   a. Renal clearance measures the volume of plasma that is cleared of drug per unit time:

   $$CL \text{ (mL/min)} = U \times V/P$$

   where **U** is the concentration of drug per milliliter of **urine, V the volume** of the urine excreted per minute, and **P** the concentration of drug per milliliter of **plasma.**

    (1) A drug excreted by **filtration alone** (e.g., insulin) will have a clearance equal to the GFR (125–130 mL/min).

    (2) A drug excreted by **filtration and complete secretion** (e.g., *para*-aminohippuric acid) will have a clearance equal to renal plasma clearance (650 mL/min).

    (3) Clearance values between 130 and 650 mL/min suggest that a drug is **filtered, secreted, and partially reabsorbed.**

  b. A variety of factors influence renal clearance, including age (some mechanisms of excretion may not be fully developed at the time of birth), other drugs, and disease.

  c. In the presence of **renal failure,** the clearance of a drug may be reduced significantly, resulting in higher plasma levels. For those drugs with a narrow TI, dose adjustment may be required.

VII. PHARMACOKINETICS

Pharmacokinetics describes changes in plasma drug concentration over time. Although it is ideal to determine the amount of drug that reaches its site of action as a function of time after administration, it is usually impractical or not feasible. Therefore, the plasma drug concentration is measured. This provides useful information, because the amount of drug in the tissues is generally related to plasma concentration.

A. Distribution and elimination

  1. *One-compartment model* (Fig. 1.7)

    a. The drug appears to distribute instantaneously after IV administration of a single dose. If the mechanisms for drug elimination, such as biotransformation by hepatic enzymes and renal secretion, are not saturated following the therapeutic dose, a semilog plot of plasma concentration versus time will be **linear.**

    b. Drug elimination is **first order;** that is, a constant fraction of drug is eliminated per unit time. For example, one-half of the drug is eliminated every 8 hours. Elimination of most drugs is a first-order process.

    c. The slope of the semilog plot is $-k$, where k is the rate constant of elimination and has units of time and the intercept on the y axis is C_0 (*Note:* C_0 is used to calculate V_d for drugs that obey a one-compartment model.)

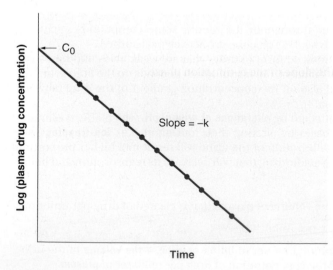

FIGURE 1.7. One-compartment model of drug distribution.

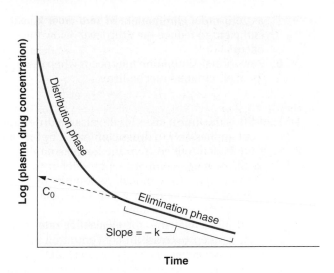

FIGURE 1.8. Two-compartment model of drug distribution.

d. The **plasma drug concentration** (C_t) **relative to the initial concentration (C_0)** at any time (t) after administration is given by

$$\ln C_t = \ln C_0 - kt$$

and the **relationship of the plasma concentrations** at any two points in time is given by

$$\ln C_2 = \ln C_1 - k (t_2 - t_1)$$

2. *Two-compartment model* (Fig. 1.8)
    a. The two-compartment model is a more common model for distribution and elimination of drugs. Initial rapid decreases in the plasma concentration of a drug are observed because of a **distribution phase,** the time required for the drug to reach an equilibrium distribution between a central compartment, such as the plasma space, and a second compartment, such as the aggregate tissues and fluids to which the drug distributes. During this phase, plasma drug concentrations decrease very rapidly because the drug is being eliminated from the body (e.g., by metabolism and renal elimination) and also because the drug is exiting the plasma space as it distributes to other tissues and fluid compartments.
    b. After distribution, a linear decrease in the log drug concentration is observed if the **elimination phase** is first order. The curve is less steep in this phase because there is no longer a net decrease in plasma levels of drug due to distribution to the tissues which has been completed.
    c. For drugs that obey a two-compartment model, the value of C_0 obtained by extrapolation of the elimination phase is used to calculate V_d, and the elimination rate constant, k, is obtained from the slope of the elimination phase.
    d. The expressions for $\ln C_t$ and CL shown above for a one-compartment model also apply during the elimination phase for drugs that obey a two-compartment model.
3. *First-order elimination*
    a. First-order elimination accounts for elimination of most drugs. It refers to the elimination of a constant fraction of drug per unit time; that is, the rate of elimination is a **linear function** of the plasma drug concentration.
    b. First-order elimination occurs when elimination systems are not saturated by the drug.
4. *Zero-order elimination*
    a. In this model, the plot of the log of the plasma concentration versus time will decrease in a concave upward manner, and a constant amount of drug will be eliminated per unit time (e.g., 10 mg of drug will be eliminated every 8 hours). This is referred to

as zero-order elimination, or **zero-order kinetics.** (Note that after an interval of time sufficient to reduce the drug level below the saturation point, first-order elimination occurs.)

   b. Zero-order elimination may occur when therapeutic doses of drugs exceed the capacity of elimination mechanisms.

B. Half-life ($t_{1/2}$)
   1. Half-life is the time it takes for the plasma drug concentration to be reduced by 50%. This concept applies only to drugs eliminated by **first-order kinetics.**
   2. Half-life is determined from the log plasma drug concentration versus time profile for drugs fitting a one-compartment model or from the elimination phase for drugs fitting the two-compartment model. As long as the dose administered does not exceed the capacity of the elimination systems (i.e., the dose does not saturate those systems), the half-life will remain constant.
   3. The half-life is related to the **elimination rate constant (k)** by the equation $t_{1/2} = 0.693/k$, (i.e., for a steep decrease in concentration k is high and $t_{1/2}$ is thus short) and to the **volume of distribution (V_d)** and **clearance (CL)** by the equation $t_{1/2} = 0.693\,V_d/CL$. This relationship emphasizes that drugs that are widely distributed in the body (i.e., a high V_d) will take a long time to be eliminated and drugs for which the body has a high capacity to remove (i.e., a high CL) will take a short time to be eliminated.
   4. For all doses in which first-order elimination occurs, >95% of the drug will be eliminated in a time interval equal to five half-lives. This applies for therapeutic doses of most drugs.

C. Multidose kinetics
   1. *Infusion and multi-dose repeat administration*
      a. If a drug is given by continuous IV infusion at a constant dose rate and elimination is first-order, it will eventually reach a constant steady-state plasma concentration when the rate of elimination becomes equal to the rate of administration.
      b. If a drug that is eliminated by first-order kinetics is administered repeatedly (e.g., one tablet or injection every 8 hours), the *average* plasma concentration of the drug will increase until a *mean* **steady-state** level is reached. (This will not occur for drugs that exhibit zero-order elimination.)
      c. The time required to reach steady state is equal to five half-lives regardless of whether administration is via continuous infusion or repeated administration. **Whenever a dose rate is changed it will take five half-lives for a new steady-state level to be reached** for any route of administration.
   2. *Steady state after repeat administration*
      a. Some fluctuation in plasma concentration will occur even at steady state.
      b. Levels will be at the high point of the steady-state range shortly after a dose is administered; levels will be at the low point immediately before administration of the next dose. Hence, steady state designates an **average plasma concentration** and the range of fluctuations above and below that level.
      c. The magnitude of fluctuations can be controlled by the **dosing interval.** A shorter dosing interval decreases fluctuations, and a longer dosing interval increases them. On cessation of multidose administration, >95% of the drug will be eliminated in a time interval equal to five half-lives if first-order kinetics applies.
   3. *Maintenance dose rate*
      a. Maintenance dose rate is the dose of a drug required per unit time to maintain a desired steady-state level in the plasma to sustain a specific therapeutic effect.
      b. To determine the dose rate required to maintain an average steady-state plasma concentration of drug, multiply the desired plasma concentration by the CL:

$$\text{Maintenance dose rate} = \text{Desired [drug]}_{plasma} \times \text{Clearance (CL)}$$
$$(\text{amount/time}) = (\text{amount/volume}) \times (\text{volume/time})$$

This yields dose rate in units of amount per time (e.g., mg/hour). One may understand this fundamental relationship in the following way: To remain at steady state, the **dose rate must equal the elimination rate;** that is, the rate at which the drug is added to the body must equal the rate at which it is eliminated. Recall that the elimination rate = $CL \times [Drug]_{plasma}$. Therefore, because the dose rate must equal the elimination rate to be at steady state, dose rate also equals $CL \times$ Desired $[drug]_{plasma}$.

   c. If one administers a drug at the maintenance dose rate, a steady-state plasma concentration of the drug will be reached in four to five half-lives. (*Note:* This is four to five half-lives, not four to five doses!).

4. ***Loading dose***
   a. A large loading dose may be needed initially when the therapeutic concentration of a drug in the plasma must be achieved **rapidly** (e.g., a life-threatening situation in which one cannot wait for five half-lives for the drug to reach the desired steady-state level). In this situation one may administer a loading dose.
   b. To calculate the loading dose, select the desired plasma concentration of drug and multiply by the V_d:

$$\text{Loading dose} = \text{Desired } [drug]_{plasma} \times V_d$$
$$\text{(amount or mass)} = \text{(mass/volume)} \times \text{(volume)}$$

   c. After administration of the loading dose (which rapidly achieves the desired plasma concentration of drug), one administers the drug at the maintenance dose rate to maintain the drug concentration at the desired steady-state level.

Review Test

Directions: Each of the numbered items or incomplete statements in this section is followed by answers or by completions of the statement. Select the ONE lettered answer or completion that is BEST in each case.

1. Somatostatin interacts with

(A) G_i-protein–coupled receptor
(B) G_q-protein–coupled receptor
(C) Ligand-activated ion channel
(D) Receptor-activated tyrosine kinase
(E) Intracellular nuclear receptor

2. Cortisol is capable of targeting intranuclear receptors secondary to its ability to

(A) Recruit intracellular kinases
(B) Undergo autophosphorylation
(C) Diffuse through lipid membranes
(D) Interact with G-protein
(E) Interact with AC

3. Which of the following parameters is used to indicate the ability of a drug to produce the desired therapeutic effect relative to a toxic effect?

(A) Potency
(B) Intrinsic activity
(C) TI
(D) Efficacy
(E) Bioavailability

4. A 64-year-old woman with a history of multiple abdominal surgeries due to Crohn's disease presents to the emergency room with obstipation and feculent emesis. A diagnosis of small bowel obstruction is made, and she is taken to the operating room for lysis of adhesions and resection of stenosed region of small bowel. Postoperatively, the patient is noted to have elevated blood pressure, and oral metoprolol is administered; however, no improvement of hypertension is observed. This is likely due to

(A) The first-pass effect
(B) Decreased passage of drug through intestine
(C) Decreased GI blood flow
(D) Destruction of drug by stomach acid
(E) Increased protein binding of the drug

5. An important feature of congestive heart failure (CHF) regarding drug action is

(A) Impaired blood flow to the intestine
(B) Increased protein binding of various drugs
(C) Increased volume of distribution
(D) Increased drug elimination
(E) Altered drug kinetics

6. Which of the following is the term used to describe the elimination rate via metabolism catalyzed by alcohol dehydrogenase when the enzyme is saturated?

(A) Zero-order kinetics
(B) First-order elimination
(C) Clearance
(D) Biotransformation
(E) Redistribution

7. A 69-year-old woman is being treated in the intensive care unit for presumed staphylococcal sepsis. To avoid problems with possible resistance, she is empirically given IV vancomycin while waiting for the culture results to come back. Vancomycin is a renally excreted drug. The patient's routine laboratory workup reveals a creatinine value of 3.2, indicating acute renal failure. What specific considerations will have to be made with regard to adjustments of the prescribed medication?

(A) She will have to be switched to an oral (per nasogastric tube) vancomycin preparation
(B) The patient will need to be water restricted to decrease the volume of distribution
(C) No changes to the current regimen will be made because the condition of the patient is life-threatening and the drug needs to be administered regardless
(D) The dose of vancomycin will need to be reduced because of increased accumulation
(E) Dosage adjustments will have to be made because the patient is currently ventilated

8. Glucuronidation reactions

(A) Are considered phase I reactions
(B) Require an active center as the site of conjugation
(C) Include the enzymatic activity of alcohol dehydrogenase
(D) Located in mitochondria are inducible by drugs
(E) Require nicotinamide adenine dinucleotide phosphate (NADPH) for the enzymatic reaction

9. A 38-year-old woman presents to her psychiatrist with a request to try a different antidepressant medication, since she doesn't feel her current medication is helping. She even felt so depressed that she started drinking heavily in the past couple of months. The doctor wants to try imipramine; however, since this drug is known to undergo an extensive first-pass effect, he orders a hepatic function panel before prescribing it, given the patient's recent history of alcohol use. What is the rationale for the doctor's decision?

(A) In the presence of hepatic dysfunction, drugs with a high first-pass metabolism reach high systemic concentrations
(B) The results of the hepatic function panel may reveal a particular susceptibility to the drug
(C) Bioavailability of imipramine is increased by the fraction of drug removed by the first pass
(D) The drug is more rapidly metabolized by the liver when hepatic aminotransferase levels are elevated
(E) Solubility of the drug is affected in the face of hepatic damage

10. A 43-year-old man who was recently fired from a well-paying job decides to commit suicide and ingests a jarful of his antiseizure medication, phenobarbital. His wife finds him at home sleeping but notices that he has diminished breathing, low body temperature, and skin reddening. She brings him to the ER, where he is appropriately diagnosed with barbiturate overdose. The patient is given bicarbonate to alkalinize his urine. How does alkalinization of urine with bicarbonate help to overcome the toxic effects of phenobarbital in this situation?

(A) It increases glomerular filtration
(B) It decreases proximal tubular secretion
(C) It decreases distal tubular reabsorption
(D) It enhances drug metabolism
(E) It decreases untoward side effects

11. Erythromycin is prescribed "qid," or four times daily, because of its short half-life. The rationale for such a frequent dosing schedule is

(A) To achieve the steady-state plasma concentration of the drug
(B) To avoid the toxicity of the drug because of its low therapeutic index (TI)
(C) To aid more complete distribution of the drug
(D) To inhibit the first-pass metabolism of the drug
(E) To ensure that the drug concentration remains constant over time

12. A 13-year-old boy suffers two tonic-clonic seizures within 1 week. He is diagnosed with epilepsy, and phenytoin therapy is started. To achieve proper drug concentrations in plasma, the patient is first given a loading dose, followed by maintenance doses. The blood level of phenytoin is frequently monitored to adjust the maintenance dose as needed. What is the rationale behind such a regimen?

(A) If the drug is administered at a maintenance dose rate, steady-state concentration will be reached after two half-lives
(B) A loading dose is administered to achieve the desired plasma concentration rapidly
(C) The maintenance dose rate usually does not equal the elimination rate, which is why the loading dose is required
(D) Loading dose of the drug does not depend on the volume of distribution, whereas the maintenance dose does
(E) The maintenance dose rate does not depend on clearance of the drug, whereas the loading dose does

13. A 78-year-old woman is started on digoxin for her congestive heart failure (CHF). Her initial dose is 0.25 mg. The C_0, obtained by extrapolation of the elimination phase, is determined to be 0.05 mg/L. What is the patient's apparent volume of distribution?

(A) 0.5 L
(B) 0.2 L
(C) 0.0125 L
(D) 1 L
(E) 5 L

14. A drug has a volume of distribution of 50 L and undergoes zero-order elimination at a rate of 2 mg/hour at plasma concentrations >2 mg/L. If a patient is brought to the ER with a plasma concentration of 4 mg/L of the drug, how long will it take (in hours) for the plasma concentration to decrease 50%?

(A) 1
(B) 2
(C) 10
(D) 25
(E) 50

15. You administer a 100-mg tablet of drug X to a patient every 24 hours and achieve an average steady-state plasma concentration of the drug of 10 mg/L. If you change the dose regimen to one 50 mg tablet every 12 hours, what will be the resulting average plasma concentration (in mg/L) of the drug after five half-lives?

(A) 2.5
(B) 5
(C) 10
(D) 20
(E) 40

16. Following IV administration, the initial rates of drug distribution to different tissues depend primarily on which of the following parameters?

(A) Blood flow to the tissues
(B) Fat content of the tissues
(C) Degree of ionization of the drug in the tissues
(D) Active transport of the drug out of different cell types
(E) Specific organ clearances

17. A drug is administered in the form of an inactive prodrug. The prodrug increases the expression of a cytochrome P-450 that converts the prodrug to its active form. With chronic, long-term administration of the prodrug, which of the following will be observed?

(A) The potency will decrease
(B) The potency will increase
(C) The efficacy will decrease
(D) The efficacy will increase

18. Which subfamily of cytochrome P-450s is responsible for the highest fraction of clinically important drug interactions resulting from metabolism?

(A) CYP1A
(B) CYP2A
(C) CYP3A
(D) CYP4A
(E) CYP5A

19. In most patients, an antibiotic is eliminated 25% by hepatic metabolism, 50% by renal filtration, and 25% by biliary excretion. If the normal maintenance dose rate = 10 mg/hour, what dose rate will you administer to a patient 12 normal with a creatinine clearance that is (assume that hepatic and biliary clearances are normal)?

(A) 2.5 mg/hour
(B) 5.0 mg/hour
(C) 6.0 mg/hour
(D) 7.5 mg/hour
(E) 20 mg/hour

20. If the oral dosing rate of a drug is held constant, what will be the effect of increasing the bioavailability of the preparation?

(A) Increase the half-life for first-order elimination
(B) Decrease the first-order elimination rate constant
(C) Increase the steady-state plasma concentration
(D) Decrease the total body clearance
(E) Increase the volume of distribution

21. You administer to a patient an oral maintenance dose of drug calculated to achieve a steady-state plasma concentration of 5 mcg/L. After dosing the patient for a time sufficient to reach steady state, the average plasma concentration of drug is 10 mcg/L. A decrease in which of the following parameters explains this higher than anticipated plasma drug concentration?

(A) Bioavailability
(B) Volume of distribution
(C) Clearance
(D) Half-life

22. Administration of an IV loading dose to a patient of drug X yields an initial plasma concentration of 100 mcg/L. The table below illustrates the plasma concentration of X as a function of time after the initial loading dose.

Time (hours)	Plasma conc. (mcg/L)
0	100
1	50
5	25
9	12.5

What is the half-life (in hours) of drug X?

(A) 1
(B) 2
(C) 4
(D) 5
(E) 9

23. Which of the following factors will determine the number of drug–receptor complexes formed?

(A) Efficacy of the drug
(B) Receptor affinity for the drug
(C) TI of the drug
(D) Half-life of the drug
(E) Rate of renal secretion

24. Which of the following is an action of a noncompetitive antagonist?

(A) Alters the mechanism of action of an agonist
(B) Alters the potency of an agonist
(C) Shifts the dose–response curve of an agonist to the right
(D) Decreases the maximum response to an agonist
(E) Binds to the same site on the receptor as the agonist

25. The renal clearance of a drug is 10 mL/min. The drug has a molecular weight of 350 and is 20% bound to plasma proteins. It is most likely that renal excretion of this drug involves

(A) Glomerular filtration
(B) Active tubular secretion
(C) Passive tubular reabsorption
(D) Both glomerular filtration and active tubular secretion
(E) Both glomerular filtration and passive tubular reabsorption

Answers and Explanations

1. **The answer is A.** Somatostatin binds to G_i-coupled protein receptor, initiating exchange of GTP for GDP, which inhibits AC and leads to reduced cAMP production. G_q-protein–coupled receptor is an example of the phospholipase C pathway, in which interaction with the ligand leads to increased phospholipase C activity and eventual activation of protein kinase C via PIP_2 and IP_3 pathway. This is exemplified by interaction of epinephrine with its receptor. Ligand-activated ion channel is an example of interaction of specific ligand with an ion channel, which permits passage of ions through the channel. Acetylcholine is an example of such an interaction. Receptor-activated tyrosine kinase is exemplified by insulin, where binding of ligand activates specific tyrosine kinase, leading to a cascade of reactions within the cell. Finally, intracellular nuclear receptor is exemplified by cortisol, which binds to it and exerts its effects on DNA replication.

2. **The answer is C.** The ability to target intracellular receptors depends on the ligand's ability to cross lipid barriers, such as the nuclear envelope. Recruitment of intracellular kinases is characterized by some receptor-activated tyrosine kinases. Autophosphorylation is a feature of many different kinases. Interactions with G-protein and AC are characteristics of membrane receptors.

3. **The answer is C.** Lithium is an example of a drug with a very low therapeutic index (TI), which requires frequent monitoring of the plasma level to achieve the balance between the desired effect and untoward toxicity. Potency of the drug is the amount of drug needed to produce a given response. Intrinsic activity of the drug is the ability to elicit a response. Efficacy of the drug is the maximal drug effect that can be achieved in a patient under a given set of conditions. Bioavailability of the drug is the fraction of the drug that reaches the bloodstream unaltered.

4. **The answer is B.** Adequate passage of drug through the small intestine is required to observe the effects of the drug, because most of the absorption takes place in the small intestine. After extensive abdominal surgery, especially that involving a resection of a portion of small bowel, the passage may be slowed, or even stopped, for a period of time. Abdominal surgery rarely results in reduced blood flow to the intestine, nor does such an operation influence protein binding, or the first-pass effect. Destruction of drug by stomach acid does not depend on intraabdominal surgery.

5. **The answer is C.** Because of the patient's edema and ascites, the apparent volume of distribution will be increased, which may require small adjustments in his usual medication doses. Edematous states do not influence gastrointestinal (GI) blood flow, nor do they affect drug–protein interactions. Drug elimination may be slowed with congestive heart failure (CHF) exacerbation, not increased. Drug kinetics are generally not changed by edematous states.

6. **The answer is A.** Alcohol is one of the drugs that follow zero-order kinetics (i.e., higher drug concentrations are not metabolized because the enzyme that is involved in the process is saturable). In first-order elimination, the rate of elimination actually depends on the concentration of the drug, multiplied by proportionality constant. Clearance is a measure of the capacity of the body to remove the drug. Biotransformation simply refers to the general mechanism of a particular drug's elimination. Redistribution is one of the possible fates of a drug, which usually terminates drug action.

7. **The answer is D.** Since vancomycin is cleared by the kidneys, renal functional status needs to be considered when prescribing such a drug, because it may accumulate and produce undesirable toxic side effects. Switching from the vancomycin to an oral preparation will reduce its bioavailability. There is no indication that the patient is in the state of increased

volume of distribution (such as edema), and water restriction will not have a noticeable effect on apparent volume of distribution. Changes to the current regimen are necessary because of the patient's acute renal failure, and this has to be done regardless of the urgency of the situation. The fact that the patient is being ventilated may indicate that she needs extra hydration because of increased insensible losses, but this has nothing to do with her vancomycin dose directly.

8. **The answer is B.** Glucuronidation reactions, which are considered phase II reactions, require an active center (a functional group) as the site of conjugation. Phase I reactions are biotransformation reactions, not conjugation reactions. Alcohol dehydrogenase is an example of a phase I reaction. Phase II reactions' enzymes are located in the endoplasmic reticulum, not mitochondria. Nicotinamide adenine dinucleotide phosphate (NADPH) is required for aromatic hydroxylation, an example of a phase I reaction.

9. **The answer is A.** First-pass metabolism simply means passage through the portal circulation before reaching the systemic circulation. In the face of liver dysfunction, drug levels may reach higher concentrations. A hepatic function panel is generally not used to deduce a patient's susceptibility to the drug. Bioavailability of drugs is decreased, not increased by the fraction removed after the first pass through the liver. Drugs are usually less rapidly metabolized when hepatic enzymes are elevated (which indicates hepatic dysfunction). Solubility of drugs has nothing to do with hepatic damage.

10. **The answer is C.** Alterations of urinary pH affect renal distal tubular reabsorption of drugs by ion trapping, which affects the ionization of weak acids and bases. Since phenobarbital is a weak acid, raising the pH of the urine will increase the % of the drug in the ionized form and "trap" it in the ultrafiltrate because charged molecules cannot be reabsorbed back across membranes in the tubule into the plasma. This "trapping" in the ultrafiltrate thus causes a net increase in elimination of the drug in the urine. Other renal mechanisms will not be affected since: a) glomerular filtration depends mainly on the size of the drug as well as protein binding and b) proximal tubular secretion will not be affected by alkalinization of urine since this process depends on the availability of transporters.

11. **The answer is A.** Dosing schedules of drugs are adjusted according to their half-lives to achieve steady-state plasma concentration. Attempting to avoid the toxicity of the drug because of its low therapeutic index (TI) represents an unlikely scenario, since to reduce toxicity of a drug with a low TI, one would reduce the dosing schedule, not increase it. Distribution of the drug is generally not affected by dosing schedule. Nor is dose scheduling affected by first-pass metabolism. Some fluctuation in plasma concentration occurs even at steady state; it is the average concentration over time that is the goal of steady state.

12. **The answer is B.** The rationale for the loading dose is to give a patient a sufficient dose of a medication to achieve the desired effect quickly, which is necessary in some situation (such as prevention of further seizures). When drug is administered at maintenance rate, steady state is achieved after about five half-lives. The maintenance dose is usually equal to the elimination rate. The loading dose depends on the volume of distribution, whereas the maintenance dose depends on the clearance of the drug.

13. **The answer is E.** To calculate the volume of distribution, use the formula in which the dose of the drug is divided by the plasma concentration. In this case, 0.25 mg is divided by 0.05 mg/L, giving the result of 5 L for volume of distribution.

14. **The answer is E.** For the plasma concentration of drug to decrease by 50%, half the drug present in the body initially must be eliminated. The amount of drug in the body initially is the volume of distribution × the plasma concentration (50 L × 4 mg/L = 200 mg). When the plasma concentration falls to 2 mg/L, the body will contain 100 mg of drug (50 L × 2 mg/L = 100 mg). Since the body eliminates the drug at a rate of 2 mg/hour, it will require 50 hours for 100 mg of the drug to be eliminated.

15. **The answer is C.** A 100 mg tablet every 24 hours is a dose rate of 4.17 mg/hour ($100/24 = 4.17$), which is the same dose rate as one 50 mg tablet every 12 hours ($50/12 = 4.17$). Thus, the average plasma concentration will remain the same, but *decreasing both* the dose and the dose interval will decrease the peak to trough variation of plasma concentration.

16. **The answer is A.** The *initial rate* of distribution of a drug to a tissue depends primarily on the rate of blood flow to that tissue. At longer times, however, a drug may undergo redistribution among various tissues, e.g., a very lipophilic drug may become concentrated in adipose tissue with time.

17. **The answer is B.** The induction of the cytochrome P-450 following chronic administration will increase the conversion of the inactive prodrug to the active form. This will shift the dose–response curve of the prodrug to the left (i.e., increase its potency) without changing its efficacy.

18. **The answer is C.** The CYP3A subfamily is responsible for roughly 50% of the total cytochrome P450 activity present in the liver and is estimated to be responsible for approximately half of all clinically important untoward drug interactions resulting from metabolism.

19. **The answer is D.** Maintenance dose rate = (clearance) × (desired plasma concentration), and the whole body clearance is the sum of all the individual organ clearances. In most patients, the hepatic metabolism, renal filtration, and biliary excretion account for 25%, 50%, and 25% of the whole body clearance, respectively. Since the creatinine clearance in this patient indicates that the renal filtration is only half normal, the renal clearance of the drug will be decreased by half. This means that the whole body clearance will be 75% of that of normal (25% hepatic, 25% renal, and 25% biliary). Therefore, the dose should also be 75% of the standard dose.

20. **The answer is C.** If the oral dosing rate is constant but the bioavailability increases, the fraction of the administered dose that reaches the general circulation unaltered increases. This, in turn, will increase the steady-state plasma concentration.

21. **The answer is C.** Steady-state plasma concentration of drug = (dose rate)/(clearance). Thus, a decrease in clearance will increase the plasma drug concentration, whereas an increase in any of the other three parameters will *decrease* the steady-state plasma concentration.

22. **The answer is C.** Inspection of the plasma concentration values indicates that the half-life of drug does not become constant until 1–9 hours after administration. The drug concentration decreases by half (from 50 to 25 mcg/L) between 1 and 5 hours (a 4-hour interval) and again decreases by half (from 25 to 12.5 mcg/L) between 5 and 9 hours (again, a 4-hour interval). This indicates the half-life of the drug is 4 hours. The rapid decrease in plasma concentration between 0 and 1 hour, followed by a slower decrease thereafter (and the constant half-life thereafter) indicates that this drug obeys a two-compartment model with an initial distribution phase followed by an elimination phase. The half-life is always determined from the elimination phase data.

23. **The answer is B.** Receptor affinity for the drug will determine the number of drug–receptor complexes formed. Efficacy is the ability of the drug to activate the receptor after binding has occurred. Therapeutic index (TI) is related to safety of the drug. Half-life and secretion are the properties of elimination and do not influence the formation of drug–receptor complexes.

24. **The answer is D.** A noncompetitive antagonist decreases the magnitude of the response to an agonist but does not alter the agonist's potency (i.e., the ED_{50} remains unchanged). A competitive antagonist interacts at the agonist binding site.

25. **The answer is E.** This drug will undergo filtration and passive reabsorption. Because the molecular weight of the drug is small, free drug will be filtered. Because 20% of the drug is bound to plasma proteins, 80% of it is free and available for filtration, which would be at a rate of 100 mL/min (i.e., 0.8×125 mL/min; 125 mL/min is the normal glomerular filtration rate [GFR]). A clearance of 10 mL/min must indicate that most of the filtered drug is reabsorbed.

2 Drugs Acting on the Autonomic Nervous System

I. THE PERIPHERAL EFFERENT NERVOUS SYSTEM

A. **The autonomic nervous system (ANS)** controls **involuntary activity** (Fig. 2.1 and Table 2.1).
1. *Parasympathetic nervous system (PNS)*
   a. Long preganglionic axons originate from neurons in the cranial and sacral areas of the spinal cord and, with few exceptions, synapse on neurons in ganglia located close to or within the innervated organ.
   b. Short postganglionic axons innervate cardiac muscle, bronchial smooth muscle, and exocrine glands.
   c. Parasympathetic innervation predominates over sympathetic innervation of salivary glands, lacrimal glands, and erectile tissue.
2. *Sympathetic nervous system (SNS)*
   a. Short preganglionic axons originate from neurons in the thoracic and lumbar areas of the spinal cord and synapse on neurons in ganglia located outside of, but close to, the spinal cord. The adrenal medulla, anatomically considered a modified ganglion, is innervated by sympathetic preganglionic axons.
   b. Long postganglionic axons innervate many of the same tissues and organs as the PNS.
   c. Innervation of **thermoregulatory sweat glands** is anatomically sympathetic, but the postganglionic nerve fibers are cholinergic and release acetylcholine (ACh) as the neurotransmitter.
3. *Enteric nervous system*
   a. Considered a third branch of the ANS.
   b. Highly organized, semiautonomous, neural complex localized in the gastrointestinal **(GI) system.**
   c. Receives preganglionic axons from the PNS and postganglionic axons from the SNS.
   d. Nerve terminals contain peptides and purines as neurotransmitters.

B. **The somatic nervous system** (Fig. 2.1) controls **voluntary activity.** This system contains long axons that originate in the spinal cord and directly innervate skeletal striated muscle.

C. **Neurotransmitters of the autonomic and somatic nervous systems** (Fig. 2.1)
1. *ACh*
   a. ACh is released by exocytosis from nerve terminals.
   b. ACh is the neurotransmitter across synapses at the ganglia of the SNS and PNS and across synapses in tissues innervated by the PNS and the somatic nervous system.
   c. ACh is synthesized in nerve terminals by the cytoplasmic enzyme choline acetyltransferase, which catalyzes the transfer of an acetate group from acetyl coenzyme A to choline that has been transported into "cholinergic" neurons by a sodium-dependent membrane carrier. Synthesized ACh is transported from cytoplasm to vesicle-associated transporters.

FIGURE 2.1. Organization of the autonomic nervous system.

    d. ACh is stored in nerve terminal vesicles that, through calcium-dependent exocytosis, are released by nerve action potentials. On release, a step blocked by **botulinum toxin,** ACh is rapidly hydrolyzed and inactivated by tissue acetylcholinesterase (AChE) and also by nonspecific butyrylcholinesterase (pseudocholinesterase) to choline and acetate.

    e. ACh is not administered parenterally for therapeutic purposes because it is hydrolyzed nearly instantly by butyrylcholinesterase.

  2. ***Norepinephrine and epinephrine*** are **catecholamines,** possessing a catechol nucleus and an ethylamine side chain.

    a. Storage and release

      (1) Norepinephrine is stored in vesicles that, through a calcium-dependent process, release their contents by exocytosis from nerve terminals at postganglionic nerve endings of the SNS (except at thermoregulatory sweat glands, where ACh is the neurotransmitter).

      (2) Norepinephrine also exists in a nonvesicular cytoplasmic pool that is released by indirectly acting sympathomimetic amines (e.g., **tyramine, amphetamine, ephedrine**) by a process that is not calcium-dependent.

      (3) Norepinephrine and some epinephrine are released from adrenergic nerve endings in the brain. In the periphery, epinephrine, along with some norepinephrine, is the major catecholamine released from adrenal medullary chromaffin cells into the general circulation, where they function as hormones.

    b. Biosynthesis of catecholamines (Fig. 2.2)

      (1) In prejunctional nerve endings, tyrosine is hydroxylated by tyrosine hydroxylase, the rate-limiting enzyme in the synthesis of catecholamines, to form dihydroxyphenylalanine (dopa); dopa is then decarboxylated by dopa decarboxylase to form dopamine.

table 2.1 Actions of the Autonomic Nervous System on Selected Effector Organs

Effector	Action of Sympathetic (Thoracolumbar) Division	Action of Parasympathetic (Craniosacral) Division
Eye (pupil)	Dilation (ex)	Constriction (ex)
Heart		
Rate	Acceleration (ex)	Slowing (in)
Contractility	Increased (ex)	Decreased (in)
Arterioles		
Skin and most others	Constriction (ex)	—
Skeletal muscle	Dilation (ex)	—
Glands		
Salivary	Viscid secretion (ex)	Watery secretion (ex)
Lacrimal	—	Secretion (ex)
Sweat	Secretion (ex)	—
Bronchial muscle	Relaxation (in)	Contraction (ex)
GI tract		
Muscle wall	Relaxation (in)	Contraction (ex)
Sphincters	Contraction (ex)	Relaxation (in)
Urinary bladder		
Fundus	Relaxation (in)	Contraction (ex)
Trigone; sphincter	Contraction (ex)	Relaxation (in)
Penis	Ejaculation (ex)	Erection (in)
Uterus	Relaxation (in)	—
Metabolism		
Liver	Gluconeogenesis (ex)	—
	Glycogenolysis (ex)	—
Kidney	Renin secretion(ex)	—
Fat cells	Lipolysis (ex)	—

ex, excitatory; in, inhibitory; —, no functionally important innervation.

(2) Dopamine is transported into vesicles, a step blocked by **reserpine,** where it is hydroxylated on the side chain by dopamine β-hydroxylase to form norepinephrine.

(3) In certain areas of the brain and in the adrenal medulla, norepinephrine is methylated on the amine group of the side chain by phenylethanolamine-*N*-methyltransferase to form epinephrine.

c. Termination

(1) The action of **norepinephrine** is terminated primarily by **active transport** from the cytoplasm into the nerve terminal by a norepinephrine transporter (**uptake 1**), a process that is inhibited by **cocaine** and tricyclic antidepressant agents such as **imipramine. Norepinephrine** is then transported by a second carrier system into storage vesicles, as is **dopamine** and **serotonin,** a process also blocked by **reserpine.**

(2) Another active transport system (**uptake 2**) is located on glia and smooth muscle cells.

(3) There is also some simple **diffusion** away from the synapse.

(4) **Norepinephrine** and **epinephrine** are also oxidatively deaminated by **mitochondrial monoamine oxidase (MAO)** in nerve terminals and effector cells, notably in the liver and intestine.

(5) Nerve cells and effector cells contain **catechol-*O*-methyltransferase (COMT),** which metabolizes catecholamines. Metabolites, including **3-methoxy-4-hydroxymandelic acid,** provide a measure of catecholamine turnover in the body.

FIGURE 2.2. Biosynthesis of catecholamines.

D. Receptors of the nervous system

1. **Cholinoceptors**

   a. **Nicotinic receptors:** Cholinoceptors that are activated by the alkaloid nicotine (Fig. 2.1)

   (1) Nicotinic receptors are localized at myoneural junctions of somatic nerves and skeletal muscle (N_M), autonomic ganglia (N_G), including the adrenal medulla, and certain areas in the brain.

   (2) Nicotinic receptors are a component of postjunctional transmembrane polypeptide that forms a **ligand-gated** (i.e., regulated) cation-selective ion channel (see Fig. 1.1A). Binding of ACh to the receptor site causes opening of the ion channel and an influx of positively charged ions (sodium and potassium) and across the cellular membrane. This influx of positive charge depolarizes the postsynaptic membrane.

   (3) In skeletal muscle, ACh interacts with nicotinic receptors to produce membrane depolarization and a propagated action potential through the transverse tubules of skeletal muscle. This results in the release of Ca^{2+} from the sarcoplasmic reticulum and, through a further series of chemical and mechanical events, **muscle contraction.** Hydrolysis of ACh by AChE results in muscle cell repolarization.

   (a) The continued presence of a nicotine agonist, like **succinylcholine,** at nicotinic receptors, or excessive cholinergic stimulation, can lead to a **"depolarizing blockade"** (phase I block), in which normal depolarization is followed by persistent depolarization. During phase I block, skeletal muscle is unresponsive to either neuronal stimulation or direct stimulation.

   (b) The selective nicotinic receptor antagonists **tubocurarine** and **trimethaphan** can block the effect of ACh at skeletal muscle and autonomic ganglia, respectively.

   b. **Muscarinic receptors:** Cholinoceptors that are activated by the alkaloid muscarine (Fig. 2.1)

(1) Muscarinic receptors are localized on numerous autonomic effector cells, including cardiac atrial muscle and cells of the sinoatrial (SA) and atrioventricular (AV) nodes, smooth muscle, exocrine glands, and vascular endothelium (mostly arterioles), although the latter does not receive parasympathetic innervation, as well as certain areas in the brain.

(2) Muscarinic receptors consist of at least five **receptor subtypes (M_1–M_5).** Muscarinic M_1-receptors are found in sympathetic postganglionic neurons; M_2-receptors are found in cardiac and smooth muscles; M_3-receptors are found in glandular cells (e.g., gastric parietal cells), and the vascular endothelium and vascular smooth muscle. M_5-receptors are found in the vascular endothelium. All five of the receptor subtypes, including M_4-receptors, are found in CNS neurons.

(3) ACh interacts with **M_1, M_3, and M_5 muscarinic cholinoceptors** to increase **phosphatidylinositol (PI) turnover** and **Ca^{2+} mobilization** (see Fig. 1.1D).

  (a) By activation of **G protein** (G_q), the interaction of ACh with M_1 and M_3 muscarinic cholinoceptors stimulates **polyphosphatidylinositol phosphodiesterase (phospholipase C),** which hydrolyzes PI to **inositol trisphosphate (IP_3)** and **diacylglycerol (DAG).**

  (b) **IP_3 mobilizes intracellular Ca^{2+}** from the endoplasmic and sarcoplasmic reticula, and activates Ca^{2+}-regulated enzymes and cell processes.

  (c) **DAG activates protein kinase C,** which results in phosphorylation of cellular enzymes and other protein substrates and the **influx of extracellular calcium** that results in activation of contractile elements in smooth muscle.

(4) ACh also interacts with **M_2 and M_4 muscarinic cholinoceptors** to **activate G proteins (G_i),** which leads to **inhibition of adenylyl cyclase** activity with decreased levels of cyclic AMP (cAMP) and to **increased K^+ conductance** with effector cell hyperpolarization.

(5) Cholinergic agonists act on **M_3 muscarinic receptors** of **endothelial cells** to promote the release of **nitric oxide (NO),** which diffuses to the **vascular smooth muscle** to activate guanylyl cyclase and increase cyclic GMP (cGMP) and to produce **relaxation.**

2. *Adrenoceptors* (Fig. 2.1)

  a. α-**Adrenoceptors**

  (1) α-Adrenoceptors are classified into two major receptor subgroups (there are subtypes of each group). $α_1$-**Receptors** are located in **postjunctional** effector cells, notably vascular smooth muscle, where responses are mainly excitatory; $α_2$-**receptors** are located primarily in **prejunctional** adrenergic nerve terminals, and also in fat cells and in the β cells of the pancreas.

  (2) α-Adrenoceptors mediate vasoconstriction ($α_1$), GI relaxation ($α_1$), mydriasis ($α_1$), prejunctional inhibition of release of norepinephrine and other neurotransmitters ($α_2$), inhibition of insulin release ($α_2$), and inhibition of lipolysis ($α_2$).

  (3) α-Adrenoceptors are distinguished from β-adrenoceptors by their interaction (in descending order of potency), with the adrenergic agonists **epinephrine = norepinephrine ≫ isoproterenol,** and by their interaction with relatively selective antagonists such as **phentolamine.**

  (4) $α_1$-**Receptors,** like muscarinic M_1 cholinoceptors, **activate guanine nucleotide-binding proteins (Gq)** in many cells, which results in activation of **phospholipase C** and stimulation of phosphoinositide (PI) hydrolysis that leads to increased formation of **IP_3** and mobilization of intracellular stores of Ca^{2+} and to increased **DAG** and activation of protein kinase C.

  (5) $α_2$-**Receptors,** like muscarinic M_2-cholinoceptors, **activate inhibitory guanine nucleotide-binding proteins (G_i), inhibit adenylyl cyclase** activity, and decrease intracellular cAMP levels and the activity of cAMP-dependent protein kinases (see Fig. 1.1C).

  b. β-**Adrenoceptors** (Fig. 2.1)

  (1) β-Adrenoceptors, located mostly in postjunctional effector cells, are classified into two major receptor subtypes, $β_1$-receptors (primarily excitatory) and $β_2$-receptors (primarily inhibitory).

(a) β_1-**Receptor subtype**
   (i) β_1-Receptors mediate increased contractility and conduction velocity, and renin secretion in the kidney (β_3-receptors mediate activation of fat cell lipolysis).
   (ii) The β_1-receptor subtype is defined by its interaction (in descending order of potency) with the adrenergic agonists **isoproterenol > epinephrine = norepinephrine** and by its interaction with relatively selective antagonists such as **atenolol.**
(b) β_2-**Receptor subtype**
   (i) β_2-Receptors mediate vasodilation and intestinal, bronchial, and uterine smooth muscle relaxation.
   (ii) The β_2-receptor subtype is defined by its interaction (in descending order of potency) with the adrenergic agonists **isoproterenol = epinephrine $\gg$ norepinephrine.**
(2) β-**Receptor activation**
   (a) β-Receptors activate **guanine nucleotide-binding proteins** (G_s; see Fig. 1.1B).
   (b) Activation **stimulates adenylate cyclase** activity and increases intracellular CAMP levels and the activity of cAMP-dependent protein kinases. Adrenoceptor-mediated changes in the activity of protein kinases (and also levels of intracellular Ca^{2+}) bring about changes in the activity of specific enzymes and structural and regulatory proteins, resulting in modification of cell and organ activity.

II. PARASYMPATHOMIMETIC DRUGS

A. **Direct-acting muscarinic cholinoceptor agonists**
   1. *Action and chemical structure*
      a. Direct-acting parasympathomimetic drugs act at muscarinic cholinoceptors to mimic many of the physiologic effects that result from stimulation of the parasympathetic division of the ANS (see Fig. 2.1).
      b. **Bethanechol** (Urecholine) and **methacholine** are choline esters with a quaternary ammonium group that are structurally similar to ACh and have substantially reduced activity at nicotinic receptors and are more resistant to hydrolysis by AChE.
   2. *Pharmacologic effects* (Tables 2.2 and 2.3)
      a. **Eye**
         (1) Direct-acting muscarinic cholinoceptor agonists contract the circular smooth muscle fibers of the ciliary muscle and iris to produce, respectively, a spasm of accommodation and an increased outflow of aqueous humor into the canal of Schlemm, resulting in a **reduction in intraocular pressure.**
         (2) These drugs contract the smooth muscle of the iris sphincter to cause **miosis.**
      b. **Cardiovascular system**
         (1) Direct-acting muscarinic cholinoceptor agonists produce a **negative chronotropic effect** (reduced SA node activity).
         (2) These drugs **decrease conduction velocity** through the AV node.
         (3) These drugs have no effect on force of contraction because there are no muscarinic receptors on, or parasympathetic innervation of, ventricles.
         (4) Direct-acting muscarinic cholinoceptor agonists produce **vasodilation** that results primarily from their action on endothelial cells to promote the release of **NO,** which diffuses to the vascular smooth muscle and produces relaxation. Vascular smooth muscle has muscarinic receptors but no parasympathetic innervation. The resulting decrease in blood pressure can result in a reflex increase in heart rate. (Intravenous infusion of low doses of ACh causes a reflex sympathetic-stimulated increase in heart rate; higher doses directly inhibit heart rate.)

t a b l e **2.2** Actions of Direct-Acting Cholinoceptor Agonists	
Effector	**Effects of Muscarinic Agonists**
Heart (rate, conduction velocity)[a]	Decrease
Arterioles (tone)	Decrease
Blood pressure	Decrease
Pupil size	Decrease
Salivation	Increase
Lacrimation	Increase
Bronchial tone	Increase
Intestine (motility)	Increase
GI secretions	Increase

Urinary bladder
  Body (tone)
  Sphincter
	
	Increase
	Decrease

[a]Responses (e.g., heart rate) may be affected by reflexes.

- c. **GI tract**
  - **(1)** Direct-acting muscarinic cholinoceptor agonists increase smooth muscle contractions and tone, with increased **peristaltic activity and motility.**
  - **(2)** These drugs increase salivation and acid secretion.
- d. **Urinary tract**
  - **(1)** Direct-acting muscarinic cholinoceptor agonists **increase contraction of the ureter and bladder smooth muscle.**
  - **(2)** These drugs increase **sphincter relaxation.**
- e. **Respiratory system** effects of direct-acting muscarinic cholinoceptor agonists include **bronchoconstriction** with increased resistance and increased bronchial secretions.
- f. **Other effects**
  - **(1)** These drugs increase the secretion of tears from lacrimal glands and increase sweat gland secretion.
  - **(2)** These drugs produce tremor and ataxia.
3. *Specific drugs and their therapeutic uses.* These drugs are used primarily for diseases of the eye, GI tract, urinary tract, the neuromuscular junction, and the heart (Table 2.4).
  - a. **Bethanechol** (Urecholine)
    - **(1)** Bethanechol is used to stimulate smooth muscle motor activity of the urinary tract to **prevent urine retention.**

t a b l e **2.3** Effects of Muscarinic Cholinoceptor and Adrenoceptor Agonists on Smooth Muscles of the Eye			
Type of Drug	**Muscle**	**Effect**	**Result**
Muscarinic agonist	Iris circular (constrictor)	Contraction	Miosis
	Ciliary circular	Contraction	Accommodation
Muscarinic antagonist	Iris circular (constrictor)	Relaxation	Mydriasis
	Ciliary circular	Relaxation	Cycloplegia
α-Adrenergic agonist	Iris radial (dilator)	Contraction	Mydriasis
	Ciliary circular	None	None

t a b l e **2.4** Selected Therapeutic Uses of Selected Direct-Acting Cholinoceptor Agonists		
Agent	**Conditions/Disorders**
Bethanechol	Prevents urine retention; postoperative abdominal distension; gastric atony
Methacholine	Diagnostic for bronchial hypersensitivity
Pilocarpine	Open-angle glaucoma; acute narrow-angle glaucoma; Sjögren syndrome

(2) It is used occasionally to stimulate GI smooth muscle motor activity for **postoperative abdominal distention** and for **gastric atony** following bilateral vagotomy (in the absence of obstruction).

(3) Bethanechol is administered PO or SC, not by IV or IM route, because parenteral administration may cause cardiac arrest.

(4) When given orally, GI effects predominate, and there are relatively minor cardiovascular effects.

(5) Bethanechol has limited distribution to the CNS.

(6) It is resistant to hydrolysis and thus has a relatively long duration of action (2–3 h).

b. **Methacholine** (Mecholyl) is occasionally used **to diagnose bronchial hypersensitivity.** Patients with no clinically apparent asthma are more sensitive to methacholine-induced bronchoconstriction than normal patients.

c. **Pilocarpine**

(1) Pilocarpine is occasionally used topically for **open-angle glaucoma,** either as eyedrops or as a sustained-release ocular insert (Ocusert). β-adrenoceptor antagonists and prostaglandin analogs are the drugs of choice to treat open-angle glaucoma. Other drug classes used include α-adrenergic receptor agonists and diuretics.

(2) When used before surgery to treat **acute narrow-angle glaucoma** (a medical emergency), pilocarpine is often given in combination with an indirectly acting muscarinic agonist such as **physostigmine.**

(3) Pilocarpine and **cevimeline** (Evoxac) increase salivary secretion. They are used to treat **Sjögren syndrome**-associated dry mouth.

(4) Pilocarpine is a tertiary amine that is well absorbed from the GI tract and enters the CNS.

d. **Carbachol** is used rarely as a treatment for open-angle glaucoma.

e. **Nicotine-based products and varenicline** (Chantix), direct-acting nicotinic receptor agonists, are approved for use in smoking cessation (Chapter 5 X D 2).

4. *Adverse effects and contraindications*

a. The **adverse effects** associated with direct-acting muscarinic cholinoceptor agonists are extensions of their pharmacologic activity. The most serious include **nausea, vomiting, sweating, salivation, bronchoconstriction, decreased blood pressure, and diarrhea,** all of which can be blocked or reversed by atropine. Systemic effects are minimal for drugs applied topically to the eye.

b. These drugs are contraindicated in the presence of **peptic ulcer** (because they increase acid secretion), **asthma, cardiac disease, and Parkinson disease.** They are not recommended in hyperthyroidism because they predispose to arrhythmia; they are also not recommended when there is mechanical obstruction of the GI or urinary tract.

B. **Indirect-acting parasympathomimetic agents**

1. *Chemical structure*

a. **Edrophonium** is an alcohol with a quaternary ammonium group.

b. **Neostigmine** and **physostigmine** are examples of carbamic acid esters of alcohols (carbamates) with either quaternary or tertiary ammonium groups.

c. **Echothiophate** and **isoflurophate** are examples of organic derivatives of phosphoric acid.

2. ***Mechanism of action*** (Fig. 2.3A and B)

    a. Indirect-acting parasympathomimetic agents **inhibit AChE** and **increase ACh levels** at both muscarinic and nicotinic cholinoceptors to mimic many of the physiologic effects that result from increased ACh in the synaptic junction and stimulation of cholinoceptors of the parasympathetic division of the ANS.

    b. ACh interacts with AChE at two sites: The N^+ of choline (ionic bond) binds to the **anionic site,** and the acetyl ester binds to the **esteratic site** (serine residue). As ACh is hydrolyzed, the serine-OH side chain is acetylated and free choline is released. Acetyl-serine is hydrolyzed to serine and acetate. The half-life $(t_{1/2})$ of acetylserine hydrolysis is 100–150 microseconds.

    c. Edrophonium (Tensilon) acts at the same sites of AChE to competitively inhibit ACh hydrolysis. It has a short duration of action (5–15 min).

    d. Neostigmine (Prostigmin), **physostigmine** (Eserine, Antilirium), and **demecarium** (Humorsol), like ACh, interact with AChE and undergo a two-step hydrolysis. However, the serine residue of the enzyme is covalently carbamylated rather than acetylated. Hydrolysis of the carbamylserine residue is much slower than that of acetylserine (30 min to 6 h).

      (1) Neostigmine, physostigmine, and demecarium also have direct agonist action at skeletal muscle nicotinic cholinoceptors.

      (2) These drugs differ in absorption as follows:

        (a) Because of its quaternary ammonium structure, **neostigmine** is **poorly absorbed** from the GI tract and has negligible distribution into the CNS.

        (b) Physostigmine is **well absorbed** after oral administration, and it enters the CNS.

    e. Echothiophate (Phospholine) and **isoflurophate** (Floropryl), irreversible and toxic organophosphate cholinesterase inhibitors, result in **phosphorylation of AChE** rather than acetylation. With time, the strength of the bond increases ("aging"), and AChE becomes irreversibly inhibited. The enzyme can be reactivated within the first 30 minutes by **pralidoxime.** Hydrolysis of the covalent alkylphosphoryl-serine bond takes days.

FIGURE 2.3. A. Hydrolysis of acetylcholine by acetylcholinesterase. **B.** Interaction of neostigmine with acetylcholinesterase.

   (1) Echothiophate is poorly absorbed from the GI tract and has negligible distribution into the CNS.

   (2) Isoflurophate is highly lipid soluble and is well absorbed across all membranes, including skin.

f. **Pralidoxime** (Protopam)

   (1) Pralidoxime is an **AChE reactivator** that must be administered IV within minutes of exposure to an AChE inhibitor because it is effective only prior to "aging."

   (2) Pralidoxime acts as an **antidote for organophosphorus insecticide and nerve gas poisoning.** It binds the anionic site and reacts with the P=O group of alkylphos-phorylated serine to cause hydrolysis of the phosphoserine bond.

   (3) This drug is most effective at the neuromuscular junction. It is ineffective in the CNS and against carbamylated AChE.

   (4) Pralidoxime produces few adverse effects in normal doses.

3. *Pharmacologic effects* (Table 2.2)

a. With the major exception of arteriole tone and blood pressure, where their effects are less pronounced, the pharmacologic effects of indirect-acting parasympathomimetic agents are similar to those of direct-acting muscarinic cholinoceptor agonists.

b. By increasing ACh at the neuromuscular junction, these drugs increase the contraction strength of skeletal muscle. The effect is more pronounced if muscle contraction is already weak, as occurs in **myasthenia gravis**.

4. *Therapeutic uses*

a. **Glaucoma**

   (1) Physostigmine is often used concurrently with **pilocarpine** for maximum effect in the treatment of **acute angle-closure glaucoma,** a medical emergency.

   (2) Direct- and indirect-acting cholinomimetics have been largely replaced for the treatment of chronic **open-angle glaucoma** by topical β-adrenergic receptor antagonists and by prostaglandin analogs.

b. **GI and urinary tract disorders**

   (1) Postoperative ileus and congenital megacolon, and urinary tract retention can be treated with direct or indirectly acting cholinomimetic drugs such as **bethanechol** and **neostigmine**.

   (2) These agents are also used to increase the tone of the lower esophageal sphincter.

c. **Myasthenia gravis**

   (1) Myasthenia gravis is an **autoimmune disease** in which antibodies complex with nicotinic receptors at the neuromuscular junction to cause skeletal muscle weakness and fatigue. AChE inhibitors, such as **pyridostigmine**, are used to increase ACh levels at the neuromuscular junction to fully activate the remaining receptors.

   (2) Myasthenia gravis can be diagnosed using the **Tensilon test,** which can also assess the adequacy of treatment with AChE inhibitors. Small doses of **edrophonium** improve muscle strength in untreated patients with myasthenia or in treated patients in whom AChE inhibition is inadequate. If there is no effect, or if muscle weakness increases, the dose of the AChE inhibitor is too high (excessive ACh stimulation at the neuromuscular junction results in a depolarizing blockade).

   (3) Atropine can be used to control excessive muscarinic stimulation by AChE inhibitors.

   (4) Tolerance may develop to long-term use of the AChE inhibitors.

d. **Alzheimer disease: Donepezil** (Aricept), **galantamine** (Reminyl), **rivastigmine** (Exelon), and **tacrine** (Cognex) are AChE inhibitors used to ameliorate the cognitive deficit associated with Alzheimer disease (see Chapter 5 VI E).

e. **Neostigmine** or **edrophonium** can be used following surgery to **reverse neuromuscular blockade** and paralysis resulting from adjunct use of nondepolarizing agents.

f. **Atropine** and **scopolamine poisoning that results in severe body temperature elevation or tachycardia** can be treated with **physostigmine,** which reverses the central and the peripheral effects of competitive muscarinic antagonists.

5. *Adverse effects and toxicity*
   a. The adverse effects associated with indirect-acting sympathomimetic agents are an extension of pharmacologic activity and arise from **excessive cholinergic stimulation.**
   b. Adverse effects include muscarinic effects similar to those of direct-acting cholinergic drugs and nicotinic effects such as **muscle weakness, cramps and fasciculations, excessive bronchial secretions, convulsions, coma, cardiovascular collapse,** and **respiratory failure.**
   c. Many lipid-soluble organophosphates are used as insecticides (e.g., malathion) or nerve gases (e.g., sarin) and may be absorbed in sufficient quantities from the skin or lungs to cause cholinergic intoxication. Treatment includes the following steps:
      (1) Maintain respiration and decontaminate to prevent further absorption.
      (2) Administer **atropine** parenterally to inhibit muscarinic effects.
      (3) Administer **pralidoxime** within minutes of exposure.

III. MUSCARINIC-RECEPTOR ANTAGONISTS

A. **Mechanism and chemical structure** (Table 2.5)
   1. Muscarinic-receptor antagonists are competitive antagonists of ACh at all muscarinic cholinoceptors.
   2. Muscarinic-receptor antagonists are either tertiary amine alkaloids (e.g., **atropine, scopolamine, tropicamide**) or quaternary amines (e.g., **propantheline [Pro-Banthine], ipratropium [Atrovent]**).
   3. **Tertiary amines** are often used for their effects on the **CNS. Quaternary amines,** which have minimal CNS actions, are often used for their effects on **peripheral systems.**

B. **Pharmacologic effects**
   1. *Eye* (Table 2.3)
      a. Muscarinic-receptor antagonists produce **cycloplegia** by blocking parasympathetic tone, leading to paralysis of the ciliary muscle and loss of accommodation.
      b. These drugs produce **mydriasis** by blocking parasympathetic tone to the iris circular (constrictor) muscle. Unopposed sympathetic stimulation of the radial muscle results in dilation of the pupil.
   2. *Cardiovascular system*
      a. Muscarinic-receptor antagonists **increase heart rate** due to cholinergic blockade at the SA node.

table 2.5 Properties of Some Cholinoceptor-Blocking Agents

Agent	Action	Muscarinic	Nicotinic	Comments
Atropine	Competitive antagonist	+		Prototype muscarinic cholinoceptor-blocking agent
Scopolamine	Competitive antagonist	+		Actions similar to those of atropine
Propantheline	Competitive antagonist	+		Peripheral-acting cholinoceptor blocking agent
Trimethaphan	Competitive, nondepolarizing antagonist		+	Peripheral-acting ganglionic blocking agent
Cisatracurium	Competitive, nondepolarizing antagonist at motor endplate		+	Neuromuscular junction blocking agent
Succinylcholine	Depolarizing agonist at motor endplate		+	Neuromuscular junction blocking agent

    b. These drugs dilate blood vessels in facial blush area (atropine flush), which is not related to the antagonist action.

  3. *GI tract*
    a. Muscarinic-receptor antagonists **decrease salivation.**
    b. These drugs **reduce peristalsis,** resulting in prolonged gastric emptying and intestinal transit.
    c. They also reduce gastric acid secretion.

  4. *Other effects*
    a. Muscarinic-receptor antagonists produce some **bronchodilation** and decrease mucus secretion.
    b. These drugs relax the ureters and bladder in the urinary tract and constrict the urinary sphincter.
    c. Tertiary amines can produce restlessness, headache, excitement, hallucinations, and delirium.
    d. These drugs produce **anhidrosis** and dry skin because of the inhibition of sympathetic cholinergic innervation of the sweat glands.

C. Pharmacologic properties
  1. Unlike quaternary ammonium drugs (10%–30% absorption), most tertiary muscarinic-receptor antagonists are well absorbed across the GI tract or mucosal surfaces and distribute throughout the body, including the brain.
  2. **Atropine** and **scopolamine** have relatively long durations of action.

D. Therapeutic uses (Table 2.6)
  1. *Eye*
    a. Shorter-acting muscarinic-receptor antagonists (e.g., homatropine, cyclopentolate [Cyclogyl], **tropicamide**) that produce mydriasis are administered topically as eyedrops or as ointments for **refractive measurements** and for **ophthalmoscopic examination** of the retina and other structures of the eye (α-adrenoceptor agonists, such as **phenylephrine,** are used for simple funduscopic examination without cycloplegia).
    b. Longer-acting muscarinic-receptor antagonists (such as **homatropine**) are generally preferred as adjuncts to **phenylephrine** to prevent synechia formation in **anterior uveitis and iritis.**
  2. *Cardiovascular system* uses are limited and include the administration of these drugs as a treatment for **acute myocardial infarction** with accompanying bradycardia and hypotension or arrhythmias (e.g., **atropine**).
  3. *Urinary tract* uses of **atropine** and other muscarinic-receptor antagonists include the administration of these drugs for symptomatic treatment of **urinary urgency** in inflammatory bladder disorder. **Oxybutynin** (Ditropan) and **trospium** (SpasMex), and the more selective M_3-receptor antagonists **darifenecin** (Enablex), **solifenacin** (Vesicare), **tolterodine** (Detrol), and **fesoterodine** (Toviaz), are additional agents in this class used to treat certain urinary tract disorders.

t a b l e **2.6**	Selected Therapeutic Use of Muscarinic Cholinoceptor Antagonists
Organ/System	**Therapeutic Use**
Eye	Refractive measurement; ophthalmologic examination, uveitis and iritis
Heart	Acute myocardial infarction
Bladder	Urinary urgency
Lung	Surgical anesthesia to suppress secretions
CNS	Motion sickness (scopolamine); Parkinson disease
Multiple organs/systems	Cholinergic poisoning

4. *Central nervous system*
   a. Antimuscarinic drugs, **benztropine, biperiden, trihexyphenidyl,** and others, are used as adjunct to levodopa therapy for some patients with **Parkinson disease** (see Chapter 5).
   b. **Scopolamine** (used orally, intravenously, or transdermally) prevents **motion sickness** by blocking muscarinic receptors in the vestibular system and in the CNS (see Chapter 8). **Scopolamine** also has additional amnestic and sedative properties.
5. *Respiratory system*
   a. **Atropine** and **scopolamine** can be used to suppress bronchiolar secretions during **surgical and spinal anesthesia** and to prevent the muscarinic effects of AChE inhibitors used to reverse muscle paralysis at the end of surgery.
   b. **Ipratropium** (Atrovent) and **tiotropium** (Spiriva) are used as an inhalant to treat reactive airway disease such as asthma and chronic obstructive pulmonary disease (COPD).
6. *Other uses:* Tertiary agents such as **atropine** are used to block peripheral and CNS effects due to cholinergic excess, especially those caused by poisoning with AChE inhibitor-containing insecticides and muscarine-containing mushrooms.

E. Adverse effects and contraindications
   1. *The adverse effects* of muscarinic-receptor antagonists are extensions of pharmacologic activity and include **mydriasis, cycloplegia, dry eyes, tachycardia, dry mouth, elevated temperature, dry skin, urine retention, agitation, hallucinations, and delirium** ("hot as a hare, dry as a bone, red as a beet, blind as a bat, mad as a hatter"). Symptomatic treatment rather than use of **physostigmine** is recommended. **Neostigmine** is used to treat poisoning with quaternary muscarinic-receptor antagonists.
   2. *Contraindications (relative)* are **glaucoma,** particularly angle-closure glaucoma, **GI and urinary tract obstruction** (e.g., prostatic hypertrophy), and **gastric ulcer.**
   3. *Drug interactions* of muscarinic-receptor antagonists include the production of additive effects when administered with other drugs with muscarinic-receptor antagonist activity (certain antidepressants, antipsychotics, and antihistamines).

IV. GANGLION-BLOCKING DRUGS

A. Mechanism and therapeutic uses (see Table 2.5)
   1. *Ganglion-blocking drugs*
      a. **Trimethaphan** (Arfonad) and **mecamylamine** (Inversine) inhibit the effect of ACh at nicotinic receptors by acting competitively (**nondepolarizing blockade**) at both sympathetic and parasympathetic autonomic ganglia.
      b. Because of a lack of selectivity and numerous adverse effects, they are used rarely in the clinical setting (hypertensive emergencies).

V. SKELETAL MUSCLE RELAXANTS

A. Classification and structure
   1. *Neuromuscular junction-blocking drugs* (see Table 2.5)
      a. Classified as either **nondepolarizing or depolarizing** types, neuromuscular junction-blocking drugs cause neuromuscular paralysis. They are structurally similar to ACh.
      b. These drugs contain one or two **quaternary nitrogens** that limit their entry into the CNS.
   2. *Spasmolytic drugs* act to reduce abnormal muscle tone without paralysis. These drugs increase or mimic the activity of γ-**aminobutyric acid (GABA)** in the spinal cord and brain or interfere with the release of calcium in skeletal muscle.

B. **Nondepolarizing agents**

1. *Mechanism*
   a. Nondepolarizing agents **competitively inhibit the effect of ACh** at the postjunctional membrane nicotinic receptor of the neuromuscular junction. There is some prejunctional inhibition of ACh release.
   b. These agents prevent depolarization of the muscle and propagation of the action potential.

2. *Pharmacologic properties*
   a. Nondepolarizing agents are administered parenterally and are generally used for long-term motor paralysis. Paralysis and muscle relaxation occur within 1–5 minutes.
   b. Nondepolarizing agents have durations of action that range from 20 to 90 minutes.
   c. Most nondepolarizing agents are metabolized by the liver or are excreted unchanged. The duration of action may be prolonged by hepatic or renal disease.
   d. Intermediate-acting steroid muscle relaxing agents (e.g., **rocuronium** [Zemuron], **vecuronium** [Norcuron]) are more commonly used than long-acting agents.

3. *Specific drugs* (Table 2.7)
   a. **Tubocurarine** (prototype) is seldom used clinically at this time.
   b. **Metocurine** (Metubine) is a derivative of tubocurarine. It has the same properties, but with less histamine release and thus less hypotension and bronchoconstriction. Metocurine has a long duration of action (>40 min).
   c. **Atracurium** (Tracrium) and **Cisatracurium** (Nimbex)
      (1) Atracurium causes some histamine release. It is **inactivated spontaneously in plasma** by nonenzymatic hydrolysis that is delayed by acidosis. Its duration of action is reduced by hyperventilation-induced respiratory alkalosis. **Laudanosine,** a breakdown product of atracurium, may accumulate to cause **seizures.**
      (2) Cisatracurium is a stereoisomer of atracurium that releases less histamine and forms less laudanosine. It has **replaced atracurium** use in clinical practice.
   d. **Mivacurium** (Mivacron) is a short-acting (10–20 min), which is rapidly hydrolyzed by plasma cholinesterase, has a slow onset of action relative to succinylcholine, and produces moderate histamine release at high doses.
   e. **Vecuronium** (Norcuron), **Rocuronium** (Zemuron), and **Pancuronium** (Pavulon)
      (1) All are steroid derivatives with **little, histaminic or ganglion-blocking activity.**
      (2) Vecuronium and rocuronium have intermediate durations of action (20–40 min). They are metabolized primarily by the liver.

| t a b l e   **2.7** | Properties of Some Skeletal Muscle Relaxants |

Nondepolarizing Agent	Duration of Action	Ganglion Blockade	Histamine Release	Cardiac Muscarinic Receptors	Comments
Tubocurarine[a]	Long	+	+ +	—	Prototype
Atracurium[a]	Intermediate	—	+	—	Inactivat.ed spontaneously in plasma; laudanosine, a breakdown product, may cause seizures
Cisatracurium[a]	Intermediate	—	—	—	Less laudanosine formed than atracurium
Mivacurium[a]	Short	—	+ +	—	Hydrolyzed by plasma cholinesterase
Pancuronium[b]	Long	—	—	+ +	Increased heart rate
Vecuronium[b]	Intermediate	—	—	—	Metabolized by liver
Depolarizing Agent					
Succinylcholine	Very short	+ +	+	+ +	Hydrolyzed by cholinesterase; malignant hyperthermia is a rare, potentially fatal complication

[a]Isoquinoline derivative.
[b]Steroid derivative.

(3) Pancuronium has a longer duration of action (120–180 min) and is used less frequently than the others. It is excreted by the kidney with only minimal hepatic metabolism.

4. *Therapeutic uses*

a. Nondepolarizing agents are used during surgery as adjuncts to general anesthetics to induce muscle paralysis and muscle relaxation. The order of muscle paralysis is small, rapidly contracting muscles (e.g., extrinsic muscles of the eye) before slower contracting muscle groups (e.g., face and extremities), followed by intercostal muscles, and then the diaphragm. Recovery of muscle function is in reverse order, and respiration often must be assisted.

b. These agents are also used for muscle paralysis in patients when it is critical to control ventilation, e.g., ventilatory failure from pneumonia, for endotracheal intubation, and to control muscle contractions during **electroconvulsive therapy.**

5. *Reversal of nondepolarizing drug blockade:* AChE inhibitors, such as **neostigmine,** are administered for pharmacologic antagonism to reverse residual postsurgical muscarinic receptor blockade and avoid inadvertent hypoxia or apnea.

6. *Adverse effects and contraindications* (Table 2.7)

a. Cardiovascular system. Tubocurarine, atacurium, mivacurium, pancuronium, and metocurine may produce cardiovascular effects such as **hypotension** or **increased heart rate** due to histamine release, ganglionic-blocking activity, or vagolytic activity.

b. Respiratory system: Some nondepolarizing agents can produce **bronchospasm** in sensitive individuals due to histamine release. Agents that release histamine are contraindicated for asthmatic patients and patients with a history of anaphylactic reactions.

7. *Drug interactions*

a. **General inhalation anesthetics,** particularly **isoflurane,** increase the neuromuscular blocking action of nondepolarizing agents. The dose of the neuromuscular junction-blocking drug may have to be reduced.

b. **Aminoglycoside antibiotics,** among others, inhibit prejunctional ACh release and potentiate the effect of nondepolarizing and depolarizing neuromuscular junction-blocking drugs.

C. Depolarizing agents (Table 2.7) include succinylcholine (Anectine), the only depolarizing drug of clinical importance.

1. *Mechanism of action*

a. Succinylcholine is a **nicotinic receptor agonist** that acts at the motor endplate of the neuromuscular junction to produce **persistent stimulation and depolarization of the muscle,** thus preventing stimulation of contraction by ACh.

b. After a single IV injection and depolarization of the muscle, there are initial muscle contractions or **fasciculations** (in the first 30–60 s) that may be masked by general anesthetics. Because succinylcholine is metabolized more slowly than ACh at the neuromuscular junction, the muscle cells remain depolarized (**depolarizing or phase I block**) and unresponsive to further stimulation, resulting in a **flaccid paralysis** (5–10 min).

c. With continuous long-term exposure (45–60 min), the muscle cells repolarize. However, they cannot depolarize again while succinylcholine is present and, therefore, remain unresponsive to ACh (**desensitizing or phase II block**).

d. AChE inhibition will enhance the initial phase I block by succinylcholine but can reverse phase II block.

2. *Pharmacologic properties*

a. Succinylcholine has a rapid onset and short duration of action. Action is rapidly terminated (5–10 min) by **hydrolysis by plasma and liver cholinesterase.**

b. Reduced plasma cholinesterase synthesis in end-stage hepatic disease or reduced activity following the use of irreversible AChE inhibitors may increase the duration of action.

3. *Therapeutic uses* of succinylcholine include the administration of the drug as an **adjunct in surgical anesthesia** to obtain muscle relaxation while using lower levels of general anesthetic, to induce **brief paralysis in short surgical procedures,** and to **facilitate intubation.**

4. *Adverse effects*
  a. **Postoperative muscle pain** at higher doses.
  b. **Hyperkalemia**
    (1) Hyperkalemia results from loss of tissue potassium during depolarization.
    (2) Risk of hyperkalemia is enhanced in patients with burns, muscle trauma, or spinal cord transections.
    (3) Hyperkalemia can be life-threatening, leading to **cardiac arrest** and circulatory collapse.
  c. **Malignant hyperthermia**
    (1) Malignant hyperthermia is a rare but often fatal complication in susceptible patients that results from a rapid increase in muscle metabolism. About 50% of patients are genetically predisposed, with mutations in the skeletal muscle Ca^{2+}-release channel of the sarcoplasmic reticulum (ryanodine receptor, RYR1).
    (2) Malignant hyperthermia is most likely to occur when succinylcholine is used with the general anesthetic **halothane.**
    (3) It is characterized by tachycardia and, among other manifestations, intense **muscle spasm** that results in a rapid and profound **hyperthermia.**
    (4) Drug treatment is with **dantrolene** (see following).
  d. **Prolonged paralysis** may result in apnea (lasting 1–4 h) in a small percentage of patients (1/10,000) with **genetically atypical or low levels of plasma cholinesterase.** Mechanical ventilation is necessary.
  e. **Bradycardia** from direct muscarinic cholinoceptor stimulation is prevented by atropine.
  f. **Increased intraocular pressure** may result from extraocular muscle contractions; use of succinylcholine may be contraindicated for penetrating eye injuries.
  g. Succinylcholine produces increased intragastric pressure, which may result in fasciculations of abdominal muscles and a danger of aspiration.

D. **Spasmolytic drugs**
  1. *These muscle relaxants* **reduce increased muscle tone** associated with a variety of nervous system disorders (e.g., **cerebral palsy, multiple sclerosis, spinal cord injury, and stroke**) that result in loss of supraspinal control and hyperexcitability of α- and γ-motoneurons in the spinal cord, causing abnormal skeletal muscle, bowel, and bladder function.
  2. *Selected drugs*
    a. **Dantrolene** (Dantrium)
      (1) Dantrolene acts directly on muscle to reduce skeletal muscle contractions.
      (2) Dantrolene is also used to treat **malignant hyperthermia.**
      (3) This drug interferes with Ca^{2+} release from the sarcoplasmic reticulum; benefit may not be apparent for a week or more.
      (4) The major adverse effects of dantrolene are **muscle weakness,** which may limit therapy, and sedation. Long-term use can result in hepatotoxicity that may be fatal. Hepatic function should be monitored during treatment.
    b. **Baclofen** (Lioresal)
      (1) Baclofen is an analog of GABA. It is a $GABA_B$-receptor agonist that hyperpolarizes neurons to inhibit synaptic transmission in the spinal cord.
      (2) Adverse effects include some drowsiness and an increased frequency of seizures in epileptic patients.
    c. **Tizandine** (Zanaflex)
      (1) Tizandine is an alpha2 adrenoceptor agonist analog of clonidine that reduces muscle spasm with less muscle weakness than baclofen, dantrolene, and diazepam.
      (2) Adverse effects include some drowsiness and hypotension and reports of hepatotoxicity.
    d. **Benzodiazepines** (see Chapter 5)
      (1) Benzodiazepines such as **diazepam** act on the spinal cord and CNS to facilitate GABA activity.
      (2) The major adverse effect is **sedation.**

e. **Botulinum toxin (Botox)**
   (1) Botulinum toxin acts by **inhibiting the release of ACh from motor nerve terminals.**
   (2) **Botulinum toxin** is used to treat local muscle spasms, spastic disorders like **cerebral palsy**, and blepharospasm- and strabismus-associated dystonia. It is also used for cosmetic reduction of facial wrinkles.

VI. SYMPATHOMIMETIC DRUGS

A. **Action and chemical structure**
   1. These drugs act either **directly** or **indirectly to activate** postjunctional and prejunctional **adrenoceptors** to **mimic** the effects of **endogenous catecholamines** such as norepinephrine and epinephrine. Their actions can generally be predicted from the type and location of the receptors with which they interact and whether or not they cross the blood–brain barrier to enter the CNS.
   2. Indirectly acting agents act within nerve endings to **increase the release of stored catecholamines,** act at the prejunctional membrane to **block the reuptake of catecholamines** that have been released from nerve endings, or act **enzymatically to prevent their biotransformation**.

B. **Pharmacologic effects** (Table 2.8)
   1. *Cardiovascular system*
      a. β_1**-Receptor agonists,** through an increased calcium influx in cardiac cells, increase the rate (chronotropic effect) and force (inotropic effect) of myocardial contraction and increase the conduction velocity (dromotropic effect) through the AV node, with a decrease in the refractory period.
      b. β_2**-Receptor agonists** cause relaxation of vascular smooth muscle that may invoke a reflex increase in heart rate.
      c. α_1**-Receptor agonists** constrict smooth muscle of resistance blood vessels (e.g., in the skin and splanchnic beds), causing increased peripheral resistance usually with an

t a b l e **2.8**	Direct Effects of Adrenoceptor Agonists			
Effector	α_1	α_2	β_1	β_2
Heart				
Rate			Increase	
Force			Increase	
Arterioles (most)	Constrict			Dilate
Blood pressure	Increase			Decrease
Intestine				
Wall	Relax	Relax		Relax
Sphincters	Contract			
Salivation				
Volume	Increase			
Amylase			Increase	
Pupil	Dilate			
Bronchial smooth muscle				Relax
Urinary bladder				
Body	Constrict			Relax
Sphincter	Constrict			
Release of NE from nerves		Decrease		

increase in blood pressure. In normotensive patients (less effect in those with hypotension), the increased blood pressure may invoke a reflex baroreceptor vagal discharge and a slowing of the heart, with or without an accompanying change in cardiac output.

    d. α_2-**Receptor agonists** reduce blood pressure by a prejunctional action on neurons in the CNS to inhibit sympathetic outflow.

  2. *Eye* (see Table 2.3)

    a. α-**Receptor agonists** contract the radial muscle of the iris and dilate the pupil (mydriasis). These drugs also increase the outflow of aqueous humor from the eye.

    b. β-**Receptor antagonists** decrease the production of aqueous humor.

  3. *Respiratory system effects* include β_2-**receptor agonist**-induced relaxation of bronchial smooth muscle and decreased airway resistance.

  4. *Metabolic and endocrine effects*

    a. β-**Receptor agonists** increase liver and skeletal muscle glycogenolysis and increase lipolysis in fat cells. α_2-**Receptor agonists** inhibit lipolysis.

    b. β-**Receptor agonists** increase, and α_2-**receptor agonists** decrease, insulin secretion.

  5. *Genitourinary tract effects* include α-**Receptor agonist** contraction of the bladder wall, urethral sphincter, prostate, seminal vesicles, and ductus deferens.

C. **Specific sympathomimetic drugs** are selected for use depending on the duration of action, route of administration, and also the specific effect on a particular tissue, which in turn depends on the tissue population of adrenoceptor subtypes.

  1. *Epinephrine and norepinephrine*

    a. Epinephrine and norepinephrine are poorly absorbed from the GI tract and do not enter the CNS to any appreciable extent. Absorption of epinephrine from subcutaneous sites is slow because of local vasoconstriction. Nebulized and inhaled solutions and topical preparations of epinephrine are available. Epinephrine and norepinephrine are most often **administered IV** (with caution to avoid cardiac arrhythmias or local tissue necrosis).

    b. These drugs are metabolized extensively by enzymes in the liver by **COMT** and **MAO**. Metabolites are excreted by the kidney.

    c. Epinephrine and norepinephrine actions at neuroeffector junctions are terminated primarily by **simple diffusion** away from the receptor site and by **active uptake** into sympathetic nerve terminals and subsequent active transport into storage vesicles. Actions are also partially terminated at neuroeffector junctions by metabolism by extraneuronal COMT and intraneuronal MAO.

    (1) **Epinephrine**

      (a) Epinephrine activates β_1-, β_2-, and α-adrenoceptors.

      (b) Epinephrine administration in humans **increases systolic pressure** as a result of positive inotropic and chronotropic effects on the heart (β_1-receptor activation) and generally results in **decreased total peripheral resistance** and **decreased diastolic pressure due to vasodilation** in the vascular bed of skeletal muscle (β_2-receptor activation) that overcomes the vasoconstriction produced in most other vascular beds, including the kidney (α-receptor activation). The mean arterial pressure may increase slightly, decrease, or remain unchanged, depending on the balance of effects on systolic and diastolic pressure.

      (c) At high doses, epinephrine causes vasoconstriction in the vascular bed of skeletal muscle (α-receptor activation).

      (d) Epinephrine **increases coronary blood flow** as a result of increased cardiac workload; it may precipitate **angina** in patients with coronary insufficiency.

      (e) Epinephrine **increases the drainage of aqueous humor** (α-receptor activation) and reduces pressure in **open-angle glaucoma**. It **dilates the pupil** (mydriasis) by contraction of the radial muscle of the eye (α-receptor activation).

      (f) Epinephrine **relaxes bronchial smooth muscle** (β_2-receptor activation).

    (2) **Norepinephrine** is rarely used therapeutically. It **activates β_1-receptors** and α **receptors**. It has little activity at β_2-receptors.

2. **Dopamine** (Intropin)
   a. Dopamine activates peripheral β_1-**adrenoceptors** to increase heart rate and contractility.
   b. Dopamine **activates** prejunctional and postjunctional dopamine D_1-**receptors** in the renal, coronary, and splanchnic vessels to reduce arterial resistance and increase blood flow. Prejunctionally, dopamine inhibits norepinephrine release.
   c. At **low doses,** dopamine has a positive inotropic effect and increases systolic pressure, with little effect on diastolic pressure or mean blood pressure.
   d. At **higher doses,** dopamine activates α-receptors and causes vasoconstriction, with a reflex decrease in heart rate.

3. β-**Adrenoceptor agonists**
   a. **Dobutamine**
      (1) Dobutamine is a **synthetic catecholamine** that is related to **dopamine** but whose activities are related to actions at α-**receptors** and β-**receptors** with no effect on dopamine receptors.
      (2) This drug increases cardiac output with limited vasodilating activity and reflex tachycardia.
      (3) Dobutamine is administered by **IV infusion** because of its short half-life ($t_{1/2}$ = 2 min).
   b. **Terbutaline** (Brethine, Bricanyl), **albuterol** (Proventil, Ventolin), **metaproterenol** (Alupent), **pirbuterol** (Maxair), **salmeterol** (Serevent), and **formoterol** (Foradil) are examples of drugs with more **selective β_2-receptor agonists** that **relax bronchial smooth muscle** with fewer cardiac effects and longer duration of action than epinephrine. Selectivity is lost at high concentrations.
   c. **Isoproterenol** (Isuprel) **activates β-receptors** with little activity on α-receptors. It dilates bronchial smooth muscle. It is infrequently used because of the availability of selective β_2-adrenoceptor agonists.

4. α-**Adrenoceptor agonists**
   a. **Phenylephrine, methoxamine** (Vasoxyl), and **metaraminol** (Aramine)
      (1) These drugs produce effects primarily by **direct α_1-receptor stimulation** that results in vasoconstriction, increased total peripheral resistance, and increased systolic and diastolic pressure. **Metaraminol** also has **indirect activity;** it is taken up and released at sympathetic nerve endings, where it acts as a false neurotransmitter. It also releases epinephrine.
      (2) These drugs are less potent but because they are not metabolized by COMT they have longer durations of action than catecholamines.
   b. **Xylometazoline** (Otrivin) and **oxymetazoline** (Afrin)
      (1) These drugs have selective action at α-receptors.
      (2) At **high doses,** these drugs may cause **clonidine-like effects** because of their action in the CNS.
   c. **Clonidine** (Catapres), **methyldopa** (Aldomet), **guanabenz** (Wytensin), and **guanfacine** (Tenex)
      (1) These antihypertensive agents directly or indirectly activate prejunctional and, possibly, postjunctional α_2-**receptors** in the **vasomotor center** of the medulla to **reduce sympathetic tone.**
      (2) These drugs reduce **blood pressure,** with a decrease in total peripheral resistance and minimal long-term effects on cardiac output and heart rate.
      (3) **Methyldopa** is a **prodrug** that is metabolized to the active agent α-**methylnorepinephrine** (and α-methyldopamine) in nerve endings. It **lowers blood pressure by reducing peripheral vascular resistance.** At higher nontherapeutic doses, it activates peripheral α-receptors to cause vasoconstriction.

5. **Other adrenoceptor agonists**
   a. **Ephedrine**
      (1) Ephedrine acts indirectly to release norepinephrine from nerve terminals and has some direct action on adrenoceptors.

(2) Ephedrine has effects similar to those of **epinephrine,** but is less potent; it has a longer duration of action because it is resistant to metabolism by COMT and MAO.

(3) This drug is effective orally and, unlike catecholamines, penetrates the brain and can produce CNS stimulation.

(4) **Ephedrine** is found in the herbal medication **ma huang.**

(5) **Pseudoephedrine** (Sudafed) is an isomer of ephedrine.

(6) After continued use, **tachyphylaxis** may develop due to ephedrine's peripheral effects.

  b. **Amphetamine, dextroamphetamine** (Dexedrine), **methamphetamine** (Desoxyn), **modafinil** (Provigil), **methylphenidate** (Ritalin), and **hydroxyamphetamine** (Paremyd) (see Chapter 5)

(1) These drugs produce effects similar to those of **ephedrine,** with indirect and some direct activity.

(2) **Dextroamphetamine** has more CNS-stimulatory activity than the *levo* isomer, which has more cardiovascular activity.

(3) These drugs are well absorbed and, except for **hydroxyamphetamine,** enter the CNS readily and have marked stimulant activity.

D. **Therapeutic uses** (Table 2.9)

  1. *Cardiovascular system*

    a. **Phenylephrine** and other direct-acting α-receptor sympathomimetic drugs are used for **short-term hypotensive emergencies** when there is inadequate perfusion of the heart and brain such as during severe hemorrhage.

    b. **Ephedrine and midodrine** (Pro-Amatine), prodrugs that are hydrolyzed to the α_1-adrenoceptor agonist desglymidodrine, are used to treat **chronic orthostatic hypotension.**

    c. **The use of sympathomimetic agents in most forms of shock is controversial and should be avoided. Further vasoconstriction may be harmful.**

(1) Low-to-moderate doses of **dobutamine** or **dopamine** may be useful in cases of **cardiogenic or septic shock** because they increase cardiac output with minimal vasoconstrictive effect on the peripheral vasculature.

(2) **Epinephrine** is used to reverse hypotension and angioedema associated with **anaphylactic shock.**

    d. **Dobutamine** is used to treat **congestive heart failure.**

    e. **Methyldopa** is used to treat **hypertension.**

    f. **Fenoldopam** (Corlopam) is a selective dopamine **D_1-receptor agonist** used to treat severe hypertension.

t a b l e **2.9**	Selected Therapeutic Uses of Adrenoceptor Agonists	
Clinical Condition/Application	**Agonist**	**Receptor**
Hypotensive emergency	Phenylephrine; methoxamine; norepinephrine	α_1
Chronic, orthostatic hypotension	Ephedrine; midodrine, phenylephrine	α_1
Anaphylactic shock	Epinephrine	α and β
Heart block, cardiac arrest	Isoproterenol; epinephrine	β_1
Congestive heart failure	Dobutamine	β_1
Infiltration nerve block	Epinephrine	α_1
Hay fever and rhinitis	Phenylephrine; OTC[a]	α_1
Asthma	Metaproterenol; terbutaline; albuterol	β_2

[a]Over-the-counter preparations.

    g. **Isoproterenol** and **epinephrine** have been used for temporary emergency treatment of **cardiac arrest** and **heart block** because they increase ventricular automaticity and rate and increase AV conduction.

    h. **Epinephrine** is commonly used in combination with local anesthetics (1:200,000) during infiltration block to reduce blood flow. α-Receptor agonist activity causes local vasoconstriction, which **prolongs local anesthetic action** and allows the use of lower doses with reduced chance of toxicity. **Phenylephrine** has also been used.

    i. **Epinephrine** is used during **spinal anesthesia** to maintain blood pressure, as is **phenylephrine,** and topically to reduce superficial bleeding.

2. *Respiratory system*

    a. **Phenylephrine** and other short- and longer acting α-**adrenoceptor agonists,** including **oxymetazoline, xylometazoline, tetrahydrozoline** (Tyzine), ephedrine, and pseudoephedrine, are used for symptomatic relief of **hay fever and rhinitis** of the common cold. Long-term use may result in ischemia and rebound hyperemia, with development of chronic rhinitis and congestion.

    b. **Albuterol, and also metaproterenol, terbutaline, pirbuterol, bitolterol** and other β_2-adrenoceptor agonists are preferred for treating symptoms of **acute asthma.** They are also used for treatment of COPD. For **chronic asthma,** these drugs, including **salmeterol** and **formoterol** with long durations of action, should be used in combination with steroids.

    c. **Epinephrine** is administered IM to treat **acute bronchospasm** and also bronchospasm, congestion, angioedema, and cardiovascular collapse of **anaphylaxis.**

3. *Eye*

    a. **Phenylephrine** facilitates **examination of the retina** because of its mydriatic effect. It is also used for minor allergic hyperemia of the conjunctiva.

    b. β-**Adrenoceptor blockers and prostaglandin analogs** are used for the treatment of **chronic open-angle glaucoma (they have supplanted the use of α_2-receptor agonists).**

4. *CNS*

    a. **Amphetamine** and related analogs (e.g., **modafinil**) are used to treat **narcolepsy** (controversial) because of their arousal effects and their ability to increase the attention span; and to treat **attention-deficit hyperactivity disorder** (e.g., **methylphenidate**).

    b. **Hydroxyamphetamine** and **phenylephrine** are used for the **diagnosis of Horner syndrome.**

    c. **Dexmedetomidine** (Precedex), a novel selective α_2-**adrenoceptor agonist** that acts centrally, is used intravenously as a **sedative** in patients hospitalized in intensive care settings.

5. *Other uses* include **tizaididine** (Zanaflex) as a **muscle relaxant.**

E. Adverse effects and toxicity

    1. The adverse effects of sympathomimetic drugs are generally extensions of their pharmacologic activity.

    2. Overdose with **epinephrine** or other pressor agents may result in **severe hypertension,** with possible **cerebral hemorrhage, pulmonary edema,** and **cardiac arrhythmia.** Milder effects include headache, dizziness, and tremor. Increased cardiac workload may result in angina or myocardial infarction in patients with coronary insufficiency.

    3. Phenylephrine should not be used to treat closed-angle glaucoma before iridectomy as it may cause **increased intraocular pressure.**

    4. Sudden discontinuation of an α_2-**adrenoceptor agonist** may cause **withdrawal symptoms** that include headache, tachycardia, and a rebound rise in blood pressure.

    5. Drug abuse may occur with amphetamine and amphetamine-like drugs.

    6. Drug interactions

        a. **Tricyclic antidepressants** block catecholamine reuptake and may potentiate the effects of norepinephrine and epinephrine.

        b. Some **halogenated anesthetic agents** and **digitalis** may sensitize the heart to β-receptor stimulants, resulting in ventricular arrhythmias.

VII. ADRENERGIC RECEPTOR ANTAGONISTS

These drugs interact with either α- or β-adrenoceptors to prevent or reverse the actions of endogenously released norepinephrine or epinephrine or exogenously administered sympathomimetic agents.

A. α-Adrenoceptor antagonists

1. **Pharmacologic effects**

   a. The pharmacologic effects of α-adrenoceptor antagonists are predominantly cardiovascular and include **lowered peripheral vascular resistance and blood pressure.** These agents prevent pressor effects of α-receptor agonists.

   b. α-Adrenoceptor antagonists convert the pressor action of sympathomimetic agents with both α- and β-adrenoceptor agonist activity to a depressor response; this is referred to as **epinephrine reversal.**

2. **Specific drugs** (Table 2.10)

table **2.10**   Therapeutic Uses of Selected Adrenoceptor Antagonists

Drug	Receptor	Features	Major Uses
Phentolamine[a]	α$_1$ and α$_2$	Short duration of action (1–2 h)	Hypertension of pheochromocytoma
Phenoxybenzamine[a]		Long duration of action (15–50 h)	Hypertension of pheochromocytoma
Prazosin[a]	α$_1$	Minimal reflex tachycardia	Mild-to-moderate hypertension (often with a diuretic or a β-adrenoceptor antagonist); severe congestive heart failure (with a cardiac glycoside and a diuretic)
Terazosin			Mild-to-moderate hypertension
Doxazosin			Mild-to-moderate hypertension
Propranolol[a]	β$_1$ and β$_2$	Local anesthetic activity	Hypertension; angina; pheochromocytoma, cardiac arrhythmias; migraine headache; hypertrophic subaortic stenosis
Timolol			Hypertension; glaucoma
Metipranolol			Glaucoma
Levobunolol			Glaucoma
Nadolol		Long duration of action (15–25 h)	a. Hypertension; angina
b. Pindolol		Partial β$_2$-receptor agonist activity[b]	Hypertension; angina
Penbutolol		Partial β$_2$-receptor agonist activity[b]; mild-to-moderate hypertension	Hypertension; angina
Carteolol		Partial β$_2$-receptor agonist activity[b]; excreted unchanged	Hypertension; angina; glaucoma
Metoprolol[a]	β$_1$>β$_2$	Patient bioavailability is variable; extended release form available	Hypertension; angina
Atenolol		Eliminated by the kidney	Hypertension; angina
Esmolol		Ultrashort acting (10 min)	Supraventriculartachycardia
Betaxolol		Long duration of action (15–25 h)	Glaucoma; hypertension
Acebutolol		Partial agonist[b]	Hypertension; ventricular arrhythmias
Labetalol[a]	β$_1$, β$_2$, and α$_1$	Partial agonist[b]; rapid blood pressure reduction; local anesthetic activity	Mild-to-severe hypertension; hypertensive emergencies

[a]Drugs listed in **boldface type** are considered prototype drugs.
[b]Lower blood pressure without significant reduction in cardiac output or resting heart rate; also do not elevate triglyceride levels or decrease high-density lipoprotein cholesterol.

a. Phentolamine (Regitine) is an intravenously administered, short-acting competitive antagonist at both α_1- and α_2-receptors. It reduces peripheral resistance and decreases blood pressure.

b. Prazosin (Minipress)

   (1) Prazosin is the prototype of competitive antagonists selective for α_1-receptors. Others include **terazosin** (Hytrin), **doxazosin** (Cardura), **tamsulosin** (Flomax), **silodosin** (Rapaflo), and **alfuzosin** (Uroxatral).

   (2) Prazosin reduces peripheral resistance and blood pressure.

   (3) This drug is administered orally. Prazosin has a **slow onset** (2–4 h) and a **long duration of action** (10 h) and is extensively metabolized by the liver (50% during first pass).

c. Labetalol (Normodyne and Trandate)

   (1) Labetalol is a **competitive antagonist** (partial agonist) that is relatively selective for α_1-receptors and also blocks β-receptors.

   (2) Labetalol reduces heart rate and myocardial contractility, decreases total peripheral resistance, and lowers blood pressure.

   (3) This drug undergoes extensive first-pass metabolism.

d. Phenoxybenzamine (Dibenzyline)

   (1) Phenoxybenzamine is a noncompetitive, irreversible antagonist with some selectivity for α_1-receptors.

   (2) Phenoxybenzamine binds covalently, resulting in a long-lasting (15–50h) blockade.

3. *Therapeutic uses* (Table 2.10)

   a. An overview

   (1) α_1-Adrenoceptor antagonists are used most often to treat hypertension and urinary obstruction of benign prostatic hypertrophy (BPH).

   (2) α_2-Adrenoceptor antagonists have no important therapeutic uses.

   b. Pheochromocytoma

   (1) Pheochromocytoma is a **tumor** of the **adrenal medulla** that secretes excessive amounts of catecholamines. Symptoms include hypertension, tachycardia, and arrhythmias.

   (2) **Phentolamine** and **phenoxybenzamine** are used to treat the tumor in the preoperative stage; they also are used for long-term management of inoperable tumors.

   (3) β-Receptor antagonists are often used to prevent the cardiac effects of excessive catecholamines after an α-receptor blockade is established.

   c. Prazosin and others in its class, and **labetalol,** are used with other drugs to treat **essential hypertension.**

   d. α_1-Adrenoceptor antagonists, such as **prazosin, terazosin, doxazosin,** and **alfuzosin,** are used to treat urinary obstruction of **BPH. Tamsulosin** and **silodosin** may have greater efficacy due to their selective action at α_{1A}-**receptors.**

   e. Other uses of α-adrenoceptor antagonists (e.g., **phentolamine**) include reversible peripheral vasospasm like **Raynaud syndrome,** and **erectile dysfunction** (in combination with **papaverine**).

4. *Adverse effects*

   a. Major adverse effects of **phentolamine** and **phenoxybenxamine** include postural hypotension and tachycardia.

   b. Prazosin, terazosin, and **doxazosin** produce postural hypotension and bradycardia on initial administration; these drugs produce no significant tachycardia.

   c. Adverse effects of **labetalol** include postural hypotension and GI disturbances. Bradycardia occurs with overdose. Labetalol produces fewer adverse effects on the bronchi and cardiovascular system than selective β-receptor antagonists.

B. β-Adrenoreceptor antagonists

   1. *Pharmacologic effects*

   a. Cardiovascular system

   (1) β-Adrenoreceptor antagonists **lower blood pressure,** possibly because of their combined effects on the heart, the renin–angiotensin system, and the CNS.

    (2) These drugs **reduce** sympathetic-stimulated increases in **heart rate** and **contractility** and **cardiac output.**

    (3) β-Adrenoreceptor antagonists **lengthen AV conduction time and refractoriness and suppress automaticity.**

    (4) Initially, they may increase peripheral resistance. However, long-term administration results in decreased peripheral resistance in patients with hypertension.

    (5) β-Adrenoreceptor antagonists reduce renin release.

  b. Respiratory system

    (1) β-Adrenoreceptor antagonists **increase airway resistance** as a result of β_2-receptor blockade.

    (2) This respiratory effect is more pronounced in asthmatics because of unopposed, compensatory, reflex sympathomimetic α-receptor activity resulting from decreased cardiac output.

  c. Eye

    (1) β-Adrenoreceptor antagonists decrease the production of aqueous humor, resulting in **reduced intraocular pressure.**

  d. Other activities

    (1) β-Adrenoreceptor antagonists **inhibit lipolysis** (β_3).

    (2) These drugs **inhibit glycogenolysis** (β_2) in the liver (they may impede recovery from the hypoglycemic effect of insulin).

    (3) These drugs decrease high-density lipoprotein levels.

    (4) Some β-adrenoceptor antagonists have local anesthetic action, including **propranolol** and **labetalol.**

2. *Specific drugs* (Table 2.10)

  a. An overview

    (1) **Propranolol** is the **prototype** β-adrenoreceptor antagonist.

    (2) These drugs have an **antihypertensive effect** that is slow to develop (the mechanism is unclear).

    (3) β-Adrenoreceptor antagonists are absorbed well after oral administration. Including **propranolol,** many have **low bioavailability** (<50%) because of extensive first-pass metabolism; marked interpatient variability is seen, particularly with **metoprolol.**

    (4) With the exceptions of **esmolol** (10 min) and **nadolol** and **betaxolol** (15–25 h), most have a $t_{1/2}$ of 3–12 hours.

  b. Propranolol (Inderal)

    (1) Propranolol is a competitive antagonist at β_1- and β_2-receptors.

    (2) Propranolol is used in **long-term treatment of hypertension,** but it is not useful for hypertensive crisis.

    (3) This drug is used to treat **supraventricular and ventricular arrhythmias** and is administered IV for the emergency treatment of arrhythmias.

    (4) This drug is cleared by hepatic metabolism and, therefore, has prolonged action in the presence of liver disease.

  c. Metoprolol (Lopressor), **betaxolol** (Betoptic), **bisoprolol** (Zebeta), **atenolol** (Tenormin), **acebutolol** (Sectral), **esmolol** (Brevibloc), and **nebivolol** (Bystolic)

    (1) These drugs are selective β_1**-receptor antagonists** that may offer some advantage over nonselective β-adrenoceptor antagonists to treat cardiovascular disease in asthmatic patients, although cautious use is still warranted.

    (2) **Atenolol** is **eliminated** primarily by the **kidney** and undergoes little hepatic metabolism; it has little local anesthetic activity; it enters the CNS poorly.

    (3) **Esmolol** is **ultrashort acting** ($t_{1/2}$ = 10 min) because of extensive hydrolysis by plasma esterases; it is administered by **IV infusion.**

  d. Labetalol (Normodyne and Trandate) and **Carvedilol** (Coreg)

    (1) Labetalol is a partial agonist that blocks β-receptors and α_1-receptors (3:1 to 7:1 ratio). Carvedilol also has mixed activity but is equiactive at β-receptors and α_1-receptors.

   (2) Labetalol reduces heart rate and myocardial contractility, decreases total peripheral resistance, and lowers blood pressure.

   (3) This drug is administered PO or IV and undergoes extensive first-pass
   metabolism.

   e. Timolol (Blocadren), **levobunolol** (Betagan), **nadolol** (Corgard), and **sotalol** (Betapace)

   (1) These drugs are **nonselective β-receptor antagonists.**

   (2) Timolol and levobunolol have excellent **ocular effects** when applied **topically for glaucoma. Metipranolol** (OptiPranolol) is also used to treat glaucoma.

   (3) Sotalol additionally prolongs the cardiac action potential and is used to treat **arrhythmias.**

   f. Pindolol (Visken), **carteolol** (Cartrol), and **penbutolol** (Levatol) are nonselective antagonists with partial β_2-receptor agonist activity.

   (1) Carteolol is **excreted unchanged.**

3. *Therapeutic uses* (see Table 2.10)

   a. Cardiovascular system (see also Chapter 4)

   (1) β-Adrenoreceptor antagonists are used to treat **hypertension,** often in combination with a diuretic or vasodilator.

   (2) These drugs reduce the incidence of **myocardial infarction.**

   (3) These drugs provide prophylaxis for **supraventricular and ventricular arrhythmias.**

   (4) β-Adrenoreceptor antagonists provide prophylaxis for **angina pectoris.** Long-term
   use of **timolol, propranolol,** and **metoprolol** may prolong survival after myocardial
   infarction.

   (5) Propranolol relieves angina, palpitations, dyspnea, and syncope in **obstructive cardiomyopathy.** This effect is thought to be related to the slowing of ventricular
   ejection and decreased resistance to outflow.

   b. Eye

   (1) Topical application of **timolol, betaxolol, levobunolol,** and **carteolol** reduces intraocular pressure in **glaucoma.**

   (2) Sufficient **timolol** can be absorbed after topical application to increase airway
   resistance and decrease heart rate and contractility.

   c. Other uses

   (1) Propranolol is used to control clinical symptoms of sympathetic overactivity in
   hyperthyroidism, perhaps by inhibiting conversion of thyroxine to triiodothyronine.

   (2) Propranolol and others may be beneficial in the prophylaxis of **migraine headache.**

   (3) Propranolol relieves acute **anxiety** and panic symptoms by inhibiting peripheral
   overactivity of the SNS.

4. *Adverse effects and contraindications*

   a. All agents

   (1) β-Adrenoreceptor antagonists should be administered with extreme caution in
   patients with preexisting compromised cardiac function because they can precipitate **heart failure** or heart block.

   (2) These drugs may augment insulin action in diabetics and **mask tachycardia** associated with hypoglycemia.

   (3) β-Adrenoreceptor antagonists may **mask** the signs of developing **hyperthyroidism.**

   (4) After abrupt withdrawal, adrenoceptor "supersensitivity" and increased risk of
   angina and **arrhythmias** may occur. **Tapered withdrawal** is recommended.

   b. Nonselective adrenoceptor antagonists

   (1) These drugs may cause **bronchoconstriction,** and thus they are contraindicated
   for asthmatics. Patients with chronic obstructive lung disease are particularly
   susceptible.

   (2) β_1-Selective antagonists should also be used cautiously to treat asthmatics
   because they have some β_2-receptor antagonist activity.

   c. Propranolol, and other β-receptor blockers, cause **sedation, sleep disturbances, and depression.**

DRUG SUMMARY TABLE

Direct-Acting Cholinoceptor Agonists
Acetylcholine (Miochol-E)
Bethanechol (Urecholine, generic)
Carbachol (generic)
Cevimeline (Evoxac)
Methacholine (Provocholine)
Pilocarpine (generic)
Varenicline (Chantix)

Indirect-Acting Cholinoceptor Agonists
Ambenonium (Mytelase)
Demecarium (Humorsol)
Donepezil (Aricept)
Echothiophate (Phospholine)
Edrophonium (Tensilon, generic)
Galantamine (Reminyl)
Neostigmine (Prostigmin, generic)
Physostigmine (Eserine, generic)
Pyridostigmine (Mestinon, Regonol)
Rivastigmine (Exelon)
Tacrine (Cognex)

Cholinesterase Regenerator
Pralidoxime (Protopam, generic)

Muscarinic Cholinoceptor Antagonists
Atropine (generic)
Clidinium (Quarzan, generic)
Cyclopentolate (Cyclogyl, generic)
Darifenacin (Enablex)
Dicyclomine (Bentyl, generic)
Fesoterodine (Toviaz)
Flavoxate (Uripas)
Glycopyrrolate (Robinul, generic)
Homatropine (generic)
Ipratropium (Atrovent, generic)
Mepenzolate (Cantil)
Methantheline (Banthine)
Oxybutynin (Ditropan, generic)
Propantheline (Pro-Banthine)
Scopolamine (generic)
Solifenacin (Vesicare)
Tiotropium (Spiriva)
Tolterodine (Detrol)
Tridihexethyl (Pathilon)
Tropicamide (generic)
Trospium (Spasmex)

Ganglion Blocking Drugs
Mecamylamine (Inversine)
Trimethaphan (Arfonad)

Skeletal Muscle Relaxants
Neuromuscular Blocking Drugs
Atracurium (generic)
Cisatracurium (Nimbex)
Mivacurium (Mivacron)
Pancuronium (Pavulon, generic)
Rocuronium (Zemuron, generic)
Succinylcholine (Anectine, generic)
Tubocurarine (generic)
Vecuronium (Norcuron, generic)

Spasmolytic Drugs
Baclofen (Lioresal, generic)
Botulinum toxin-type A (Botox)
Botulinum toxin-type B (Myobloc)
Dantrolene (Dantrium)

Sympathomimetic Drugs
Albuterol (Proventil, Ventolin, generic)
Amphetamine (generic)
Apraclonidine (Lopidine)
Bitolterol (Tornalate)
Brimonidine (Alphagan)
Clonidine (Catapres, generic)
Dexmedetomidine (Precedex)
Dextroamphetamine (Dexedrine, generic)
Dipivefrin (Propine)
Dobutamine (Dobutrex, generic)
Dopamine (Intropin, generic)
Ephedrine (generic)
Epinephrine (generic)
Fenoldopam (Corlopam)
Formoterol (Foradil)
Guanabenz (Wytensin, generic)
Guanfacine (Tenex)
Hydroxyamphetamine (Paredrine)
Isoproterenol (Isuprel, generic)
Levalbuterol (Xopenex)
Metaproterenol (Alupent, generic)
Metaraminol (Aramine)
Methamphetamine (Desoxyn)
Methoxamine (Vasoxyl)
Methyldopa (Aldomet, generic)

Methylphenidate (Ritalin, generic)
Midodrine (Pro-Amatine)
Modafinil (Provigil)
Naphazoline (Privine)
Norepinephrine (generic)
Oxymetazoline (generic)
Phenylephrine (generic)
Pirbuterol (Maxair)
Pseudoephedrine (Sudafed)
Salmeterol (Serevent)
Terbutaline (Brethine, generic)
Tetrahydrozoline (generic)
Xylometazoline (Otrivin, generic)

Adrenergic Receptor Antagonists
Alpha-Receptor Blockers
Alfuzosin (Uroxatral)
Doxazosin (Cardura, generic)
Phenoxybenzamine (Dibenzyline)
Phentolamine (Regitine)
Prazosin (Minipress, generic)
Silodosin (Rapaflo)
Tamsulosin (Flomax)
Terazosin (Hytrin, generic)
Tolazoline (Priscoline)

Beta-Receptor Blockers
Acebutolol (Sectral, generic)
Atenolol (Tenormin, generic)
Betaxolol (Kerlone)
Bisoprolol (Zebreta, generic)
Carteolol (Cartrol)
Carvedilol (Coreg)
Esmolol (Brevibloc)
Labetalol (Normodyne, Trandate, generic)
Levobunolol (Betagan)
Metipranolol (OptiPranolol)
Metoprolol (Lopressor, generic)
Nadolol (Corgard, generic)
Nebivolol (Bystolic)
Penbutolol (Levatol)
Pindolol (Visken, generic)
Propranolol (Inderal, generic)
Sotalol (Betapace, generic)
Timolol (Blocadren. generic)

Review Test

Directions: Each of the numbered items or incomplete statements in this section is followed by answers or by completions of the statement. Select the ONE lettered answer or completion that is BEST in each case.

1. Botulinum toxin causes paralysis by

(A) Inhibiting choline acetyltransferase
(B) Blocking transport of choline into neurons
(C) Blocking release of acetylcholine from storage vesicles
(D) Inhibiting acetylcholinesterase
(E) Blocking the synapse at ganglia

2. Which of the following neurotransmitters interacts with guanethidine?

(A) Acetylcholine
(B) Epinephrine
(C) Dopamine
(D) Norepinephrine
(E) Serotonin

3. What is the mechanism of action of cocaine?

(A) Propagation of action of norepinephrine by inhibiting its active transport from the synapse
(B) Oxidative deamination of norepinephrine in nerve terminals and the effector cells
(C) Inhibition of metabolism of norepinephrine in nerve terminals
(D) Potentiation of tyrosine hydroxylase, the rate-limiting enzyme in the synthesis of norepinephrine
(E) Promotion of release of norepinephrine from adrenergic nerve endings

4. What intracellular effect does albuterol, a β_2-agonist, produce?

(A) Allows passage of sodium through a ligand-gated ion channel
(B) Activates G_s-protein, resulting in stimulation of adenylyl cyclase
(C) Activates G_q-protein, resulting in increase of phosphatidylinositol and calcium mobilization

(D) Activates G_i-protein, resulting in inhibition of adenylyl cyclase
(E) Binds to μ-receptors in specific areas of the brain

5. What class of medications does bethanechol belong to?

(A) Nicotinic blockers
(B) α-Agonists
(C) β_1-Blockers
(D) β_2-Blockers
(E) Muscarinic agonists

6. A 38-year-old farmer is brought to the ER by his wife with symptoms of sudden difficulty breathing, sweatiness, and anxiety. He was spraying insecticide when this happened. It has been 25 minutes since the symptoms started. The patient is emergently intubated and given atropine and another medication that acts to reactivate acetylcholinesterase. What medication is it?

(A) Physostigmine
(B) Propranolol
(C) Pralidoxime
(D) Phenylephrine
(E) Pancuronium

7. Oxybutynin works by

(A) Inhibiting acetylcholinesterase at muscarinic and nicotinic receptors
(B) Causing a neuromuscular blockade
(C) Antagonizing α_1-adrenoceptors
(D) Binding to muscarinic receptors
(E) Activating β_2-adrenoceptors

8. A 78-year-old man with Parkinson disease experiences worsening of his symptoms. He is already taking levodopa. Since the disease is characterized by degeneration of dopaminergic neurons, leading to the lack of inhibition of cholinergic neurons, the addition of which medication is likely to help alleviate the patient's symptoms?

(A) Benztropine
(B) Reserpine
(C) Doxazocin
(D) Timolol
(E) Tubocurarine

9. A 66-year-old woman with a long history of heavy smoking presents to her doctor with complaints of shortness of breath and chronic coughing that has been present for about 2 years and has been worsening in frequency. The doctor decides to prescribe a bronchodilator agent that has minimal cardiac side effects, since the patient also has an extensive cardiac history. Which medication did the doctor likely prescribe?

(A) Albuterol
(B) Prazosin
(C) Atenolol
(D) Ipratropium
(E) Pseudoephedrine

10. From the list below, choose the depolarizing neuromuscular blocker most likely to be used in "rapid sequence intubation," a procedure that is done when the stomach contents have a high risk of refluxing and causing aspiration.

(A) Baclofen
(B) Succinylcholine
(C) Neostigmine
(D) Homatropine
(E) Pralidoxime

11. Ephedra (ephedrine) causes increased blood pressure by

(A) Indirect action on cholinergic receptors
(B) Blockade of adrenergic receptors
(C) Stimulation of release of epinephrine
(D) Inhibition of reuptake of catecholamines
(E) Direct action on dopamine receptors

12. A 34-year-old carpenter presents to the ER after an accident in which he inadvertently chopped off the tip of his index finger. He is taken to the OR for reattachment of the digit, and after sedation, a local anesthetic is administered around the site of the injury. The local anesthetic used in the procedure did not contain any epinephrine, as it usually does for most surgical procedures. The reason for this is

(A) Epinephrine causes increased blood loss during delicate surgery
(B) Epinephrine causes swelling of the tissues, making surgery more challenging
(C) Epinephrine is contraindicated in emergency surgery
(D) Epinephrine causes vasoconstriction, which can lead to vascular ischemia in digits
(E) Epinephrine can cause hypotension when administered with sedative agents

13. A 7-year-old boy is brought in by his parents for complaints of hyperactivity at school. He is also inattentive and impulsive at home. After a detailed interview, the physician decides to give the boy amphetamine-containing medication for presumed attention hyperactivity disorder. Amphetamine

(A) Inhibits epinephrine reuptake
(B) Indirectly acts on norepinephrine receptors
(C) Blocks effects of norepinephrine
(D) Directly acts on cholinoreceptors
(E) Inhibits serotonin reuptake

14. Which of the following medications is used to prevent premature labor?

(A) Tamsulosin
(B) Cevimeline
(C) Atracurium
(D) Tolterodine
(E) Terbutaline

15. What significant side effect of terazosin should the doctor warn a 69-year-old patient about?

(A) Bronchospasm
(B) Postural hypotension
(C) Heart failure
(D) Sedation
(E) Drug abuse

16. A floor nurse pages you about a patient who is having chest pain. You order an electrocardiogram and rush to see the patient. He describes the pain as tight pressure and is demonstrably sweating and gasping for air. The ECG comes back with acute ST-segment elevations in inferior leads, and you diagnose a myocardial infarction. You start giving the patient oxygen and give him sublingual nitroglycerin and morphine for pain. You also give him another medication, which you have read may prolong his survival in this dire situation. What class of medication is it?

(A) β-Blocker
(B) α-Agonist
(C) Muscarinic agonist
(D) Neuromuscular blocker
(E) Dopamine agonist

17. A 35-year-old woman presents to your office for a regular check-up. Her only complaint is recurrent migraine headaches, which have increased in frequency over the years. On examination, her blood pressure is elevated at 150/70. You decide to start her on antihypertensive therapy that is also used for prophylaxis of migraines. Which medication is it?

(A) Clonidine
(B) Prazosin
(C) Hydrochlorothiazide
(D) Propranolol
(E) Verapamil

18. In contrast to propranolol, metoprolol

(A) Is used for the management of hypertension
(B) Has greater selectivity for β_2-adrenoceptors
(C) May be beneficial for the acute treatment of migraine headache
(D) Is less likely to precipitate bronchoconstriction in patients with asthma

19. Intravenous administration of epinephrine to a patient results in a severe decrease in diastolic pressure and an increase in cardiac output. Which of the following drugs might the patient have previously taken that could account for this unexpected effect?

(A) Propranolol
(B) Atropine
(C) Phenylephrine
(D) Prazosin

20. Which of the following drugs is used to diagnose myasthenia gravis?

(A) Atropine
(B) Neostigmine
(C) Bethanechol
(D) Edrophonium
(E) Pralidoxime

21. Pilocarpine reduces intraocular pressure in patients with glaucoma because it

(A) Activates nicotinic cholinoceptors
(B) Blocks muscarinic cholinoceptors

(C) Selectively inhibits peripheral activity of sympathetic ganglia
(D) Inhibits acetylcholinesterase

22. Prolonged apnea may occur following the administration of succinylcholine to a patient with a hereditary deficiency of which of the following enzymes?

(A) Glucose-6-phosphate dehydrogenase
(B) Plasma cholinesterase
(C) Monoamine oxidase
(D) Cytochrome $P450_{3A}$
(E) Acetylcholinesterase

23. Dantrolene is used to treat malignant hyperthermia caused by succinylcholine because dantrolene

(A) Blocks Ca^2 release from sarcoplasmic reticulum
(B) Induces contraction of skeletal muscle
(C) Increases the rate of succinylcholine metabolism
(D) Inhibits succinylcholine binding to nicotinic receptors
(E) Acts centrally to reduce fever

24. A drug that acts at prejunctional α_2-adrenoceptors and is used to treat hypertension is

(A) Clonidine
(B) Metaproterenol
(C) Dobutamine
(D) Dopamine

25. Drug X causes an increase in blood pressure and a decrease in heart rate when administered to a patient intravenously. If an antagonist at ganglionic nicotinic receptors is administered first, drug X causes an increase in blood pressure and an increase in heart rate. Drug X most likely is

(A) Propranolol
(B) Norepinephrine
(C) Isoproterenol
(D) Terbutaline
(E) Curare

26. Poisoning with an insecticide containing an acetylcholinesterase inhibitor is best managed by administration of which one of the following agents?

(A) Physostigmine
(B) Bethanechol
(C) Propranolol
(D) Pilocarpine
(E) Atropine

27. Receptor actions of acetylcholine are mimicked by nicotine at which one of the following sites?

(A) Adrenal medullary chromaffin cells
(B) Urinary bladder smooth muscle cells
(C) Iris circular (constrictor) muscle
(D) Heart sinoatrial pacemaker cells

28. Muscarinic cholinoceptor agonists may cause vasodilation through the release of endothelial

(A) Histamine
(B) Norepinephrine
(C) Acetylcholine
(D) Nitric oxide

29. Emergency treatment of acute heart failure is best managed with which of the following drugs?

(A) Metaproterenol
(B) Phenylephrine
(C) Dobutamine
(D) Norepinephrine
(E) Isoproterenol

30. Which one of the following agents, when applied topically to the eye, would cause both mydriasis and cycloplegia?

(A) Phenylephrine
(B) Carbachol
(C) Prazosin
(D) Atropine

31. Neostigmine would be expected to reverse which one of the following conditions?

(A) Paralysis of skeletal muscle induced by a competitive, nondepolarizing muscle relaxant
(B) Paralysis of skeletal muscle induced by a depolarizing muscle relaxant
(C) Cardiac slowing induced by stimulation of the vagus nerve
(D) Miosis induced by bright light

32. The direct cardiac effects of dobutamine would be blocked by which one of the following agents?

(A) Prazosin
(B) Metoprolol
(C) Clonidine
(D) Isoproterenol

33. Topical application of timolol to the eye would be expected to induce which of the following?

(A) Miosis
(B) Mydriasis
(C) Decreased formation of aqueous humor
(D) Increased outflow of aqueous humor

34. Phenylephrine is used to treat patients with nasal mucosa stuffiness because it causes vasoconstriction by

(A) Blocking nicotinic cholinoceptors
(B) Blocking β-adrenoceptors
(C) Stimulating α-adrenoceptors
(D) Stimulating muscarinic cholinoceptors

Answers and Explanations

1. **The answer is C.** Botulinum toxin blocks calcium-dependent exocytosis of acetylcholine from storage vesicles, producing paralysis. Common sources of botulinum toxin include canned home goods and, in cases of infant botulism, honey. The condition is life-threatening, and urgent care is necessary. Choline acetyltransferase is an enzyme catalyzing synthesis of acetylcholine from an acetate and choline. Sodium-dependent transport of choline can be blocked by hemicholinium. Enzyme acetylcholinesterase is responsible for catalyzing hydrolysis of acetylcholine. Acetylcholine synapses at the ganglia of many neurons and tissues, and this step is not blocked by botulinum toxin.

2. **The answer is D.** Guanethidine blocks the release of norepinephrine from storage vesicles into the nerve terminals. Acetylcholine release can be blocked by botulinum toxin. Epinephrine, dopamine, and serotonin release can be blocked by other agents (beyond the scope of this chapter), but not by guanethidine.

3. **The answer is A.** Cocaine is a potent inhibitor of norepinephrine uptake, a process that normally terminates norepinephrine's action. Oxidative deamination of norepinephrine in nerve terminals and the effector cells describes the action of monoamine oxidase, which is targeted by certain antidepressant medications. Inhibition of metabolism of norepinephrine in nerve terminals describes catechol-O-methyltransferase, which is found in nerve and other effector cells. Potentiation of tyrosine dehydroxylase would, in fact, cause excessive amounts of norepinephrine to accumulate; however, this enzyme is not affected by cocaine. Norepinephrine release can be blocked, not promoted, by agents such as bretylium and guanethidine.

4. **The answer is B.** β_2-agonists, like albuterol, activate G_s-protein, which results in stimulation of adenylyl cyclase, with subsequent increase in intracellular CAMP. Passage of sodium via ligand-gated ion channel is manifested by nicotinic acetylcholine receptors. Activation of G_q-protein resulting in increase in phosphatidylinositol and calcium mobilization refers to the mechanism of action of muscarinic receptor types M_1 and M_3, as well as α_1-adrenoceptors. Activation of G_q-protein resulting in increase in phosphatidylinositol and calcium mobilization refers to mechanism of action of M_2-cholinoceptors and α_2-adrenoceptors. Finally, binding to μ-receptors in the specific areas of the brain describes the action of opioid agents.

5. **The answer is E.** Bethanechol is a type of muscarinic receptor agonist that is used clinically to ameliorate urinary retention. Nicotinic blockers such as trimethaphan are rarely used in clinical practice because of the lack of selectivity. α-Agonists such as epinephrine can be used in the management of acute bronchospasm (anaphylaxis). β_1-Blockers do not have direct effects on bronchial smooth muscle. β_2-Agonists such as albuterol are used for the treatment of asthma.

6. **The answer is C.** Acetylcholinesterase reactivator pralidoxime has to be given within 30 minutes of exposure to insecticide because of the effects of "aging" (i.e., strengthening of the alkylphosphoryl-serine bond formed between AChE and organophosphate). Physostigmine is a cholinesterase inhibitor that is occasionally used in atropine or scopolamine poisoning. Propranolol is a β-blocker used for hypertension as well as other indications. Phenylephrine is an α-agonist used for hypotensive emergencies. Pancuronium is a nondepolarizing inhibitor of acetylcholine that is used for muscle paralysis.

7. **The answer is D.** Oxybutynin acts by binding to muscarinic receptors located on the detrusor muscle of the bladder, suppressing involuntary contraction of the muscle. Neuromuscular blockers such as succinylcholine are used for anesthesia. α_1-Antagonists such as terazosin are used for benign prostatic hypertrophy. β_2-Agonists such as terbutaline can be used to suppress premature labor.

8. **The answer is A.** Benztropine, an antimuscarinic agent, is used as an adjunct for the treatment of Parkinson disease. Reserpine is a norepinephrine uptake inhibitor occasionally used for the treatment of hypertension. Doxazocin, an α-blocker, is used for benign prostatic hyperplasia. Timolol is a β-blocker used for glaucoma. Tubocurarine is a neuromuscular blocker used in anesthesia.

9. **The answer is D.** Ipratropium bromide is used extensively for chronic obstructive pulmonary disease (COPD), which is the most likely diagnosis in this case. It acts by antagonizing muscarinic receptors in bronchial smooth muscle, thereby causing bronchodilation. Albuterol is also used for the treatment of COPD; however, it can cause adverse cardiac effects such as tachycardia and is not recommended in this case. Prazosin is an α-blocker used for benign prostatic hypertrophy (BPH). Atenolol is a β-blocker used for hypertension. Pseudoephedrine is an α-agonist used for nasal congestion.

10. **The answer is B.** Succinylcholine is a depolarizing neuromuscular blocker that is used in rapid-sequence intubation, as well as other procedures. It quickly relaxes all muscles in the body, allowing a prompt intubation to prevent the reflux of gastric contents into the trachea. Baclofen is a centrally acting skeletal muscle relaxant used for spasticity. Neostigmine is an indirect-acting cholinergic agonist used for the treatment of myasthenia gravis and reversal of neuromuscular blockade. Homatropine is an antimuscarinic agent used for induction of mydriasis for ophthalmologic examinations. Pralidoxime is an acetylcholinesterase reactivator used for organophosphate poisoning.

11. **The answer is C.** Ephedrine acts indirectly to release norepinephrine from nerve terminals, causing effects similar to those of catecholamines, including elevated blood pressure. This potentially dangerous agent has been removed from the OTC market because of an increasing number of deaths being reported as caused by this agent. An example of an indirect-acting cholinergic agonist is edrophonium, which is used for diagnosis of myasthenia gravis. Some adrenoceptor blockers, such as atenolol, are used for the treatment of hypertension. Catecholamine reuptake inhibition is a property of some antidepressant medications. Dopamine receptor agonists are used in the treatment of Parkinson disease.

12. **The answer is D.** Epinephrine is contraindicated as an anesthetic adjuvant for surgeries involving most facial structures, digits, and the penis, because of the risk of vascular compromise. This agent causes decreased blood loss for most other surgeries because of vasoconstriction. Although local anesthetic agents such as Marcaine or Xylocaine can cause mild local tissue swelling, epinephrine does not; either way, it is not a contraindication for hand surgery. Epinephrine causes elevated blood pressure when administered systemically; however, it has no systemic side effects when administered locally.

13. **The answer is B.** Amphetamine and similar compounds are stimulants used for treatment of attention-deficit/hyperactivity disorder (ADHD) in which they are thought to act centrally to increase attention span. Currently, there is no medication on the U.S. market that inhibits reuptake of epinephrine. Blocking of the effects of norepinephrine will not alleviate symptoms of ADHD. Direct-acting cholinoceptor agonists are not used in the treatment of ADHD. Serotonin reuptake inhibitors are used for depression and some other conditions.

14. **The answer is E.** Terbutaline, a β_2-agonist, is used to suppress premature labor because of its ability to stop uterine contractions. Tamsulosin, an α_1-blocker, is used for benign prostatic hypertrophy. Cevimeline, a cholinergic agonist, is used for Sjögren syndrome. Atracurium a nondepolarizing muscular blocker, is used for anesthesia. Tolterodine, a muscarinic blocker, is used for urinary incontinence.

15. **The answer is B.** α_1-Adrenoceptor agonists such as terazosin may cause significant postural hypotension and should be prescribed carefully in the elderly population. Bronchospasm is a possible side effect of β-blockers. β-Blockers can also produce heart failure in some patients. Sedation is common with the use of some agents such as propranolol. Drug abuse can be observed in patients using centrally acting adrenoreceptor agonists such as amphetamine.

16. **The answer is A.** β-Blockers such as atenolol are now part of management of acute myocardial infarction, along with oxygen, nitroglycerin, and morphine. They reduce sympathetic activity and heart contractility, thereby reducing the oxygen demand. α-Agonists such as phenylephrine are used in the management of hypotension due to shock. Muscarinic agonists such as pilocarpine can be used in the management of glaucoma. Neuromuscular blockers such as atracurium are used in anesthesia. Dopamine agonists are used in the management of Parkinson disease.

17. **The answer is D.** The β-blocker propranolol is a good choice for an antihypertensive medication; however, it is also successfully used for other indications, such as prophylaxis of migraine headaches, situational anxiety, and hyperthyroidism-induced palpitations. The other choices are all acceptable antihypertensive medications, but from this list, only propranolol is used for migraine prophylaxis.

18. **The answer is D.** Metoprolol is more selective at β_1-adrenoceptors, which are more abundant in the heart than in the lungs. Like propranolol, it may be beneficial in the prophylaxis of migraine.

19. **The answer is D.** Prazosin is the only drug listed that blocks postjunctional α_1-adrenoceptors and inhibits epinephrine-mediated vasoconstriction.

20. **The answer is D.** Edrophonium, which will increase muscle strength in untreated myasthenic patients, is the preferred acetylcholinesterase inhibitor (Tensilon test) because it has a short duration of action.

21. **The answer is B.** Pilocarpine is a muscarinic cholinoceptor agonist.

22. **The answer is B.** Plasma cholinesterase is responsible for the rapid inactivation of succinylcholine.

23. **The answer is A.** In patients with malignant hyperthermia, a rare hereditary disorder, an impaired sarcoplasmic reticulum is unable to sequester calcium. The sudden release of calcium results in extensive muscle contraction that can be reduced with dantrolene.

24. **The answer is A.** Clonidine acts at prejunctional α_2-adrenoceptors and is used to treat hypertension. Metaproterenol is a selective β_2-adrenoceptor agonist. Dobutamine is a relatively selective β_1-adrenoceptor agonist. Dopamine activates both prejunctional and postjunctional dopamine receptors and also β_1-adrenoceptors.

25. **The answer is B.** In the absence of a nicotinic receptor antagonist, norepinephrine may result in a reflex baroreceptor-mediated increase in vagal activity. The presence of such an agent unmasks the direct stimulant effect of norepinephrine on heart rate.

26. **The answer is E.** Atropine blocks the effects of increased acetylcholine resulting from cholinesterase inhibition. Physostigmine indirectly activates cholinoceptors; bethanechol and pilocarpine directly activate cholinoceptors. Propranolol is a β-adrenoceptor antagonist.

27. **The answer is A.** Nicotinic cholinoceptors are found in adrenal medullary chromaffin cells. At the other sites, acetylcholine activates muscarinic cholinoceptors.

28. **The answer is D.** The release of nitric oxide activates guanylate cyclase, increasing guanosine 3',5'-monophosphate (cyclic GMP) and sequestering calcium. This leads to a relaxation of vascular smooth muscle.

29. **The answer is C.** Dobutamine, a relatively selective β_1-adrenoceptor agonist, increases cardiac output and lowers peripheral resistance. Metaproterenol has a relatively more selective action on the respiratory system than the cardiovascular system. Phenylephrine and norepinephrine increase peripheral resistance. Isoproterenol increases heart rate.

30. **The answer is D.** Atropine produces both mydriasis and cycloplegia (the inability to accommodate for near vision). Phenylephrine causes mydriasis without cycloplegia. Carbachol causes pupillary constriction. Prazosin is an α-adrenoceptor antagonist.

31. **The answer is A.** Acetylcholine accumulation due to neostigmine inhibition of cholinesterase will reverse the action of the competitive neuromuscular blocking agents.

32. **The answer is B.** The β_1-adrenoceptor antagonist metoprolol blocks the β_1-adrenoceptor activity of dobutamine.

33. **The answer is C.** β-Adrenoceptor blocking agents such as timolol reduce aqueous humor formation.

34. **The answer is C.** Phenylephrine activates α-adrenoceptors, producing vasoconstriction.

chapter 3 | Drugs Acting on the Renal System

I. DIURETICS

A. Introduction

1. *Function.* Diuretics **increase urine production** by acting on the kidney (Fig. 3.1). Most agents affect water balance indirectly by altering electrolyte reabsorption or secretion. Osmotic agents affect water balance directly.

2. *Effects.* Natriuretic diuretics produce **diuresis**, associated with increased sodium (Na^+) excretion, which results in a concomitant loss of water and a reduction in extracellular volume.

3. *Therapeutic uses.* Diuretic agents are generally used for the management of edema, hypertension, **congestive heart failure (CHF)**, and abnormalities in body fluid distribution.

4. *Side effects.* Diuretics can cause electrolyte imbalances such as hypokalemia, hyponatremia, and hypochloremia and disturbances in acid–base balance.

B. Thiazide diuretics

1. *Mechanism.* Thiazide diuretics are **absorbed from the gastrointestinal (GI) tract** and produce diuresis within 1–2 hours. They are **secreted into the lumen** of the proximal tubule via organic anion carriers. They exert effects only after reaching the lumen.

   a. These agents inhibit active reabsorption of sodium chloride (NaCl) in the distal convoluted tubule by interfering with Na^+-Cl^- cotransporter (**NCC**), a specific Na^+/Cl^- transport protein (Fig. 3.2), resulting in the net excretion of Na and an accompanying volume of water.

      (1) These agents increase excretion of Cl^-, Na^+, potassium (K^+), and, at high doses, HCO_3^-.

      (2) They **reduce excretion of calcium** (Ca^{2+}).

   b. **True thiazide** diuretics are derivatives of sulfonamides (sulfonamide diuretics). Many also **inhibit carbonic anhydrase**, resulting in diminished bicarbonate (HCO_3^-) reabsorption by the proximal tubule.

2. *Specific agents*

   a. **Prototype** true thiazides include **chlorothiazide** and **hydrochlorothiazide**. Other agents include methyclothiazide. Chlorothiazide is the only thiazide available for parenteral use.

   b. **Thiazide-like drugs** such as **metolazone**, **chlorthalidone**, and **indapamide** have properties generally similar to those of the thiazide diuretics (Table 3.1). However, unlike thiazides, these agents may be effective in the presence of some renal impairment. Indapamide has proven especially useful in diabetic patients with hypertension, where it reduces the risk of cardiovascular disease.

3. *Therapeutic uses*

   a. Thiazide diuretics are the preferred class of diuretic for the treatment of **essential hypertension** when renal function is normal; they are often used in combination with other antihypertensive agents to enhance their blood pressure-lowering effects. They reduce plasma volume and total peripheral resistance.

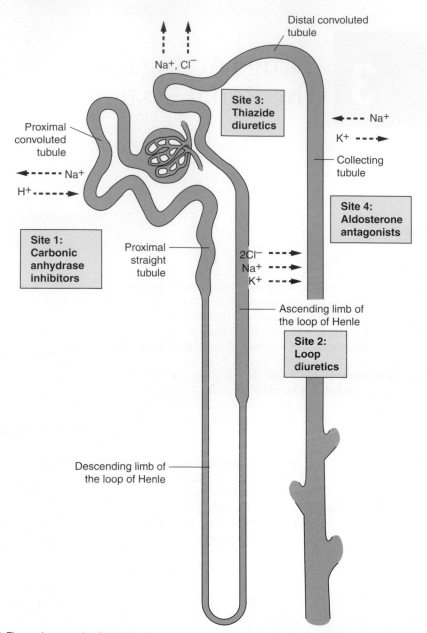

FIGURE 3.1. The nephron can be divided into four sites anatomically and pharmacologically. Site 1 is the proximal tubule, site of action of carbonic anhydrase inhibitors. Site 2 is the ascending limb of the loop of Henle, site of action of the loop diuretics. Site 3 is the distal convoluted tubule, site of action of the thiazides. Site 4 is the collecting tubule, site of action of aldosterone antagonists. Cl^-, chloride; H^+, hydrogen; K^+, potassium; Na^+, sodium.

      b. These agents reduce the formation of new calcium stones in **idiopathic hypercalciuria**.

      c. Thiazide diuretics may be useful in patients with diabetes insipidus that is not responsive to antidiuretic hormone (ADH).

      d. These agents are often used in combination with a potassium-sparing diuretic to manage **mild cardiac edema**, **cirrhotic** or **nephrotic edema**, and **edema produced by hormone imbalances**. They are frequently used in the treatment of **Ménière disease**.

    4. ***Adverse effects and contraindications.*** Thiazide diuretics should be used cautiously in the presence of renal or hepatic diseases such as cirrhosis, and they should be used only as an ancillary treatment in nephrotic syndrome.

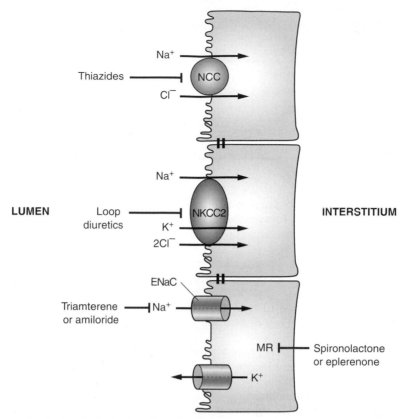

FIGURE 3.2. The molecular targets of thiazide and loop diuretics are transmembrane cotransporters, whereas the molecular target of amiloride is a specific Na^+ channel.

a. Thiazide diuretics produce electrolyte imbalances such as **hypokalemia, hyponatremia,** and **hypochloremic alkalosis.** These imbalances are often accompanied by central nervous system (CNS) disturbances, including dizziness, confusion, and irritability; muscle weakness; cardiac arrhythmias; and by decreasing plasma K^+, **increased sensitivity to digitalis.** Diets low in Na^+ and high in K^+ are recommended; K^+ supplementation may be required.

b. These agents often **elevate serum urate,** presumably as a result of competition for the organic anion carriers (which also eliminates uric acid). Gout-like symptoms may appear.

c. Thiazide diuretics can cause **hyperglycemia** (especially in patients with diabetes), **hypertriglyceridemia, hypercholesterolemia,** and hypersensitivity reactions (sulfa groups).

C. Loop diuretics

1. *Mechanism.* Loop diuretics are absorbed by the GI tract and are eliminated by filtration and tubular secretion; some elimination occurs via the hepatic-biliary route. They are administered either orally or parenterally. Diuresis occurs within 5 minutes of intravenous (IV) administration and within 30 minutes of oral administration.

a. Loop diuretics inhibit active NaCl reabsorption in the thick ascending limb of the loop of Henle by inhibiting **NKCC2,** another specific $Na^+/K^+/2Cl^-$ cotransporter. Because of the high capacity for NaCl reabsorption in this segment, agents active at this site markedly increase water and electrolyte excretion and are referred to as **high-ceiling diuretics.**

b. Loop diuretics cause increased renal prostaglandin production, which accounts for some of their activity. Nonsteroidal anti-inflammatory drugs (NSAIDs) can reduce the effectiveness of loop diuretics.

c. These agents reduce reabsorption of Cl^- and Na^+; they **increase Ca^{2+} excretion** and loss of K^+ and magnesium (Mg^{2+}).

t a b l e **3.1**	Thiazide Diuretics and Related Agents		
Drug	Chemical Class	Potency	Half-Life (h)
Chlorothiazide	Benzothiadiazide	0.1	2
Hydrochlorothiazide	Benzothiadiazide	1.0	3
Metolazone	Quinazoline	5	5
Chlorthalidone	Quinazoline	10	26
Indapamide	Indoline	20	16

2. ***Specific agents.*** Prototype drugs include furosemide and bumetanide, as well as ethacrynic acid and torsemide. **Furosemide, torsemide, and bumetanide contain a sulfhydryl group**, but **ethacrynic acid does not**; an important consideration for sulfa-sensitive patients.

3. ***Therapeutic uses***
   a. Loop diuretics are used in the treatment of **CHF** by reducing **acute pulmonary edema** and edema refractory to other agents. They are synergistic with thiazide diuretics when coadministered.
   b. These agents are used to treat **hypertension**, especially in individuals with **diminished renal function**. They reduce the plasma volume and also the total peripheral resistance.
   c. They are also used to treat acute **hypercalcemia** and **halide poisoning**.
   d. These drugs are often effective in producing diuresis in patients responding maximally to other types of diuretics.

4. ***Adverse effects and contraindications***
   a. Loop diuretics produce **hypotension** and **volume depletion**, as well as **hypokalemia**, because of enhanced secretion of K^+. They may also produce **alkalosis** due to enhanced H^+ secretion. Mg^{2+} **wasting** can also occur; therapy is often instituted gradually to minimize electrolyte imbalances and volume depletion.
   b. Loop diuretics can cause dose-related **ototoxicity**, more often in individuals with renal impairment. These effects are more pronounced with ethacrynic acid than with furosemide. These agents should be administered cautiously in the presence of renal disease or with the use of other ototoxic agents such as **aminoglycosides**.
   c. These agents can cause hypersensitivity reactions. Ethacrynic acid produces GI disturbances.

D. **Potassium-sparing diuretics**
   1. ***Mechanism***
      a. Potassium-sparing diuretics reduce Na^+ **reabsorption** and reduce K^+ **secretion** in the distal part of the nephron (collecting tubule).
      b. These are not potent diuretics when used alone; they are primarily used in combination with other diuretics.
   2. ***Selected drugs***
      a. **Antagonists of the mineralocorticoid** (aldosterone) **receptor** include **eplerenone**, which is highly receptor selective, and **spironolactone**, which binds to other nuclear receptors such as the androgen receptor.
         (1) ***Mechanism.*** These agents inhibit the action of aldosterone by competitively binding to the mineralocorticoid receptor and preventing subsequent cellular events that regulate K^+ and H^+ secretion and Na^+ reabsorption. An important action is a reduction in the biosynthesis of ENaC, the Na^+ channel in the principal cells of the collecting duct.
            (a) These agents are active only when endogenous mineralocorticoid is present; the effects are enhanced when hormone levels are elevated.
            (b) These agents are **absorbed** from the **GI tract** and are **metabolized** in the **liver**; therapeutic effects are achieved only after several days.

(2) ***Therapeutic uses.*** These drugs are generally used in combination with a thiazide or loop diuretic to treat **hypertension, CHF**, and **refractory edema**. They are also used to induce diuresis in clinical situations associated with hyperaldosteronism, such as in **adrenal hyperplasia** and in the presence of **aldosterone-producing adenomas** when surgery is not feasible.

(3) ***Adverse effects and contraindications***

    (a) These agents can cause **hyperkalemia, hyperchloremic metabolic acidosis**, and arrhythmias. Spironolactone is associated with **gynecomastia** and can also cause menstrual abnormalities in women.

    (b) These drugs are **contraindicated in renal insufficiency**, especially in diabetic patients. They must be used cautiously in the presence of liver disease. They are contraindicated in the presence of other potassium-sparing diuretics and should be used with extreme **caution** in individuals taking an **angiotensin-converting enzyme inhibitor**.

b. Amiloride and triamterene

  (1) ***Mechanism.*** Amiloride and triamterene bind to and block ENaC and thereby decrease absorption of Na^+ and excretion of K^+ in the cortical collecting tubule, independent of the presence of mineralocorticoids.

    (a) These drugs produce diuretic effects 2–4 hours after oral administration.

    (b) **Triamterene** increases urinary excretion of Mg^{2+} but amiloride does not; triamterene and amiloride are metabolized in the liver. Both drugs are **secreted** in the **proximal tubule**.

  (2) ***Therapeutic uses.*** These agents are used to manage **CHF, cirrhosis**, and **edema** caused by secondary hyperaldosteronism. They are available in combination products containing thiazide or loop diuretics (e.g., triamterene/hydrochlorothiazide, amiloride/hydrochlorothiazide) to treat hypertension.

  (3) ***Adverse effects and contraindications.*** Amiloride and triamterene produce **hyperkalemia**, the most common adverse effect, and ventricular arrhythmias. Dietary potassium intake should be reduced. Minor adverse effects include nausea and vomiting. The use of these drugs is contraindicated in the presence of diminished renal function.

E. Carbonic anhydrase inhibitors

  1. ***Mechanism.*** Carbonic anhydrase inhibitors inhibit carbonic anhydrase in all parts of the body. In the kidney, the effects are predominantly in the proximal tubule.

    a. These drugs reduce HCO_3^- reabsorption and concomitant Na^+ uptake. They also inhibit excretion of hydrogen (H^+) and coupled Na^+ uptake.

    b. Carbonic anhydrase inhibitors are **absorbed** from the **GI tract** and are **secreted** by the **proximal tubule**. Urine pH changes are observed within 30 minutes.

  2. ***Prototype drugs*** include **acetazolamide** and **methazolamide**. These agents are **sulfonamide derivatives**, forerunners of thiazide diuretics. (Thiazides separate natriuresis from carbonic anhydrase inhibition.)

  3. ***Therapeutic uses.*** Carbonic anhydrase inhibitors are rarely used as diuretics.

    a. These drugs are most useful in the treatment of **glaucoma**. They serve to decrease the rate of HCO_3^- formation in the aqueous humor and consequently reduce ocular pressure.

    b. Carbonic anhydrase inhibitors are sometimes used as adjuvants for the treatment of **seizure disorder**, but the development of tolerance limits their use.

    c. These agents may be used to produce a desired alkalinization of urine to **enhance renal secretion of uric acid and cysteine**.

    d. They may be used for prophylaxis and treatment of **acute mountain sickness**.

  4. ***Adverse reactions and contraindications***

    a. Adverse reactions include **metabolic acidosis** due to reduction in bicarbonate stores. Urine alkalinity decreases the solubility of calcium salts and increases the propensity for renal calculi formation. **Potassium wasting** may be severe.

    b. Following large doses, carbonic anhydrase inhibitors commonly produce drowsiness and paresthesias.

    c. The use of these drugs is contraindicated in the presence of **hepatic cirrhosis**.

F. **Agents influencing water excretion**

1. ***Osmotic agents*** include **mannitol, glycerin, urea, and hypertonic saline**. These agents are easily filtered, poorly reabsorbable solutes that alter the diffusion of water relative to sodium by "binding" water. As a result, net reabsorption of Na^+ is reduced. **They are commonly used to reduce intracranial pressure due to trauma and intraocular pressure prior to a surgical procedure.**

   a. **Mannitol** and **urea** are administered intravenously.

      (1) ***Therapeutic uses***

         (a) **Mannitol** is used in **prophylaxis of acute renal failure** resulting from physical trauma or surgery. Even when filtration is reduced, sufficient mannitol usually enters the tubule to promote urine output.

         (b) **Mannitol** may also be useful for reducing cerebral edema and intraocular pressure.

         (c) Parenteral **urea** is approved for the reduction of intracranial and intraocular pressure.

      (2) ***Adverse effects and contraindications***. Because the osmotic forces that reduce intracellular volume ultimately expand extracellular volume, serious adverse effects may occur in patients with CHF. Minor adverse effects include headache and nausea.

   b. **Glycerin** is administered orally. This drug is used primarily for **ophthalmic procedures**. Topical anhydrous glycerin is useful for **corneal edema**.

2. ***Agents that influence the action of ADH (vasopressin)*** influence the permeability of the luminal surface of the medullary collecting duct to water by causing water-specific water channels called aquaporin II to be inserted into the plasma membrane (Fig. 3.3). Under conditions of dehydration, ADH levels increase to conserve body water. Agents that **elevate** or mimic ADH are **antidiuretic;** agents that **lower** or antagonize ADH action are **diuretic**. Vasopressin binds to three receptors: V_{1a} in the vasculature, V_{1b} in the brain, and V_2 in renal collecting ducts.

   a. Vasopressin or analogs

      (1) ***Therapeutic uses***. These agents are useful in the management of **neurohypophyseal diabetes insipidus. Desmopressin** (DDAVP), one of the most useful analogs, is also used to treat **nocturnal enuresis**. Studies have suggested that vasopressin and its analogs are useful to maintain blood pressure in patients with **septic shock** and to increase **clotting factor VIII** in some patients with Type I von Willebrand's disease.

      (2) ***Adverse effects and contraindications***. These drugs can produce serious **cardiac-related adverse effects**, and they should be used with caution in individuals with coronary artery disease. Hyponatremia occurs in ~5% of patients.

   b. Chlorpropamide, acetaminophen, indomethacin, and clofibrate

      (1) ***Mechanisms***

         (a) **Chlorpropamide, acetaminophen,** and **indomethacin** enhance the action of ADH, at least partially by reducing the production of prostaglandins in the kidney.

         (b) **Clofibrate** increases the release of ADH centrally.

      (2) ***Therapeutic uses***. These agents are useful as antidiuretics in diabetic patients.

   c. **ADH antagonists** include the vaptans: **conivaptan,** a mixed V_{1a} and V_2 antagonist, and **tolvaptan**, a V_2 selective antagonist.

      (1) ***Therapeutic uses***. **Conivaptan** is approved for the treatment of **hypervolemic hyponatremia and syndrome of inappropriate ADH (SIADH). Tolvaptan** is approved for treating **hyponatremia** associated with CHF, cirrhosis, and SIADH. The vaptans may be more effective in treating hypervolemia in heart failure than diuretics.

   d. **Nonreceptor** antagonists of ADH action include **demeclocycline** and **lithium carbonate**. They may be useful in the treatment of **(SIADH)** secretion as seen in some lung cancers.

FIGURE 3.3. The mechanism of action of ADH includes ligand binding to the V_2 receptor, which is coupled to increased cAMP production. This ultimately causes an increase in the insertion of the water-specific transporter aquaporin II into the apical plasma membrane.

G. Other diuretics

1. *Xanthine diuretics* act by increasing cardiac output and promoting a higher glomerular filtration rate. They are seldom used as diuretics, but diuresis occurs under other clinical applications (e.g., for bronchodilatation). The mechanism of this action is antagonism of adenosine receptors.

2. *Acidifying salts* (e.g., **ammonium chloride**) decrease pH and increase luminal concentrations of Cl^- and Na^+. They are sometimes used in combination with high-ceiling diuretics to counteract alkalosis.

II. NONDIURETIC INHIBITORS OF TUBULAR TRANSPORT

A. **Nondiuretic inhibitors** influence transport of organic anions, including the endogenous anion uric acid, and cations. Transport takes place in the proximal tubule; organic compounds enter a cell by Na^+-facilitated diffusion and are excreted from the cell into the lumen by a specific organic ion transporter. *Para*-**aminohippurate**, not used clinically, is a classic compound used to study these phenomena.

B. Uricosuric agents

1. ***Mechanism.*** Uricosuric agents **increase excretion of uric acid**. Paradoxically, because of the balance among uptake into a cell, excretion from the cell, and reabsorption from the lumen, low doses of these agents often decrease urate excretion, whereas high doses increase urate excretion.

2. ***Therapeutic uses.*** These drugs are often used in the prophylactic treatment of gout.

3. ***Selected drugs***
   a. Probenecid
      (1) ***Mechanism.*** Probenecid is absorbed from the GI tract and is secreted by the proximal tubule.
         (a) Probenecid **inhibits secretion of organic anions** (e.g., from the plasma to the tubular lumen). The predominant organic ion transporters in the kidney are OAT-3 and OAT-1. Probenecid was developed to **decrease secretion of penicillin** (an organic acid) and thus prolong elimination of this antibiotic. This is affected by inhibiting **OATs**. Other drugs whose secretion is inhibited by probenecid include **indomethacin** and **methotrexate**.
         (b) At higher doses, probenecid also **decreases reabsorption of uric acid by inhibiting URAT1, a urate transport protein**. This results in a net increase in urate excretion and accounts for the drug's usefulness in treating gout.
      (2) ***Therapeutic uses.*** Probenecid is used to **prevent gout** in individuals with normal renal function. It is also used as an **adjuvant to penicillin therapy** when prolonged serum levels following a single dose are required or to enhance antibiotic concentrations in the CNS.
      (3) ***Adverse effects and contraindications***. The most common adverse effects of probenecid are hypersensitivity reactions and gastric irritation.
   b. **Allopurinol and febuxostat (see Chapter 6)**
      (1) ***Mechanism.*** These agents are not uricosuric, rather they **inhibit xanthine oxidase**, which is involved in the synthesis of uric acid. The result is **decreased production of uric acid. Febuxostat** may be more selective for xanthine oxidase than allopurinol.
      (2) ***Therapeutic uses.*** These drugs are used in the prophylactic treatment of gout and should **not be used to treat an acute attack. Colchicine or an NSAID is used for acute attacks**.

▆ DRUG SUMMARY TABLE

Diuretics—Thiazides
Chlorothiazide (Diuril, generic)
Hydrochlorothiazide (Esidrix, Oretic, others)
Methyclothiazide (Aquatensin, Enduron)
Polythiazide (Renese)

Diuretics—Thiazide-like
Metolazone (Zaroxolyn)
Chlorthalidone (Hydone, Thalitone)
Indapamide (Lozol)

Diuretics—Loop
Furosemide (Lasix, Delone, generic)
Bumetanide (Bumex)
Ethacrynic acid (Edecrin)
Torsemide (Demadex, generic)

Diuretics—Potassium-sparing
Spirolactone (Aldactone, generic)
Amiloride (Midamor, generic)

Triamterene (Dyrenium)
Eplerenone (Inspra)

Carbonic Anhydrase Inhibitors
Acetazolamide (Diamox)
Methazolamide (GlaucTabs)
Dichlorphenamide (Daranide)

Osmotic Diuretics
Mannitol (Osmitrol)
Urea (generic)
Glycerin (generic)

Antidiuretic Hormone Agonists
Desmopressin (DDAVP)
Lysine vasopressin (generic)
Vasopressin (Pitressin)

Antidiuretic Antagonists
Conivaptan (Vaprisol)
Tolvaptan (Samsca)

Demeclocycline (Declomycin)
Lithium carbonate (generic)

Uricosuric Agents
Probenecid (generic)

Urate Synthesis Inhibitors
Allopurinol (Aloprim, Zyloprim)
Febuxostat (Uloric)

Other Antigout Agents
Colchicine (generic)
Pegloticase (Krystexxa)

Review Test

Directions: Each of the numbered items or incomplete statements in this section is followed by answers or by completions of the statement. Select the ONE lettered answer or completion that is BEST in each case.

1. A 35-year-old woman presents to your office for a regular check-up. She has no complaints. On examination, her blood pressure is slightly elevated at 145/85. She is physically fit and follows a healthy diet. You decide to start her on antihypertensive therapy and prescribe hydrochlorothiazide. How does this agent work?

(A) Inhibits reabsorption of sodium chloride in the early distal convoluted tubule

(B) Decreases net excretion of chloride, sodium, and potassium

(C) Increases excretion of calcium

(D) Inhibits reabsorption of sodium chloride in the thick ascending limb of the loop of Henle

(E) Interferes with potassium secretion

2. A 7-year-old boy is brought to the clinic by his mother. He complains of sharp pain in his flanks, as well as dysuria and frequency. The doctor orders a 24-hour urine calcium test, and the results come back abnormal. After additional work-up, the child is diagnosed with idiopathic hypercalciuria. What is a common type of medication used for this aliment?

(A) Loop diuretics

(B) Carbonic anhydrase inhibitors

(C) Thiazide diuretics

(D) Potassium-sparing diuretics

(E) Osmotic diuretics

3. A 45-year-old man with a history of medication-controlled hypertension presents to your office with complaints of a painful, swollen big toe on the left foot. You suspect gout and check his uric acid levels, which are elevated. From looking at the list of the medications the patient is taking, you realize that one of the medications may be the cause of his current symptoms. Which medication might that be?

(A) Acetazolamide

(B) Amiloride

(C) Spironolactone

(D) Hydrochlorothiazide

(E) Mannitol

4. A 57-year-old man with a history of heavy alcohol use is being admitted for a first episode of congestive heart failure (CHF), which likely resulted from untreated alcoholic cardiomyopathy. The cardiologist decides to start the patient on diuretic therapy. Which class of diuretics is preferred in this scenario?

(A) Loop diuretics, because they exert their action at the distal convoluted tubule

(B) Loop diuretics, because the thick ascending limb is an area of high capacity for NaCl reabsorption

(C) Thiazide diuretics, because they exert their action at the thick ascending limb of the loop of Henle

(D) Thiazide diuretics, because they increase cardiac output

(E) Thiazide diuretics, because they increase peripheral vascular resistance

5. A 66-year-old woman suffers a myocardial infarction while in the hospital and immediately goes into respiratory distress. On examination, you realize the patient has flash pulmonary edema as a result of her infarction. Along with the management of the myocardial infarction, you start the patient on furosemide therapy to treat pulmonary edema. What is the mechanism of action of this agent?

(A) Inhibition of action of aldosterone by binding to its receptor in principal cells of the collecting duct

(B) Reduction of bicarbonate reabsorption and concomitant sodium uptake

(C) Inhibition of active reabsorption of sodium chloride at the distal convoluted tubule

(D) Alteration of the diffusion of water relative to sodium, thereby reducing sodium reabsorption

(E) Inhibition of active reabsorption of sodium chloride at the thick ascending limb of the loop of Henle

6. An 87-year-old woman who is taking multiple medications for her "heart disease" is prescribed gentamicin for diverticulitis. After a few days of taking the antibiotic, she complains of dizziness and tinnitus. What "heart medication" might she be on?

(A) Spironolactone
(B) Hydrochlorothiazide
(C) Mannitol
(D) Ethacrynic acid
(E) Urea

7. A 54-year-old man develops congestive heart failure (CHF) after suffering his second myocardial infarction. His physician puts him on a regimen of several medications, including furosemide. On follow-up, the patient is found to have hypokalemia, likely secondary to furosemide use. The addition of which medication would likely resolve the problem of hypokalemia, while helping to treat the underlying condition, CHF?

(A) Allopurinol
(B) Hydrochlorothiazide
(C) Spironolactone
(D) Acetazolamide
(E) Ethacrynic acid

8. A 60-year-old previously healthy fit man presents to your office with new-onset hypertension. Since this is an unusual age to present with essential hypertension, you order an extensive work-up. The results show low levels of potassium, high levels of aldosterone, and low levels of renin. The patient is diagnosed with Conn syndrome, or hyperaldosteronism. A computed tomographic (CT) scan of the abdomen reveals bilateral adrenal hyperplasia, which renders this patient inoperable. You decide to start the patient on spironolactone therapy. How does this medication work?

(A) It is an agonist of the mineralocorticoid receptor

(B) It interferes with the action of the mineralocorticoid receptor

(C) It promotes sodium reabsorption

(D) It increases the synthesis of sodium channels in the principal cells

(E) It is only active when endogenous mineralocorticoids are absent

9. A 45-year-old woman with a long history of alcohol abuse is being treated for cirrhosis-associated ascites. Her internist decided to give her amiloride, a diuretic helpful in edema caused by cirrhosis. What common side effect should be monitored in this patient?

(A) Hypernatremia
(B) Hypocalcemia
(C) Hyperphosphatemia
(D) Hypermagnesemia
(E) Hyperkalemia

10. A 57-year-old man develops progressive vision loss with a sensation of pressure behind his eyes. His ophthalmologist diagnoses the patient with glaucoma. To prevent further progression of the disease and to alleviate current symptoms, the physician starts the patient on acetazolamide therapy. What is the mechanism of action of this medication?

(A) Potentiates carbonic anhydrase in all parts of the body

(B) Reduces reabsorption of bicarbonate

(C) Increases excretion of hydrogen

(D) Increases rate of formation of bicarbonate in the aqueous humor

(E) Increases uptake of sodium in the proximal tubule

11. A 50-year man with mild hypertension complains of discomfort in his chest. He has slightly enlarged fat deposits in his breasts with prominent nipples. Which of the following medications might be causing this adverse effect?

(A) Amiloride
(B) Spironolactone
(C) Metolazone
(D) Hydrochlorothiazide
(E) Acetazolamide

12. Since his hypertension is under control, you decide to switch this patient to a drug that has the same mechanism of action but will avoid this adverse effect. Which of the following drugs would you use?

(A) Amiloride
(B) Eplerenone
(C) Chlorthalidone
(D) Aldosterone
(E) Allopurinol

Answers and Explanations

1. **The answer is A.** Thiazide diuretics inhibit active reabsorption of sodium chloride in the early distal convoluted tubule of the nephron by interfering with the Na/Cl cotransporter, resulting in net excretion of sodium and water. These agents increase net excretion of chloride, sodium, and potassium. They decrease excretion of calcium. Inhibiting reabsorption of sodium chloride in the thick ascending limb of the loop of Henle describes the mechanism of action of loop diuretics. Interfering with potassium secretion refers to mechanism of action of potassium-sparing diuretics.

2. **The answer is C.** Thiazide diuretics decrease excretion of calcium and thus can be used for idiopathic hypercalciuria. Loop diuretics stimulate tubular calcium excretion and can thus be used to treat hypercalcemia. Carbonic anhydrase inhibitors, potassium-sparing diuretics, and osmotic diuretics do not have a significant impact on net calcium balance.

3. **The answer is D.** Hydrochlorothiazide, a thiazide diuretic, can precipitate a gouty attack in predisposed individuals. This is because these agents increase serum uric acid as a result of competition for the organic acid carrier. Loop diuretics can have this effect too. Acetazolamide is a carbonic anhydrase inhibitor; this agent does not have a significant impact on the levels of uric acid. Amiloride and spironolactone are potassium-sparing diuretics, and they do not have a significant impact on the levels of uric acid either. The same is true for mannitol, an osmotic diuretic.

4. **The answer is B.** Loop diuretics are used in cases of congestive heart failure (CHF) and pulmonary edema because they result in fast and significant diuresis. These agents exert their action at the thick ascending limb of the loop of Henle, which is the area of highest capacity for NaCl reabsorption. Thiazide diuretics actually decrease cardiac output initially, because of decrease blood volume. As well, thiazides decrease peripheral vascular resistance, because they relax arteriolar smooth muscle.

5. **The answer is E.** Loop diuretics inhibit active NaCl reabsorption in the thick ascending limb of the loop of Henle by inhibiting a specific $Na^+/K^+/2Cl^-$ cotransporter. Inhibition of action of aldosterone by binding to its receptor in principal cells of the collecting duct describes the mechanism of action of potassium-sparing diuretics. Reduction of bicarbonate reabsorption and concomitant sodium uptake refers to carbonic anhydrase inhibitors. Inhibition of active reabsorption of sodium chloride at the distal convoluted tubule describes thiazide diuretics. Finally, alteration of the diffusion of water relative to sodium, thereby reducing sodium reabsorption, refers to osmotic diuretics.

6. **The answer is D.** Ototoxicity, as demonstrated by tinnitus and dizziness, is a common side effect of loop diuretics, especially ethacrynic acid. This effect is magnified when aminoglycoside antibiotics are added to the regimen. Spironolactone is not associated with tinnitus. Hydrochlorothiazide can cause gout in susceptible individuals. Mannitol and urea are osmotic diuretics and are not indicated in patients with heart disease, especially congestive heart failure (CHF).

7. **The answer is C.** Spironolactone is commonly added to the regimen of anti-congestive heart failure (CHF) medications, since it counteracts the loss of potassium caused by the loop diuretics such as furosemide. This agent is also effective in reducing the symptoms of refractory edema. Allopurinol is not used to treat CHF. Hydrochlorothiazide will exacerbate hypokalemia caused by the loop diuretics. Acetozolamide will not counteract hypokalemia. Ethacrynic acid is an example of another loop diuretic.

8. **The answer is B**. Spironolactone interferes with the action of the mineralocorticoid receptor. Spironolactone prevents cellular events that regulate potassium and hydrogen secretion and sodium reabsorption. Spironolactone is an antagonist of mineralocorticoid receptors. It decreases the synthesis of sodium channels in the principal cells of the collecting ducts. This agent is only active when endogenous mineralocorticoids are present.

9. **The answer is E**. Hyperkalemia, a potentially life-threatening side effect, should be recognized as a possible result of amiloride use. Hyponatremia, not hypematremia, can be observed with amiloride. This agent does not affect calcium or phosphorus balance to a significant degree. Triamterene, another potassium-sparing diuretic, can cause increased urinary excretion of magnesium; amiloride is not known to produce this effect.

10. **The answer is B**. Acetazolamide belongs to a class of medications termed carbonic anhydrase inhibitors. These agents reduce bicarbonate reabsorption in the proximal tubule. They inhibit carbonic anhydrase in all parts of the body, including the aqueous humor, which makes these agents very useful in the treatment of glaucoma. Acetazolamide inhibits excretion of hydrogen and concomitant sodium uptake.

11. **The answer is B**. Spironolactone antagonizes the action of the mineralocorticoid, progesterone, and androgen receptors. Inhibition of androgen receptors can lead to gynecomastia and breast tenderness, most often in men.

12. **The answer is B**. Eplerenone has diuretic actions base on its antagonism of the mineralocorticoid receptor. Compared with spironolactone, it is much more specific for this receptor and is not associated with gynecomastia.

chapter 4

Drugs Acting on the Cardiovascular System

I. AGENTS USED TO TREAT CONGESTIVE HEART FAILURE (CHF)

A. An overview
   1. *CHF* results when the output of the heart is insufficient to supply adequate levels of oxygen for the body. Impaired contractility and circulatory congestion are both components of failure. Compensatory elevation in angiotensin II production results in sodium retention and vasoconstriction and increases both matrix formation and remodeling.
   2. *Therapeutic agents* (Fig. 4.1)
      a. Increase cardiac contractility.
      b. Reduce preload (left ventricular [LV] filling pressure) and aortic impedance (systemic vascular resistance).
      c. Normalize heart rate and rhythm.

B. Drugs that inhibit the activity of the renin–angiotensin system
   1. *An overview*
      a. Drugs that either interfere with the biosynthesis of angiotensin II (angiotensin-converting enzyme [ACE] inhibitors), or act as antagonists of angiotensin receptors (**angiotensin receptor blockers [ARBs]**), are indicated in all patients with LV dysfunction, whether symptomatic or asymptomatic. ACE inhibitors are becoming increasingly important in the treatment of CHF and have been shown to prevent or slow the progression of heart failure in patients with ventricular dysfunction. Agents that inhibit **renin activity** are useful for treating hypertension.
      b. Principles of the renin–angiotensin system (Fig. 4.2).
   2. Several parameters regulate the **release of renin** from the kidney cortex. Reduced arterial pressure, decreased sodium delivery to the cortex, increased sodium at the distal tubule, and stimulation of sympathetic activity all increase renin release.
   3. Renin cleaves the protein angiotensinogen and **releases the decapeptide angiotensin** I. Angiotensin I is converted enzymatically (mostly in the lung) to an octapeptide, **angiotensin II** (**AgII** or Ag1-8), by the activity of **ACE;** further metabolism produces the heptapeptide (**Ag2-8**). Angiotensin II stimulates the **release of aldosterone.** Angiotensin I can also be metabolized by **ACE2 to Ag1-7. The actions of Ag1-7 oppose those of AgII.**
   4. Angiotensin II is a potent vasoconstricting agent and **causes sodium and water retention via release of aldosterone**.
   5. The actions of angiotensin II are mediated by AT1, AT2, and AT4 receptors located in most tissues. The pressor actions of angiotensin II are mediated by AT1 receptors. Ag1-7 acts via the Mas receptor.
   6. Angiotensin II can be produced locally (e.g., in the myocardium, kidney, adrenals, or in vessel walls by the action of non-ACE pathways) by the action of chymases and cathepsins.

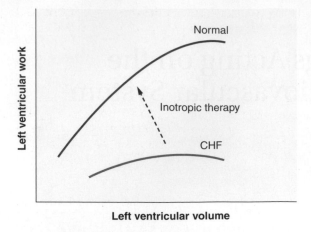

FIGURE 4.1. Pharmacologic goal in treating heart failure.

7. Because angiotensin I is produced via pathways other than the ACE pathway, angiotensin II receptor antagonists may be more effective and specific in reducing angiotensin II actions.

C. ACE inhibitors
   1. *Mechanism.* ACE inhibitors inhibit the production of angiotensin II from angiotensin I (see Fig. 4.2) by blocking the activity of ACE1; they do not inhibit ACE2. Blocking ACE1 also **diminishes the breakdown of the potent vasodilator bradykinin.**
      a. These agents **counteract** elevated peripheral vascular resistance and sodium and water retention resulting from angiotensin II and aldosterone.

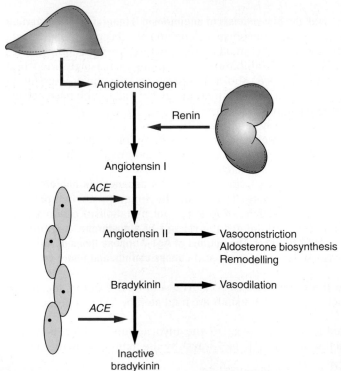

FIGURE 4.2. Major features of the renin–angiotensin system.

   b. ACE inhibitors are becoming increasingly important in the treatment of CHF and have been shown to prevent or slow the progression of heart failure in patients with ventricular dysfunction.

   c. ACE inhibitors increase cardiac output and induce systemic arteriolar dilation (reduce afterload).

   d. ACE inhibitors **cause venodilation** and **induce natriuresis,** thereby reducing preload.

   e. These drugs are especially useful for **long-term therapy.**

2. ***Therapeutic uses.*** ACE inhibitors are very useful in the treatment of **CHF, reducing risk of recurrent post-myocardial infarction (MI), reducing the progression of renal disease in diabetic nephropathy,** and treating **hypertension.** These agents have the advantage of producing minimal electrolyte disturbances and fewer adverse effects than many other agents used to treat hypertension.

3. ***Selected drugs*** (see Table 4.1 for a complete listing)

   a. Enalapril is a prodrug that is deesterified in the liver to produce **enalaprilat,** which inhibits ACE.

   (1) Therapeutic uses. Enalapril is a first-line drug in the treatment of CHF and is used to treat mild-to-severe hypertension. Diuretics enhance its activity.

   (2) Adverse effects and contraindications. Blood dyscrasias and aplastic anemia are rare but serious adverse effects of enalapril. Renal function may be impaired.

   b. Captopril, the first ACE inhibitor and the only sulfur-containing ACE inhibitor, is absorbed from the gastrointestinal (GI) tract and is metabolized to disulfide conjugates. Drug absorption is decreased ~30% by food. It does not enter the central nervous system (CNS). Captopril produces adverse effects that include rash, taste disturbance, pruritus, weight loss, and anorexia.

   c. Lisinopril is an ACE inhibitor that permits once-a-day dosing. The bioavailability of lisinopril is not affected by food.

4. ***Adverse effects*** common to all ACE inhibitors include a dry cough and, rarely, angioedema, especially of the face (both due to increased bradykinin levels), hypotension, and hyperkalemia.

D. Angiotensin II receptor blockers (ARBs)

1. ***Mechanism of action***

   a. The actions of angiotensin II are mediated by receptors that are 7-transmembrane proteins that couple to numerous signal transduction pathways. AT1 receptors are responsible for the pressor actions, increased aldosterone biosynthesis, and the proliferative and fibrotic actions of angiotensin II. In general, AT2 receptors antagonize the action of AT1 receptors. In several clinical trials, ARBs have proved as effective as ACE inhibitors in reducing mortality from CHF or following an MI.

t a b l e **4.1**	Commonly Used ACE Inhibitors and ARBs	
ACE Inhibitors	**ARBs**	**AT1/AT2 Affinity**
Captopril	Losartan (p)[a]	1,000
Enalapril (p)	Valsartan	20,000
Fosinopril (p)	Irbesartan	8,500
Lisinopril	Candesartan (p)	10,000
Quinapril (p)	Telmisartan	3,000
Benazepril (p)	Eprosartan	1,000
Moexipril (p)	Olmesartan (p)	12,500
Perindopril (p)		
Ramipril (p)		
Trandolapril (p)		

[a]p denotes prodrug, active metabolite produced by deesterification.

2. *ARBs: prototype drug—valsartan*
   a. **Mechanism.** Valsartan is an imidazole derivative with high affinity for AT1 receptors (about 20,000-fold higher than for AT2 receptors).
      (1) Oral doses are absorbed rapidly. Peak levels of the drug are obtained in about 3 hours, and it has a half-life of about 6 hours.
      (2) Valsartan is excreted in the feces, probably via biliary excretion.
   b. **Therapeutic uses.** In clinical trials, valsartan was about as effective as captopril in patients with LV dysfunction following an MI. Valsartan is as effective as ACE inhibitors in reducing blood pressure and is available in combination with hydrochlorothiazide for patients refractory to monotherapy.
   c. **Adverse effects and contraindications. Dizziness and hyperkalemia** can occur with valsartan. Since ARBs do not lead to accumulation of kinins, the incidence of both the nonproductive cough and angioedema associated with ACE inhibitors is reduced.
   d. All other ARBs (see Table 4.1) have the same mechanism of action and adverse effect profile but have subtle pharmacokinetic differences. They vary markedly in their relative affinity for AT1 and AT2 receptors.
3. *Renin inhibitors—Aliskiren* is a small molecule **direct inhibitor of renin**. It is administered orally and is eliminated mostly unchanged in the urine. Clinical trials suggest it is about as effective as ACE inhibitors or ARBs for reducing blood pressure. Diarrhea, angioedema, and hyperkalemia have been reported. The incidence of cough is reduced compared with ACE inhibitors. Aliskiren should **not** be combined with ACE inhibitors or ARBs in patients with renal impairment or diabetes due to an increase in the risk of serious adverse effects.

E. **Cardiac glycosides**
1. *Cardiac glycosides* are used for the treatment of **CHF** and **certain arrhythmias** (atrial fibrillation and flutter and paroxysmal atrial tachycardias). However, their overall use has diminished in the absence of data supporting a reduction in mortality.
2. The only cardiac glycoside used in the U.S. is **digoxin** (Lanoxin).
3. *Structure.* Cardiac glycosides are cardenolides that contain a lactone ring and a steroid (aglycone) moiety attached to sugar molecules.
4. *Mechanism*
   a. Cardiac glycosides **inhibit Na^+/K^+-ATPase,** resulting in increased intracellular Na^+ and decreased intracellular K^+. Increased Na^+ reduces the normal exchange of intracellular Ca^{2+} for extracellular Na^+ and yields somewhat elevated intracellular Ca^{2+} (Fig. 4.3).

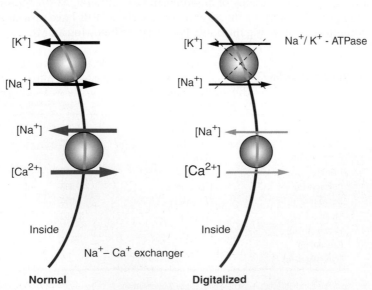

FIGURE 4.3. Changes in myocardial ion concentration following digitalis treatment.

  b. There are **multiple isoforms** of Na^+/K^+-ATPase; the cardiac **isoform** has the highest affinity for digitalis.

  c. Following treatment, each action potential produces a greater release of Ca^{2+} to activate the contractile process. The net result is a **positive inotropic effect.**

5. *Effects.* Cardiac glycosides have both direct effects on the heart and indirect effects mediated by an **increase in vagal tone.**

  a. Cardiac effects

  (1) Under normal cardiac conditions, digitalis treatment results in an increase in systemic vascular resistance and the constriction of smooth muscles in veins (cardiac output may decrease).

  (2) In the failing heart, the capacity to develop force during systole is compromised, and increased end-diastolic volume is required to achieve the same amount of work. Heart rate, ventricular volume, and pressure are elevated, whereas stroke volume is diminished.

  (a) Under these conditions, cardiac glycosides **increase stroke volume** and **enhance cardiac output.** Concomitantly, blood volume, venous pressure, and end-diastolic volume **decrease**.

  (b) The congested heart becomes smaller with treatment, and efficiency of contraction is increased (restored toward normal). **Improved circulation** reduces sympathetic activity and permits further improvement in cardiac function as a result of decreased systemic arterial resistance and venous tone.

  (3) Improved renal blood flow augments the elimination of Na^+ and water.

  b. Neural effects

  (1) Cardiac glycosides **increase vagal activity,** resulting in inhibition of the sinoatrial (SA) node and delayed conduction through the atrioventricular (AV) node.

  (2) Cardiac glycosides decrease sympathetic tone.

6. *Pharmacologic properties*

  a. Digoxin distributes to most body tissues and **accumulates in cardiac tissue.** The concentration of the drug in the heart is twice that in skeletal muscle and at least 15 times that in plasma.

  b. The **dose** of digoxin must be **individualized.** The initial loading (digitalizing) dose is often selected from prior estimates and adjusted for the patient's condition. The **maintenance dose** is based on the daily loss of the drug.

  c. Dosing levels for the treatment of CHF are generally lower than those required to decrease the ventricular response in atrial fibrillation.

  d. Digoxin has somewhat variable oral absorption; it can be given **orally** or **intravenously.** The peak effect after an intravenous (IV) dose occurs in 1.5–2 hours; the half-life ($t_{1/2}$) of digoxin is approximately 1.5 days. The maintenance dose of digoxin is approximately 35% of the loading dose.

  e. Because of a relatively rapid clearance, lack of compliance may quickly diminish therapeutic effects.

  f. Digoxin is **eliminated** by the **renal route;** the $t_{1/2}$ is prolonged in individuals with impaired renal function. Digoxin dosage can be adjusted on the basis of creatinine clearance.

7. *Adverse effects and toxicity*

  a. Narrow therapeutic index

  (1) Cardiac glycosides can cause fatal adverse effects.

  (2) These drugs induce virtually every type of arrhythmia.

  (3) Digoxin affects all excitable tissues; the most common site of action outside the heart is the GI tract (anorexia, nausea, vomiting, and diarrhea can occur), resulting either from direct action or through stimulation of the chemoreceptor trigger zone.

  (4) The use of digoxin may result in disorientation and visual disturbances.

  b. Toxicity is treated primarily by discontinuing the drug.

  (1) Potassium may help in alleviating arrhythmias.

  (2) **Antidigoxin antibodies** (digoxin immune FAB) (Digibind) and hemoperfusion are antidotes useful in acute toxicity.

(3) Antiarrhythmic agents such as phenytoin and lidocaine may be helpful in treating acute digoxin-induced arrhythmias.

(4) The first manifestation of digoxin overdose is frequently fatigue or a flu-like symptom.

c. Drug interactions

(1) Drugs that bind digitalis compounds, such as cholestyramine and neomycin, may interfere with therapy. Drugs that enhance hepatic metabolizing enzymes, such as phenobarbital, may lower the concentrations of the active drug.

(2) The risk of toxicity is increased by the following:

(a) Hypokalemia
Reduced K^+ results in increased phosphorylation of the Na^+/K^+-ATPase, and this **increases digoxin binding**. Thus, hypokalemia enhances the effects of these drugs and greatly increases the risk of toxicity. Hypokalemia may be seen with **thiazide** or other potassium-lowering diuretics.

(b) Hypercalcemia and calcium channel-blocking (CCB) agents (e.g., verapamil)
(i) CCB agents cause toxicity by adding to the drug effects on Ca^{2+} stores.
(ii) Hypocalcemia renders digitalis less effective.

(c) **Quinidine** displaces digoxin from tissue-binding sites. The $t_{1/2}$ of digoxin is prolonged because of decreased renal elimination.

F. Other inotropic agents

1. *Inamrinone lactate (formerly known as amrinone) and milrinone, the "inodilators"*

a. Inamrinone lactate and milrinone reduce LV filling pressure and vascular resistance and enhance cardiac output.

b. Inamrinone lactate and milrinone act by inhibiting phosphodiesterases in cardiac and vascular muscle, especially phosphodiesterase Type 3. This causes an increase in cyclic AMP (cAMP), thereby activating calcium channels leading to elevated intracellular Ca^{2+} levels and enhanced excitation contraction.

c. These drugs are used in patients who do not respond to digitalis; they are most effective in individuals with elevated LV filling pressure.

d. Inamrinone lactate and milrinone produce considerable **toxicity on extended administration;** they are administered intravenously only for short-term therapy. The most common **adverse effects** are transient thrombocytopenia and **hypotension**. Fever and GI disturbances occur occasionally.

e. Fewer and **less severe adverse effects** are seen with **milrinone** than with inamrinone.

2. *Dobutamine* hydrochloride is a **synthetic catecholamine** derivative that increases contractility; it acts primarily on myocardial β_1-adrenoceptors with lesser effects on β_2- and α-adrenoceptors. Dobutamine hydrochloride increases cAMP-mediated phosphorylation and the activity of Ca^{2+} channels.

a. Moderate doses of dobutamine hydrochloride do not increase heart rate.

b. Dobutamine hydrochloride does not activate dopamine receptors.

c. This drug is administered only by the IV route.

d. Dobutamine hydrochloride is used in **short-term therapy** in individuals with **severe chronic cardiac failure** and for inotropic support after an MI and cardiac surgery. It does not substantially increase peripheral resistance and, thus, is not useful in cardiac shock with severe hypotension.

e. Combined infusion therapy with **nitroprusside** or **nitroglycerin** may improve cardiac performance in patients with advanced heart failure.

f. Dobutamine hydrochloride produces tachycardia and hypertension, but it is less arrhythmogenic than **isoproterenol.**

3. *Dopamine* is a neurotransmitter and a metabolic precursor of the catecholamines. It can increase myocardial contractility and renal blood flow.

4. *Nesiritide (Natrecor)*

a. Nesiritide is a recombinant B-type natriuretic peptide approved for short-term use for acute decompensated heart failure.

b. Nesiritide increases cGMP and thereby produces vasodilation. It reduces pulmonary capillary wedge pressure and increases stroke volume.

    c. Nesiritide is a peptide that must be given parenterally; $t_{1/2}$ is about 18 minutes.

    d. Adverse effects include headache, nausea, and hypotension.

    e. Data supporting a reduction in mortality with nesiritide are lacking.

G. Diuretics (see Chapter 3)

    1. Diuretics reduce LV filling pressure and decrease LV volume and myocardial wall tension (lower oxygen demand).

    2. Diuretics are frequently combined with an ACE inhibitor in **mild CHF;** they are also used for **acute pulmonary edema.**

H. Vasodilators

    1. *Cardiac effects.* Vasodilators reduce arterial resistance or increase venous capacitance; the net effect is a reduction in vascular pressure. In response to failures of pump function, sympathetic tone increases during the resting state, causing excessive venoconstriction and ultimately reduces cardiac output. Thus, vasodilators can be effective in CHF, and they are particularly useful when heart failure is associated with hypertension, congestive cardiomyopathy, mitral or aortic insufficiency, or ischemia.

    2. *Therapeutic use*

        a. Vasodilators are used to treat **severe, decompensated CHF** refractory to diuretics and digitalis.

        b. Agents used in **short-term therapy** include **nitroprusside,** which has a direct balanced effect on arterial and venous beds, and **nitroglycerin,** which has more effect on venous beds than on arterial beds. Nitroglycerin is not as effective as nitroprusside in enhancing cardiac output.

        c. Agents used in **long-term therapy** include the direct-acting vasodilators **isosorbide dinitrate** and **hydralazine,** and **prazosin,** an α_1-adrenergic blocking agent that produces arterial and minor venous dilation. **Carvedilol,** a combined α- and nonselective β-adrenoreceptor antagonist, has been shown in several clinical trials to reduce morbidity and mortality in mild-to-severe heart failure.

II. ANTIARRHYTHMIC DRUGS

A. Causes of arrhythmias. Arrhythmias may be due to both improper impulse generation and impulse conduction. These manifest as abnormalities of rate or regularity or as disturbances in the normal sequence of activation of atria and ventricles.

    1. *Altered automaticity.* Altered automaticity can arise from the following:

        a. **Sinus node (sinus tachycardia and bradycardia). Increased vagal activity** can impair nodal pacemaker cells by elevating K^+ conductance, leading to hyperpolarization. **Increased sympathetic activity** increases the rate of phase 4 depolarization. Intrinsic disease can produce faulty pacemaker activity **(sick sinus syndrome).**

        b. **Ectopic foci** are areas within the conduction system that may, in the diseased state, develop high rates of intrinsic activity and function as pacemakers.

        c. **Triggered automaticity** results from delayed after-polarizations that reach threshold and are capable of initiating an impulse.

    2. *Abnormal impulse conduction in conduction pathways*

        a. Heart blocks may produce **bradyarrhythmias.**

        b. Reentry circus conduction may produce **tachyarrhythmias.**

B. Goals of therapy (Table 4.2)

    1. Therapy aims to restore normal pacemaker activity and modify impaired conduction that leads to arrhythmias.

    2. Therapeutic effects are achieved by sodium- or calcium-channel blockade, prolongation of effective refractory period, or blockade of sympathetic effects on the heart. Many antiarrhythmic drugs affect depolarized tissue to a greater extent than they affect normally polarized tissue.

t a b l e **4.2** Some Antiarrhythmic Drugs			
Group	Prototype Drug	Mechanism	Uses
Class IA	Quinidine Procainamide Disopyramide	Moderate block of Na^+ channels; prolong action potentials	Suppress ventricular arrhythmias
Class IB	Lidocaine Mexiletine	Weakly block Na^+ channels; shorten action potentials	Suppress ventricular arrhythmias
Class IC	Flecainide	Strongly blocks Na^+ and K^+ channels	Treat severe ventricular tachyarrhythmias
Class II	Propranolol Atenolol Nadolol	Blocks β-adrenoceptors	Suppress some ventricular arrhythmias; inhibit AV node
Class III	Amiodarone	Prolongs refractory period	Suppress ventricular arrhythmias
Class IV	Verapamil	Blocks Ca^+ channel	Treat reentrant supraventricular tachycardia; suppress AV node conduction
Class V	Adenosine	Muscarinic antagonist	Treat paroxysmal atrial tachycardia
Others			
Atropine	Atropine	Increases vagal tone	Increase heart rate in bradycardia and heart blocks
Digitalis	Digoxin	P_1-receptor antagonist	Inhibit AV node; treat atrial fibrillation

^{a}p denotes prodrug, active metabolite produced by deesterification.

C. Treatment of tachyarrhythmias: class I drugs

1. *Mechanism.* Class I drugs block fast Na^+ channels, thereby reducing the rate of phase 0 depolarization, decreasing conduction velocity, prolonging the effective refractory period, increasing the threshold of excitability, and reducing the rate of phase 4 depolarization (see Fig. 4.4). These drugs also have local anesthetic properties.
   a. **Class IA drugs** prolong the refractory period and slow conduction.
   b. **Class IB agents** shorten the duration of the refractory period.
   c. **Class IC drugs** slow conduction.
2. *Class IA*
   a. Quinidine (Quinidex, Duraquin, Cardioquin)
      (1) Effects and pharmacologic properties
         (a) At therapeutic levels, direct **electrophysiologic effects** predominate, including depression of the pacemaker rate and depressed conduction and excitability, prolongation of Q–T interval, and heart block. At low doses, **anticholinergic** (vagolytic) **effects** predominate; they may increase conduction velocity in the AV node and accelerate heart rate.
         (b) Quinidine is administered **orally** and is rapidly absorbed from the **GI tract.**
         (c) Quinidine is **hydroxylated in the liver** and has a $t_{1/2}$ of approximately 5–12 hours, which is longer in hepatic or renal disease and in heart failure.
      (2) Therapeutic uses
         (a) Quinidine is used for **supraventricular and ventricular arrhythmias,** especially if caused by ectopia, and it is used to maintain **sinus rhythm** after conversion of atrial flutter or fibrillation by **digoxin, propranolol,** or **verapamil.**
         (b) Quinidine is used to prevent frequent premature ventricular complexes and ventricular tachycardia. Paradoxical tachycardia may be seen.
         (c) As the dextrorotary isomer of **quinine,** quinidine also exhibits antimalarial, antipyretic, and oxytoxic actions.

Class IA   Class IB   Class IC

Class III   Class IV

FIGURE 4.4. Changes in ventricular action potential produced by some antiarrthymic drugs.

(3) Adverse effects
  (a) Quinidine depresses all muscles, which can lead to skeletal muscle weakness, especially in individuals with myasthenia gravis.
  (b) Quinidine can produce severe hypotension and shock after rapid infusion.
  (c) This drug can produce **cinchonism** (ringing of the ears and dizziness) and diarrhea.
  (d) Quinidine may induce thrombocytopenia, most probably as a result of platelet-destroying antibodies developed in response to the circulating protein–quinidine complexes.
  (e) Quinidine can cause ventricular arrhythmias. **Quinidine syncope** (dizziness and fainting) may occur as a result of ventricular tachycardia; this condition is associated with a prolonged Q–T interval.
  (f) GI disturbances including abdominal pain, diarrhea, nausea, and esophagitis are common with quinidine.
(4) Drug interactions
  (a) Quinidine increases digoxin plasma levels and the risk of **digoxin toxicity.**
  (b) The $t_{1/2}$ of quinidine is reduced by agents that induce drug-metabolizing enzymes **(phenobarbital and phenytoin).**
  (c) Quinidine may enhance the activity of **coumarin** anticoagulants and other drugs metabolized by hepatic microsomal enzymes.
  (d) The cardiotoxic effects of quinidine are exacerbated by hyperkalemia.
b. Procainamide (Pronestyl, Procan)
  (1) Procainamide has actions similar to those of quinidine, but it is safer to use intravenously and produces fewer adverse GI effects.
  (2) Procainamide is acetylated in the liver to N-acetylprocainamide (NAPA) at a genetically determined rate. "Slow acetylators" have earlier onset and a greater prevalence of drug-induced **lupus-like syndrome** than "fast acetylators." NAPA is also active as an antiarrhythmic.
  (3) Procainamide is eliminated by the kidney; its $t_{1/2}$ is approximately 3–4 hours. Dose reduction is required in renal failure.
  (4) Procainamide has a high incidence of adverse effects with long-term use. It is more likely than quinidine to produce severe or irreversible heart failure.
  (5) Procainamide often causes drug-induced lupus-like syndrome (with symptoms resembling systemic lupus erythematosus).

    c. Disopyramide (Norpace)

      (1) Disopyramide has action similar to that of quinidine but has the longest $t_{1/2}$ of its class.

      (2) Disopyramide is approved for the treatment of ventricular arrhythmias; it is generally reserved for cases refractory or intolerant to quinidine or procainamide.

      (3) Disopyramide produces pronounced anticholinergic effects, including dry mouth, blurred vision, constipation, urine retention, and (rarely) acute angle-closure glaucoma. It may worsen heart block and adversely affect sinus node function.

3. *Class IB*

    a. Lidocaine (Xylocaine)

      (1) Lidocaine acts exclusively on the sodium channel (both activated and inactivated), and it is highly selective for damaged tissues.

      (2) Lidocaine is a second-line choice (behind amiodarone, see following) for the treatment of ventricular arrhythmias; it is ineffective in the prevention of arrhythmias subsequent to MI. It does not slow conduction and, thus, has little effect on atrial function.

      (3) Lidocaine undergoes a large first-pass effect. It is administered via the IV or IM route, and its $t_{1/2}$ is approximately 1.5–2 hours.

      (4) Lidocaine is administered in a loading dose followed by infusion. The dose must be adjusted in CHF or hepatic disease.

      (5) Lidocaine has a low level of cardiotoxicity; the most common adverse effects are neurologic. In contrast to quinidine and procainamide, lidocaine has little effect on the autonomic nervous system.

    b. Mexiletine (Mexitil)

      (1) Mexiletine is an agent similar in action to lidocaine, but can be administered orally.

      (2) Mexiletine is used primarily for long-term treatment of ventricular arrhythmias associated with previous MI.

4. *Class IC*

    a. Flecainide (Tambocor) and encainide (Enkaid)

      (1) Flecainide is orally active; it is used for ventricular tachyarrhythmias and maintenance of sinus rhythm in patients with paroxysmal atrial fibrillation and/or atrial flutter.

      (2) These agents block sodium channels and potassium channels. These actions decrease the maximal rate of phase 0 depolarization, slow His-Purkinje conduction and cause QRS widening and shorten the action potential of Purkinje fibers without affecting the surrounding myocardial tissue.

      (3) Encainide has been removed from the U.S. market but is available for use in patients already treated with the drug (compassionate use).

      (4) The use of these drugs is limited by their propensity to cause proarrhythmic actions; cautious use is recommended in patients with sinus node dysfunction, post-MI, and CHF.

    b. Propafenone (Rythmol)

      (1) Propafenone has a spectrum of action similar to that of quinidine but does not prolong the ventricular action potential.

      (2) Propafenone possesses β-adrenoceptor antagonist activity.

      (3) This drug is approved for the treatment of supraventricular arrhythmias and suppression of life-threatening ventricular arrhythmias.

      (4) Propafenone may cause bradycardia, CHF, or new arrhythmias.

D. Treatment of tachyarrhythmias: class II drugs

    1. *Mechanism.* Class II drugs are β-**adrenoceptor antagonists,** including **propranolol,** which act by reducing sympathetic stimulation. They inhibit phase 4 depolarization, depress automaticity, prolong AV conduction, and decrease heart rate (except for agents that have sympathomimetic activity) and contractility.

2. *Major drugs* (see Table 4.2)
   a. **Propranolol** (Inderal, generic), a nonselective β-adrenoceptor antagonist, and the more selective β_1-adrenoceptor antagonists acebutolol (Sectral) and esmolol (Brevibloc) are used to treat ventricular arrhythmias. Esmolol is ultrashort acting, is administered by infusion, and is used to titrate block during surgery.
   b. **Propranolol, metoprolol** (Lopressor), **nadolol** (Corgard), and **timolol** (Blocadren) are frequently used to prevent recurrent MI.
3. *Therapeutic uses*
   a. Class II drugs are used to treat **tachyarrhythmias** caused by increased sympathetic activity. They are also used for a variety of other arrhythmias, including atrial flutter and atrial fibrillation.
   b. These drugs **prevent reflex tachycardia** produced by vasodilating agents. They are sometimes used for digitalis toxicity.
4. *Adverse effects.* The adverse effects of class II drugs include **arteriolar vasoconstriction** and **bronchospasm.** Bradycardia, heart block, and myocardial depression may occur. **Atropine** or **isoproterenol** may be used to alleviate bradycardia.

E. **Treatment of tachyarrhythmias: class III drugs.** Class III drugs prolong the action potential duration and effective refractory period. These drugs act by interfering with outward K^+ currents or slow inward Na^+ currents.
   1. *Amiodarone (Cordarone) and dronedarone (Multaq)*
      a. Amiodarone is structurally related to thyroxine. It **increases refractoriness,** and it also depresses sinus node automaticity and slows conduction.
      b. The **long half-life** of amiodarone (14–100 days) increases the risk of toxicity.
      c. The plasma concentration of amiodarone is not well correlated with its effects. Although electrophysiologic effects may be seen within hours after parenteral administration, effects on abnormal rhythms may not be seen for several days. The antiarrhythmic effects may last for weeks or months after the drug is discontinued.
      d. Amiodarone is used for the treatment of refractory life-threatening ventricular arrhythmias in preference to lidocaine; additional uses include the treatment of atrial and/or ventricular arrhythmias including conversion of atrial fibrillation and the suppression of arrhythmias in patients with implanted defibrillators; it also possesses antianginal and vasodilatory effects. Amiodarone is a first-line agent for patients unresponsive to CPR.
      e. Dronedarone is chemically similar to amiodarone but lacks an iodine atom. It is approved for the treatment of permanent atrial fibrillation and flutter that cannot be converted to normal sinus rhythm.
      f. Amiodarone produces dose-related and cumulative **adverse effects** (especially **GI-related** effects) in about 70% of patients. Serious noncardiac adverse effects include pulmonary fibrosis and interstitial pneumonitis. Other adverse effects include photosensitivity, "gray man syndrome," corneal microdeposits, and thyroid disorders (due to iodine in the drug preparation).
   2. *Ibutilide (Corvert)*
      a. Ibutilide is a class III antiarrhythmic agent indicated for rapid conversion of atrial fibrillation or atrial flutter to normal sinus rhythm.
      b. Ibutilide must be administered by IV infusion.
      c. Ibutilide blocks slow inward Na^+ currents and prolongs the action potential duration, thereby causing a slowing of the sinus rate and AV conduction velocity.
   3. *Sotalol (Betapace, Sorine)*
      a. Solatol prolongs the cardiac action potential, increases the duration of the refractory period, and has nonselective β-adrenoceptor antagonist activity.
      b. Uses include treatment of atrial arrhythmias or life-threatening ventricular arrhythmias, and treatment of sustained ventricular tachycardia.
      c. Its adverse effects include significant proarrhythmic actions, dyspnea, and dizziness.

4. *Dofetilide (Tikosyn)*
   a. Dofetilide is approved for the conversion and maintenance of normal sinus rhythm in atrial fibrillation or atrial flutter.
   b. Dofetilide is a potent inhibitor of rapid component of the delayed rectifying K^+-channels (I_{Kr}) and has no effect on conduction velocity.
   c. Adverse effects include serious arrhythmias and conduction abnormalities.

F. Treatment of tachyarrhythmias: class IV drugs
   1. *Mechanism*
      a. Class IV drugs selectively block L-type calcium channels.
      b. These drugs prolong nodal conduction and effective refractory period and have predominate actions in nodal tissues.
   2. *Verapamil (Calan, Isoptin)*
      a. Verapamil is a phenylalkylamine that blocks both **activated and inactivated slow calcium channels.** Tissues that depend on L-type calcium channels are most affected, and it has equipotent activity on the AV and SA nodes and in cardiac and vascular muscle tissues.
      b. Although verapamil is excreted primarily by the kidney, dose reduction is necessary in the presence of hepatic disease and in the elderly. Bioavailability following oral administration is about 20%; much lower doses are required when administered intravenously.
      c. Verapamil is useful in reentrant **supraventricular tachycardia,** and it can also reduce ventricular rate in **atrial flutter** and **fibrillation.**
      d. Verapamil has **negative inotropic action** that limits its use in damaged hearts; it can lead to AV block when given in large doses or in patients with partial blockage. Verapamil can precipitate sinus arrest in diseased patients, and it causes peripheral vasodilation.
      e. The **adverse cardiac effects** of verapamil, including sinus bradycardia, transient asystole, and other arrthythmias, may be exacerbated in individuals taking β-**adrenoceptor antagonists;** this can be reversed by atropine, β-adrenoceptor agonists, or calcium. Verapamil should not be used in patients with abnormal conduction circuits as in Wolff-Parkinson-White syndrome.
   3. Diltiazem (Cardiazem)
      a. Similar in effects to verapamil, although it is a benzothiazapine. It affects both cardiac and vascular smooth muscle. Its inotropic effects are less than with verapamil. Diltiazem's inhibitory effects on conduction through the AV node make it useful for certain supraventricular arrhythmia.

G. Treatment of tachyarrhythmias: class V drugs
   1. *Adenosine (Adeno-jec, Adenocard)*
      a. Adenosine acts through specific **purinergic (P_1)** receptors.
      b. Adenosine causes an increase in potassium efflux and decreases calcium influx. This hyperpolarizes cardiac cells and decreases the calcium-dependent portion of the action potential.
      c. Adenosine is the drug of choice for the treatment of **paroxysmal supraventricular tachycardia,** including those associated with Wolff-Parkinson-White syndrome.
      d. Adverse effects are relatively minor, including flushing, dizziness, and headache.
   2. *Digoxin* can control ventricular response in atrial flutter or fibrillation.

H. Treatment of bradyarrhythmias
   1. *Atropine*
      a. Atropine **blocks the effects of acetylcholine.** It elevates sinus rate and AV nodal and SA conduction velocity, and it decreases refractory period.
      b. Atropine is used to treat **bradyarrhythmias** that accompany MI.
      c. Atropine produces adverse effects that include dry mouth, mydriasis, and cycloplegia; it may induce arrhythmias.

2. *Isoproterenol (Isuprel)*
  a. Isoproterenol **stimulates β-adrenoceptors** and increases heart rate and contractility.
  b. Isoproterenol is used to **maintain adequate heart rate** and cardiac output in patients with AV block.
  c. Isoproterenol may cause tachycardia, anginal attacks, headaches, dizziness, flushing, and tremors.

III. ANTIANGINAL AGENTS

A. Goal of therapy. The goal of therapy with antianginal agents is to restore the balance between oxygen supply and demand in the ischemic region of the myocardium.

B. Types of angina
  1. *Classic angina (angina of exercise).* Classic angina occurs when oxygen demand exceeds oxygen supply, usually because of diminished coronary flow.
  2. *Vasospastic (Prinzmetal's, or variant) angina.* Vasospastic angina results from reversible coronary vasospasm that decreases oxygen supply and occurs at rest. Some individuals have **mixed angina,** in which both exercise-induced and resting attacks may occur.

C. Nitrates and nitrites
  1. *Structure and mechanism*
    a. Nitrates and nitrites are polyol esters of nitric acid and nitrous acid, respectively, and relax vascular smooth muscle.
    b. Nitrates and nitrites activate guanylate cyclase and increase cyclic guanine nucleotides. This activates cGMP-dependent kinases, ultimately leading to dephosphorylation of myosin light chain and relaxation of the contractile apparatus.
    c. These drugs dilate all vessels. Peripheral venodilation decreases cardiac preload and myocardial wall tension; arterial dilation reduces afterload. Both of these actions lower oxygen demand by decreasing the work of the heart. Redistribution of coronary blood flow to ischemic regions is increased in nitrate-treated patients.
    d. Nitrates and nitrites ameliorate the symptoms of classic angina predominantly through the improvement of hemodynamics. Variant angina is relieved through the effects on coronary circulation.
    e. Nitrates and nitrites form nitrosothiol in smooth muscle by reaction with glutathione. The use of nitroglycerine for more than a few hours is associated with significant tolerance to the drug. This is thought to be due to depletion of enzymes responsible for bioactivation of the drug.
  2. *Bioavailability and selected drugs.* These drugs have a large first-pass effect due to the presence of high-capacity organic nitrate reductase in the liver, which inactivates drugs. Sublingual administration avoids this effect. Nitrates have a $t_{1/2}$ of <10 minutes.
    a. Nitroglycerin (Cellegesic, Nitrek, others)
      (1) Nitroglycerin is preferably administered sublingually for rapid delivery and short duration.
      (2) Sustained-delivery systems (Transderm-Nitro, Nitrodisc) are available and are used to maintain blood levels. Aerosol, topical, IV, and oral preparations are also available.
    b. **Amyl nitrite** is a **volatile liquid** that is **inhaled.** An unpleasant odor and extensive cutaneous vasodilation render it **less desirable** than **nitroglycerin.**
    c. Isosorbide dinitrate (Isordil, Sorbitrate, others)
      (1) Isosorbide dinitrate has active initial metabolites.
      (2) This drug is administered orally or sublingually; it has better oral bioavailability and a longer half-life (up to 1 h) than nitroglycerin. Timed-release oral preparations are available with durations of action up to 12 hours.
      (3) Isosorbide mononitrate (Imdur, Monoker) has comparable actions with a longer plasma half-life.

3. *Therapeutic uses*
   a. Sublingual **nitroglycerin** is most often used for severe, recurrent **Prinzmetal's angina.**
   b. Continuous infusion or slowly absorbed preparations of nitroglycerin (including the transdermal patch) or derivatives with longer half-lives have been used for **unstable angina** and for **CHF in the presence of MI.**
4. *Adverse effects*
   a. Nitrates and nitrites produce **vasodilation,** which can lead to orthostatic hypotension, reflex tachycardia, throbbing headache (may be dose limiting), blushing, and a burning sensation.
   b. Large doses produce **methemoglobinemia** and cyanosis.

D. β-Adrenoceptor antagonists
   1. β-Adrenoceptor antagonists decrease heart rate, blood pressure, and contractility, resulting in **decreased myocardial oxygen requirements.** Combined therapy with nitrates is often preferred in the treatment of angina pectoris because of the decreased adverse effects of both agents.
   2. β-Adrenoceptor antagonists are contraindicated in the presence of bradycardia, AV block, and asthma.

E. Calcium channel-blocking agents (CCB)
   1. *Mechanism.* CCB agents produce a blockade of L-type (slow) calcium channels, which decreases contractile force and oxygen requirements. Agents cause **coronary vasodilation** and **relief of spasm;** they also dilate peripheral vasculature and decrease cardiac afterload.
   2. *Pharmacologic properties*
      a. CCB agents can be administered orally. When administered intravenously, they are effective within minutes.
      b. These drugs are useful for **both variant and chronic stable angina** and are also used in instances where nitrates are ineffective or when β-adrenoceptor antagonists are contraindicated.
      c. Serum lipids are not increased.
      d. These drugs produce **hypotension; edema** is a common adverse effect.
   3. *Selected drugs*
      a. Verapamil (Calan, Isoptin)
         (1) Verapamil produces slowed conduction through the AV node (predominant effect); this may be an unwanted effect in some situations (especially in the treatment of hypertension).
         (2) Verapamil may produce AV block when used in combination with β-adrenoceptor antagonists. The toxic effects of verapamil include myocardial depression, heart failure, and edema.
         (3) Verapamil also has peripheral vasodilating effects that can reduce afterload and blood pressure.
         (4) The peripheral effects of verapamil can produce headache, reflex tachycardia, and fluid retention.
      b. Nifedipine (Adalat, Procardia), isradipine (DynaCirc), nisoldipine (Sular), and nicardipine (Cardene)
         (1) These dihydropyridine calcium-channel blockers have predominant actions in the peripheral vasculature; they decrease afterload and to a lesser extent preload, and lower blood pressure.
         (2) These drugs have **significantly less direct effect on the heart** than verapamil.
      c. Diltiazem (Cardizem)
         (1) Diltiazem, a benzothiazepine, is intermediate in properties between verapamil and the dihydropyridines.
         (2) Diltiazem is used to treat variant (Prinzmetal's) angina, either naturally occurring or drug-induced and stable angina.

F. Dipyridamole (Persantine)
   1. Dipyridamole is a nonnitrate coronary vasodilator that interferes with the metabolism of the vasodilator **adenosine,** presumably by inhibiting adenosine deaminase. It potentiates the effect of **PGI$_2$** (prostacyclin, epoprostenol) and dilates resistance vessels, and inhibits platelet aggregation.
   2. Dipyridamole may be used for **prophylaxis of angina pectoris,** but the efficacy of this drug is not proved.
   3. Dipyridamole produces adverse effects that include the worsening of angina, dizziness, and headache.

IV. ANTIHYPERTENSIVE DRUGS

A. Principles of blood pressure regulation
   1. Blood pressure is regulated by the following:
      a. Cardiac output.
      b. Peripheral vascular resistance.
      c. Volume of intravascular fluid (controlled at the kidney).
   2. Baroreflexes adjust moment-to-moment blood pressure. Carotid baroreceptors respond to stretch, and their activation inhibits sympathetic discharge.
   3. The **renin–angiotensin system** provides tonic, longer term regulation of blood pressure. Reduction in renal perfusion pressure results in increased reabsorption of salt and water. Decreased renal pressure stimulates **renin production** and leads to enhanced levels of **angiotensin II.** This agent, in turn, causes resistance vessels to constrict and stimulates aldosterone synthesis, which ultimately increases the absorption of sodium and water by the kidney.

B. Goal of therapy
   1. The goal of the therapy is to **reduce elevated blood pressure,** which would ultimately lead to **end-organ damage, increased risk of stroke, and MI.**
   2. This goal is achieved through the use of various drug classes, and treatment often involves a **combination of agents** (Table 4.3).

C. Diuretics increase sodium excretion and lower blood volume and reduce total peripheral resistance.
   1. *Thiazide diuretics*
      a. Thiazide diuretics are effective in lowering blood pressure 10–15 mmHg.
      b. When administered alone, thiazide diuretics can provide relief for **mild or moderate hypertension.**
      c. Thiazide diuretics are used in combination with sympatholytic agents or vasodilators in **severe hypertension.**
   2. *Loop diuretics* are used in combination with sympatholytic agents and vasodilators for hypertension refractory to thiazide treatment.
   3. *Potassium-sparing diuretics* are used to avoid potassium depletion, especially when administered with cardiac glycosides.

D. Adrenoceptor antagonists
   1. β-*Adrenoceptor antagonists* (see Table 2.1)
      a. Propranolol (Inderal)
         (1) Propranolol antagonizes catecholamine action at both β$_1$- and β$_2$-receptors. It produces a sustained reduction in peripheral vascular resistance.
         (2) Blockade of cardiac β$_1$-adrenoceptors reduces heart rate and contractility. β$_2$-adrenoceptor blockade increases airway resistance and decreases catecholamine-induced glycogenolysis and peripheral vasodilation.

table 4.3	Some Antihypertensive Drugs		
Class	Drug	Adverse Effects	Therapeutic Use
Diuretics			
Thiazide and thiazide-related agents	Chlorothiazide, hydrochlorothiazide, chlorthalidone, metolazone, indapamide	Hypokalemia, hyperuricemia, hypersensitivity reactions, hyperglycemia	Alone to treat moderate hypertension; in combination with other classes of drugs to treat severe hypertension
Loop	Furosemide, bumetanide, ethacrynic acid	Hypokalemia, hypotension, volume depletion, hypomagnesemia, hyperuricemia, hyperglycemia, hypocalcemia	In the presence of azotemia
Potassium-sparing agents	Triamterene, spironolactone, amiloride	Hyperkalemia	Used in combination with a thiazide or loop diuretic
Peripheral sympatholytics			
β-Adrenergic antagonists	Nonselective (β$_1$ and β$_2$): propranolol, timolol, nadolol, pindolol, penbutolol, carteolol; β$_1$-selective: acebutolol, atenolol, metoprolol	Most adverse effects are mild, rarely requiring withdrawal of drug: fatigue, depression, reduced exercise tolerance, bradycardia, CHF, bronchoconstriction in presence of asthma, gastrointestinal disturbances, masked hypoglycemia, increased triglycerides, decreased low-density lipoprotein cholesterol	All grades of hypertension; may be combined with a diuretic for additive effects, or with a diuretic plus an α-adrenoceptor antagonist for resistant hypertension; also diminish cardiac oxygen demand
α$_1$- and β-Adrenoceptor antagonists	Carvedilol, labetalol	Similar to propranolol; more likely to cause orthostatic hypotension and sexual dysfunction	
α$_1$-Adrenoceptor antagonists	Prazosin, terazosin, doxazosin	First-dose syncope, orthostatic hypotension, palpitations, anticholinergic effects	As single agents in mild-to-moderate hypertension; may be useful with a diuretic and a β-adrenoceptor antagonist
Inhibitors of renin–angiotensin			
Angiotensin-converting enzyme (ACE) inhibitors	Captopril, enalapril, lisinopril, ramipril, quinapril	Hyperkalemia, rash, dysgeusia, cough; individuals with high plasma renin activity may experience excessive hypotension	Mild-to-severe hypertension
Angiotensin II receptor antagonists	Losartan potassium	Hyperkalemia	Similar to ACE inhibitors
Renin inhibitor	Aliskiren	Dizziness	Similar to ARBs
Calcium-channel blockers	Verapamil, diltiazem, nicardipine, nifedipine, Isradipine, felodipine	Negative inotropic effects, peripheral edema	Broad range of hypertensive patients; cautious use in presence of heart failure
Central sympatholytics	Methyldopa, clonidine, guanabenz	Dry mouth, sedation, lethargy, depression	Chronic hypertension
Adrenergic neuronal blocking drugs	Guanadrel	Orthostatic hypotension; severe hypotension in presence of pheochromocytoma	Severe refractory hypertension
	Reserpine	GI disturbances, mental depression	Mild-to-moderate hypertension
Vasodilators			
Arteriolar vasodilators	Hydralazine, minoxidil	Lupuslike syndrome may occur with hydralazine; minoxidil may cause severe volume retention	Sometimes for hypertension refractory to β-blocker/thiazide diuretic combination; in combination with a diuretic and often a β-blocker
Arteriolar and venule vasodilator	Sodium nitroprusside	Excessive decrease in blood pressure may occur	Emergency situations where rapid reduction in blood pressure is desired

(3) Blockade of β-adrenoceptors in the CNS decreases sympathetic activity.
(4) Propranolol also decreases renin release.
(5) Propranolol is used in mild-to-moderate hypertension.
  b. Nadolol (Corgard), timolol (Blocadren), carteolol (Cartrol), pindolol (Visken), and penbutolol (Levatol)
(1) These drugs are similar in action to propranolol and block both $β_1$- and $β_2$-adrenoceptors.
(2) Nadolol has an extended duration of action.
(3) Pindolol, carteolol, and penbutolol have partial agonist activity (sympathomimetic).
  c. Metoprolol (Lopressor), atenolol (Tenormin), acebutolol (Sectral), bisprolol (Zebeta)
(1) These drugs are relatively **selective for $β_1$-adrenoceptors**.
(2) Acebutolol has partial agonist activity.
  d. Abrupt discontinuation of β-adrenoceptor blockers can worsen angina and increase risk of MI. Dose should be gradually reduced over a period of several weeks.
2. **α-*Adrenoceptor antagonists***
  a. α-Adrenoceptor antagonists **lower total peripheral resistance** by preventing stimulation (and consequent vasoconstriction) of α-receptors, which are located predominantly in resistance vessels of the skin, mucosa, intestine, and kidney. These drugs **reduce pressure** by dilating resistance and conductance vessels.
  b. The effectiveness of these drugs diminishes in some patients because of tolerance.
(1) Prazosin (Minipress), terazosin (Hytrin), and doxazosin (Cardura)
  (a) These drugs are $α_1$-selective antagonists.
  (b) These drugs are used in treating **hypertension,** especially in the presence of CHF but their use has diminished because no evidence of reduced cardiovascular events was found in a large clinical trial with doxazosin.
  (c) Prazosin, terazosin, and doxazosin are often administered with a diuretic and a β-adrenoceptor antagonist.
  (d) These drugs may produce initial orthostatic hypotension. Other adverse effects are minimal.
(2) Phentolamine (Regitine) and phenoxybenzamine (Dibenzyline)
  (a) Phentolamine and phenoxybenzamine antagonize $α_1$- and $α_2$-adrenoceptors.
  (b) These drugs are used primarily in treating **hypertension** in the presence of **pheochromocytoma.** Phentolamine is administered parenterally; phenoxybenzamine is administered orally.
3. ***Labetalol (Normodyne, Trandate) and carvedilol (Coreg)***
  a. Labetalol is an $α_1$- and β-adrenoceptor antagonist.
  b. Labetalol reduces heart rate and contractility, slows AV conduction, and decreases peripheral resistance.
  c. Labetalol is available for both oral and IV administration.
  d. Labetalol is useful for treating hypertensive emergencies and in the treatment of **hypertension of pheochromocytoma.**
  e. Labetalol does not cause reflex tachycardia.
  f. Carvedilol has a significantly greater ratio of β to α antagonist activity than labetalol.

E. Agents that affect the renin–angiotensin system
1. ***ACE inhibitors*** (see section B)
  a. ACE inhibitors reduce vascular resistance and blood volume; they lower blood pressure by decreasing total peripheral resistance.
  b. ACE inhibitors include **captopril** (Capoten), **enalapril** (Vasotec), **lisinopril** (Prinivil, Zestril), **ramipril** (Altace), **fosinopril** (Monopril), **benazepril** (Lotensin), **moexipril** (Univasc), **quinapril** (Accupril), perindopril (Aceon), and trandolapril (Mavik).
  c. These drugs are useful in treating **mild-to-severe hypertension.** Recent studies have established beneficial effect in patients with angina, CHF, cardiac ischemia, and post-MI.
  d. ACE inhibitors may be less effective in African Americans than in Caucasians.

2. *Angiotensin II receptor antagonists, losartan potassium (Cozaar), valsartan (Diovan)* (see Table 4.1)
   a. These drugs block angiotensin II type-1 (AT-1) receptors.
   b. The effects of these drugs are similar to those seen with ACE inhibitors.
   c. These drugs are effective as monotherapy for hypertension.

3. *Inhibitors of renin activity, aliskiren (Tekturna)*
   a. Aliskiren is a small molecule inhibitor of renin and thereby reduces the production of all angiotensins.
   b. Initial clinical trials have combined aliskiren with a diuretic or an ARB and its effectiveness seems comparable to ARBs. Aliskiren should *not* be combined with an ACE inhibitor or an ARB in patients with compromised kidney function.
   c. Adverse effects are fewer compared with ACE inhibitors but include diarrhea, headache, and dizziness.

F. **Calcium channel-blocking agents**
   1. CCB agents inhibit the entry of calcium into cardiac and smooth muscle cells by blocking the L-type Ca^{2+}-channel; they lower blood pressure by reducing peripheral resistance.
   2. CCBs used for the treatment of hypertension include verapamil, nifedipine, nicardipine, nisoldipine (Sular), isradipine (DynaCirc), amlodipine (Norvasc), felodipine (Plendil), and diltiazem.
   3. CCBs are effective in the treatment of **mild-to-moderate hypertension.**
   4. When combined with a β-adrenoceptor antagonist, these agents may lower blood pressure to a greater extent than when either class of drug is administered separately.
   5. Short-acting preparations of the dihydropyridines such as nifedipine have been associated with an increase in cardiovascular mortality and events, including MI and increased anginal attacks.

G. **Other drugs**
   1. *Centrally acting sympathomimetic agents* reduce peripheral resistance, inhibit cardiac function, and increase pooling in capacitance venules.
      a. Methyldopa (Aldomet)
         (1) Methyldopa has an active metabolite, α-methylnorepinephrine, a potent false neurotransmitter.
         (2) Methyldopa activates presynaptic inhibitory α-adrenoceptors and postsynaptic $α_2$-receptors in the CNS and **reduces sympathetic outflow**. It decreases total peripheral resistance.
         (3) Methyldopa reduces pressure in standing and supine positions.
         (4) Methyldopa is used to treat mild-to-moderate hypertension; it can be added to the regimen when a diuretic alone is not successful.
         (5) Methyldopa produces adverse effects that include drowsiness, dry mouth, and GI upset. Sexual dysfunction may occur and reduce compliance.
      b. Clonidine (Catapres)
         (1) Clonidine stimulates postsynaptic $α_2$-adrenoceptors in the CNS and causes reduction in total peripheral resistance.
         (2) Clonidine is frequently combined with a diuretic.
         (3) Clonidine commonly produces drowsiness and lethargy, dry mouth, and constipation.
         (4) This drug is available as a transdermal patch (Catapres-TTS) that allows weekly dosing.
      c. Guanabenz acetate (Wytensin)
         (1) Guanabenz acetate activates central $α_2$-adrenoceptors and inhibits sympathetic outflow from the brain, which results in reduced blood pressure.
         (2) This drug is used in mild-to-moderate hypertension, most commonly in combination with a diuretic.
         (3) Guanabenz acetate most commonly produces sedation and dry mouth as adverse effects but with reduced frequency compared with clonidine.

2. *Adrenergic neuronal blocking drugs*
   a. Reserpine
      (1) Reserpine eliminates norepinephrine release in response to nerve impulse by preventing vesicular uptake. It depletes norepinephrine from sympathetic nerve terminals in the periphery and in the adrenal medulla.
      (2) Reserpine is used in mild-to-moderate hypertension.
      (3) Reserpine most commonly produces GI disturbances. Mental depression, sometimes severe, may result, especially with high doses; the use of reserpine is contraindicated in patients with a history of depression.
3. *Vasodilators*
   a. Vasodilators relax smooth muscle and lower total peripheral resistance, thereby lowering blood pressure.
   b. The use of vasodilators is declining as a result of newer modalities, such as ACE inhibitors and CCB agents, which are more effective with fewer adverse effects.
      (1) Hydralazine (Apresoline)
         (a) Hydralazine reduces blood pressure directly by **relaxing arteriolar muscle.** This effect is probably mediated by *increasing levels of HIF-1(hypoxia inducible factor 1) which regulates a number of downstream target genes that lead to decreased Ca^{2+} influx.*
         (b) Hydralazine elicits the baroreceptor reflex, necessitating **coadministration** with a **diuretic** to counteract sodium and water retention and a β-blocker to prevent tachycardia.
         (c) This drug is used to treat **chronic hypertension** and in **hypertensive crises** accompanying acute glomerular nephritis or eclampsia.
         (d) Hydralazine may cause a lupus-like syndrome.
      (2) Minoxidil (Loniten)
         (a) Minoxidil has effects similar to hydralazine. Minoxidil acts to increase K$^+$ efflux, which hyperpolarizes cells and reduces the activity of L-type (voltage-sensitive) calcium channels, and it may stimulate the production of nitric oxide. Minoxidil vasodilates predominantly arteriolar vessels.
         (b) Minoxidil also elicits the **baroreceptor reflex,** necessitating the use of a β-**adrenoceptor antagonist** and a **diuretic.**
         (c) Minoxidil is useful for long-term therapy of **refractory hypertension.**
         (d) Minoxidil produces **hirsutism,** an advantage in formulations that are now used to reduce hair loss in both males and females.
      (3) Sodium nitroprusside (Nipride, Nitropress)
         (a) Sodium nitroprusside dilates both resistance and capacitance vessels; it increases heart rate but not output.
         (b) This drug is frequently used in **hypertensive emergencies** because of its rapid action. Continuous infusion is necessary to maintain its effects.
         (c) Sodium nitroprusside is usually administered with **furosemide.**
         (d) On initial infusion, sodium nitroprusside may cause excessive vasodilation and hypotension.
         (e) Sodium nitroprusside can be converted to cyanide and thiocyanate. The accumulation of cyanide and **risk of toxicity** are minimized by concomitant administration of **sodium thiosulfate** or hydroxocobalamin.
      (4) Diazoxide (Hyperstat)
         (a) Diazoxide is used intravenously to reduce blood pressure rapidly, usually in an emergency situation.
         (b) Diazoxide is administered with **furosemide** to prevent fluid overload.
         (c) This drug is **declining in use** because of its unpredictable action and adverse effects.
4. *Fenoldopam (Corlopam)* is a selective **agonist at dopamine DA$_1$ receptors** that increases renal blood flow while reducing blood pressure. Administered by infusion, it is a useful drug in the control of emergency hypertension.

5. *Specialized vasodilators*
   a. Drugs used to treat pulmonary hypertension
      (1) **Ambrisentan (Letairis) is a selective endothelin A receptor antagonist used to treat pulmonary hypertension.** Plasma endothelin-1 is elevated in patients with pulmonary hypertension. Ambrisentan is administered orally. Peripheral edema is a common adverse effect of endothelin receptor antagonists.
      (2) **Bosentan** antagonizes both endothelin A and B receptors and reduces pulmonary hypertension. Headache and edema are common side effects.
      (3) The use of both ambrisentan and bosentan is controlled by access programs.
      (4) Prostaglandin I_2 and PGI_2 analogs such as epoprostanol and the phosphodiesterase type 5 inhibitors sildenafil and tadalfil are approved for the treatment of pulmonary hypertension.
   b. Drugs used to treat erectile dysfunction
      (1) Drugs in this class include **sildenafil** citrate (Viagra, Revatio), **tadalafil** (Cialis), and **vardenafil** hydrochloride (Levitra).
      (2) Viagra was originally developed as an antianginal and antihypertensive agent but proved very effective in treating erectile dysfunction.
      (3) These agents specifically **inhibit phosphodiesterase type 5,** the class of enzymes that are responsible for the breakdown of cGMP. The type 5 isoform is expressed in reproductive tissues and the lung. Inhibition of the breakdown of cGMP enhances the vasodilatory action of NO in the corpus callosum and in the pulmonary vasculature.
      (4) These agents are useful in the treatment of erectile dysfunction, and sildenafil citrate is approved for the treatment of pulmonary hypertension.
      (5) The most common adverse effects of the phosphodiesterase type 5 inhibitors are headache, flushing, ocular disturbances, and abdominal pain. The most serious adverse effects are cardiovascular: arrhythmias, heart block, cardiac arrest, stroke, and hypotension.
      (6) These drugs are contraindicated in patients taking nitrates, because of exacerbation of the effects of these drugs, or in patients taking α_1-adrenoceptor antagonists such as doxazosin.

V. DRUGS THAT LOWER PLASMA LIPIDS

A. An overview
   1. Dietary or pharmacologic reduction of elevated plasma cholesterol levels can reduce the risk of atherosclerosis and subsequent cardiovascular disease. The exact factors linking elevated cholesterol levels to heart disease are not yet known.
   2. The association between cardiovascular disease and elevated plasma triglycerides is less dramatic, but it is becoming more recognized. In addition, **elevated triglycerides** can produce life-threatening pancreatitis.
   3. *Hyperlipoproteinemias*
      a. **Cholesterol** is a nonpolar, poorly water-soluble substance, transported in the plasma in particles that have a hydrophobic core of cholesteryl esters and triglycerides surrounded by a coat of phospholipids, free cholesterol (nonesterified), and one or more apoproteins. These lipoprotein particles vary in the ratio of triglyceride to cholesteryl ester as well as in the type of apoprotein; they are identified as **low-density lipoprotein (LDL)** particles, **very-low-density lipoprotein (VLDL)** particles, **intermediate-density lipoprotein (IDL)** particles, and **high-density lipoprotein (HDL)** particles.
      b. Diseases of plasma lipids can be manifest as an elevation in triglycerides or as an elevation in cholesterol. In several of the complex or combined hyperlipoproteinemias, both **triglycerides and cholesterol can be elevated.**

B. Drugs useful in treating hyperlipidemias
  1. *Inhibitors of cholesterol biosynthesis (statins)*
    a. These drugs include **lovastatin** (mevinolin) (Mevacor), **simvastatin** (Zocor), **pravastatin** (Pravachol), **atorvastatin** (Lipitor), and **rosuvastatin** (Crestor) (see Table 4.1).
    b. Drugs that inhibit cholesterol biosynthesis are quite effective at lowering LDL cholesterol and total cholesterol.
      (1) Mechanism
        (a) These drugs function as competitive inhibitors of 3-hydroxy-3-methylglu-tarylcoenzyme A reductase (HMG-CoA reductase), the rate-limiting enzyme in cholesterol biosynthesis. Reduced cholesterol synthesis results in a compensatory increase in the hepatic uptake of plasma cholesterol mediated by an increase in the number of LDL receptors.
        (b) These drugs **reduce total cholesterol** by as much as 30%–50%; LDL cholesterol can be reduced by as much as 60% (rosuvastatin).
      (2) Therapeutic uses. Inhibitors of cholesterol biosynthesis are effective in reducing cholesterol levels in familial and nonfamilial hypercholesterolemias.
      (3) Recent clinical trials have established that statins interfere with osteoclast-mediated bone resorption and may reduce osteoporosis. These drugs may also interfere with intracellular localization of certain oncogenes and thereby reduce the incidence of some cancers. They also have weak anti-inflammatory activity and reduce stroke risk.
      (4) The adverse effects of these drugs include **myositis,** rhabdomyolysis, anxiety, irritability, **hepatotoxicity,** and **elevations in aminotransferases**. However, yearly liver function tests are no longer recommended.
  2. *Nicotinic acid (niacin) (Nicobid, Nicolar)*
    a. Mechanism
      (1) **Nicotinic acid** can exert cholesterol- and triglyceride-lowering effects at high concentrations (nicotinamide cannot do this). This is distinct from the role of this molecule as a vitamin, in which nicotinic acid is converted to nicotinamide and is used for the biosynthesis of the cofactors NAD and NADP.
      (2) Nicotinic acid reduces plasma VLDL by inhibiting the synthesis and esterification of fatty acids in the liver and reducing lipolysis in adipose tissue; it markedly decreases plasma triglyceride levels. As the substrate VLDL concentration is reduced, the concentrations of IDL and LDL also decrease, thereby reducing plasma cholesterol levels. HDL levels increase significantly because of reduced catabolism.
      (3) In much smaller doses, nicotinic acid can also be used as a vitamin supplement in the treatment of pellagra.
    b. Adverse effects
      (1) Nicotinic acid commonly produces flushing and an itching or burning feeling in the skin, which may reduce compliance. This is mediated by prostaglandins and histamine release and can be diminished by taking aspirin 30 minutes before taking nicotinic acid.
      (2) Nicotinic acid produces hepatic effects, including increased transaminase activities; hyperglycemia; GI disturbances and peptic ulcer; renal effects that include elevated plasma uric acid; and macular edema.
  3. *Fibric acid analogs*
    a. Fenofibrate (Antara, Triglide, Lofibra)
      (1) Mechanism
        (a) Fibrates stimulate the activity of peroxisome proliferating activating receptor α, a class of nuclear receptor. Activation of these receptors alters the transcription of a number of genes involved in triglyceride metabolism including lipoprotein lipase and apolipoprotein CIII. This **increases** the **peripheral catabolism of VLDL** and **chylomicrons,** resulting in a reduction in the plasma concentration of VLDL, most notably in triglycerides.
        (b) Fibrates **reduce hepatic synthesis of cholesterol,** which further reduces plasma triglycerides.

(2) Therapeutic uses

    (a) Fenofibrate can be used to treat **hyperlipidemia** of several etiologies, especially hypertriglyceridemia due to dysbetalipoproteinemia, a defect in apolipoprotein E that impairs clearance of chylomicron remnants and VLDL.

    (b) Fenofibrate is ineffective in primary chylomicronemia (caused by a deficiency in lipoprotein lipase) and has little effect on reducing plasma cholesterol levels.

    (c) Fenofibrate has antidiuretic action in individuals with mild or moderate **diabetes insipidus.**

(3) Adverse effects and contraindications

    (a) Fenofibrate produces cholelithiasis and cholecystitis, GI intolerance, nausea, mild diarrhea, and myalgia.

    (b) This drug frequently causes dermatologic reactions and drowsiness, as well as decreased libido in a small percentage of men.

    (c) Fenofibrate can **displace** other albumin-bound drugs, most notably the **sulfonylureas** and **warfarin.**

    (d) Fenofibrate must be used cautiously in individuals with impaired renal or hepatic function.

b. Gemfibrozil (Lopid)

  (1) Gemfibrozil is a fibrate that is more effective than fenofibrate in some circumstances and has some unique biologic activities.

  (2) The therapeutic uses of gemfibrozil are identical to those of fenofibrate; it may be more active in reducing triglycerides than fenofibrate.

4. *Ezetimibe (Zetia)*

  a. Ezetimibe acts within the intestine to reduce cholesterol absorption. Cholesterol is absorbed from the small intestine by a process that includes specific transporters including the Niemann-Pick C1-Like 1 (NPC1L1) protein which is important for sterol absorption in the gut. Ezetmibe binds to and inhibits the function of NPC1L1 thereby reducing cholesterol absorption.

  b. Ezetimibe used alone produces a reduction in plasma cholesterol of about 18% and about a 10% decline in triglyceride levels. When combined with a statin, reductions in plasma cholesterol as high as 72% have been reported in clinical trials.

  c. Ezetimibe appears to be well tolerated, with the most common adverse effects being fatigue, abdominal pain, and diarrhea.

5. *Bile acid sequestrants.* These agents include **cholestyramine** (Questran), **colestipol** (Colestid), and **colesevelam** (WelChol)

  a. Structure and mechanism

    (1) Bile acid sequestrants are large copolymers (resins) of hydrocarbons that can bind bile salts. Cholestyramine and colestipol exchange a chloride anion for a bile acid.

    (2) These resins are hydrophilic, but they are not absorbed across the intestine.

    (3) In the intestine, the resins bind bile salts and prevent enterohepatic reutilization of bile acids. In addition, they impair the absorption of dietary cholesterol.

  b. **Therapeutic uses.** Bile acid sequestrants are effective in **reducing plasma cholesterol** (10%–20%) in patients with some normal LDL receptors. This excludes patients who completely lack functional LDL receptors because of a genetic defect (homozygous familial hypercholesterolemia).

  c. Adverse effects

    (1) These agents are generally quite safe, because they are not absorbed in the intestine.

    (2) Bile acid sequestrants produce GI disturbances (constipation, nausea, and discomfort), which may reduce compliance. Colesevelam has fewer GI side effects than the other resins.

    (3) These drugs interfere with the absorption of anionic drugs (e.g., digitalis and warfarin).

DRUG SUMMARY TABLE

ACE Inhibitors
Captopril (generic)
Enalapril (Vasotec, generic)
Fosinopril (Monopril, generic)
Lisinopril (Prinivil, Zestril, generic)
Quinapril (Accupril)
Benazepril (Lotensin, generic)
Moexipril (Univasc, generic)
Perindopril (Aceon)
Ramipril (Altace)
Trandolapril (Mavik)

Angiotensin-Receptor Blockers
Losartan (Cozaar)
Valsartan (Diovan)
Irbesartan (Avapro)
Candesartan (Atacand)
Telmisartan (Micardis)
Eprosartan (Teveten)
Olmesartan (Benicar)
Azilsartan (Edarbi)

Renin Inhibitor
Aliskiren (Tekturna)

Antianginal Agents
Nitroglycerin (Cellegesic)
Amyl nitrite (generic)
Isosorbide dinitrate (Isordil)
Nifedipine (Adalat)
Isradipine (DynaCirc)
Nisoldipine (Sular)
Nicardipine (Cardene)
Diltiazem (Cardizem)
Dipyridamole (Persantine)

Antihypertensive Agents
Hydrochlorothiazide
Furosemide
Spironolactone
Eplerenone (Inspra)
Nadolol (Corgard)
Timolol (Blocadren)

Drugs Used in CHF
Digoxin (Lanoxin)
Dobutamine
Dopamine
Nesiritide (Natrecor)

Antiarrhythmics
Inamrinone
Milrinone
Quinidine (Quinidex)
Procainamide (Pronestyl)
Disopyramide (Norpace)
Lidocaine (Xylocaine)
Mexiletine (Mexitil)
Flecainide (Tambocor)
Encainide (Enkaid)
Propafenone (Rythmol)
Propranolol (Inderal)
Acebutolol (Sectral)
Esmolol (Brevibloc)
Metoprolol (Lopressor)
Nadolol (Corgard)
Timolol (Blocadren)
Carteolol (Cartrol)
Pindolol (Visken)
Penbutolol (Levatol)
Metoprolol (Lopressor)
Atenolol (Tenormin)
Acebutolol (Sectral)
Bisprolol (Zebeta)
Labetalol (Normodyne)
Carvedilol (Coreg)
Terazosin (Hytrin)
Prazosin (Minipress)
Doxazosin (Cardura)
Phentolamine (Regitine)
Phenoxybenzamine (Dibenzyline)
Methyldopa (Aldomet)
Clonidine (Catapres)
Guanabenz acetate (Wytensin)
Reserpine
Amiodarone (Cordarone)
Ibutilide (Corvert)

Antihypertensive Agents
Hydralazine (Apresoline)
Minoxidil (Loniten)
Sodium nitroprusside (Nipride)
Diazoxide (Hyperstat)

Specialized Vasodilators
Ambrisentan (Letaris)
Bosentan (Trader)
Sildenafil citrate (Viagra, Revatio)
Tadalafil (Cialis)
Vardenafil hydrochloride (Levitra)
Solatol (Betapace)
Dofetilide (Tikosyn)
Bretylium (Bretylol)
Verapamil (Calan)
Adenosine (Adeno-jec)
Atropine (generic)
Isoproterenol (Isuprel)

Lipid-Lowering Drugs
Lovastatin (Mevacor)
Simvastatin (Zocor)
Pravastatin (Pravachol)
Pitavastatin (Livalo)
Fluvastatin (Lescol)
Atorvastatin (Lipitor)
Rosuvastatin (Crestor)
Nicotinic acid (Nicobid)
Fenofibrate (Antara)
Gemfibrozil (Lopid)
Ezetimibe (Zetia)
Cholestyramine (Questran)
Colestipol (Colestid)
Colesevelam (WelChol)

Review Test

Directions: Each of the numbered items or incomplete statements in this section is followed by answers or by completions of the statement. Select the ONE lettered answer or completion that is BEST in each case.

1. A patient with a long history of cardio-vascular disease develops worsening ventricular arrhythmias. Which of the following drugs is most likely to be the cause of the arrhythmia?

(A) Quinidine
(B) Propanolol
(C) Dobutamine
(D) Methyldopa

2. A patient is admitted into the emergency room and manifests ventricular tachycardia following an acute myocardial infarction (MI). This arrhythmia is life-threatening and must be controlled immediately. Which of the following drugs would be best to quickly control the condition?

(A) Dobutamine
(B) Digitalis
(C) Quinidine
(D) Lidocaine
(E) Atropine

3. A woman who is undergoing an endo-crine work-up to diagnose the cause of a large multinodular goiter develops atrial fibrillation. Which of the following would be best to treat this arrhythmia?

(A) Verapamil
(B) Propranolol
(C) Digitalis
(D) Bretylium
(E) Tocainide

4. A 57-year-old man with atrial flutter is initially treated with quinidine to control the arrhythmia. He is released from the hospital, and while his condition improves, sporadic arrhythmias continue. Which of the following drugs might be used as an adjunct to quinidine in the treatment of the atrial flutter?

(A) Digitalis
(B) Lidocaine
(C) Procainamide

(D) Nifedipine
(E) Propranolol

5. A 16-year-old boy is brought to the hospital by ambulance following a car accident causing serious head injuries. His blood pressure is 220/170 mmHg. Fundoscopy reveals retinal damage, and you administer nitroprusside via infusion. Control of the hypertension requires 72 hours and you notice the patient becoming increasingly fatigued and nauseous. The mostly likely cause of these symptoms is

(A) Production of thiocyanate from nitroprusside
(B) Negative inotropic activity of nitroprusside
(C) Renal precipitation of nitroprusside
(D) Accumulation of nitroprusside because of its long half-life
(E) Production of hydroxocobalamin

6. A 66-year-old man presents to your office with a 5-month history of dry cough. He denies any other symptoms. His past medical history includes a recent myocardial infarction (MI), after which he was placed on several medications. He does not smoke, nor has he had a history of asthma. You decide that a medication side effect is the most likely cause of this patient's symptoms. Which medication might this be?

(A) Lisinopril
(B) Nitroglycerin
(C) Lovastatin
(D) Digoxin
(E) Quinidine

7. Since the side effects of the medication you prescribed preclude the patient in the above scenario from taking it, you switch him to therapy with an agent that is said to produce similar mortality benefits, while working via a slightly different mechanism of action. What agent is it?

(A) Furosemide
(B) Captopril
(C) Losartan
(D) Esmolol
(E) Ezetimibe

8. A 54-year-old woman is diagnosed with congestive heart failure (CHF). You prescribe captopril, a medication proven to reduce her mortality. This agent delivers several benefits to patients with CHF. Which of the following effects is caused by this drug?

(A) It has a high affinity for angiotensin II receptors
(B) It promotes increased peripheral vascular resistance
(C) It decreases cardiac output and increases afterload
(D) It causes venodilation and induces natriuresis
(E) It increases preload

9. A 76-year-old man has suffered from atrial fibrillation for many years. This condition has been under good control with amiodarone and diltiazem until recently, when he started experiencing palpitations and came back to see you. You decide to start the patient on digoxin therapy. How does this medication work?

(A) It decreases intracellular sodium and increases intracellular potassium
(B) It lowers intracellular calcium
(C) It decreases stroke volume and cardiac output
(D) It diminishes elimination of sodium and water
(E) It increases vagal activity and decreases sympathetic tone

10. A 47-year-old woman is admitted for the treatment of acute myocardial ischemia. Her prior medication included digoxin for atrial fibrillation. She also suffers from hypertension, for which she is currently not taking anything. Before you discharge her home, you decide to add a medication that works well for hypertension. While she is still on the floor she develops a dangerous arrhythmia, which you are fortunately able to treat promptly. Which medication you added likely increased the effects of digoxin that this patient was already taking?

(A) Valsartan
(B) Hydrochlorothiazide

(C) Hydralazine
(D) Tadalafil
(E) Lovastatin

11. A 55-year-old woman is admitted to the surgical intensive care unit after having a coronary artery bypass grafting of four of her coronary vessels. Overnight she develops hypotension, and her cardiac output, as measured by the Swan-Ganz catheter, is significantly lower than it had been post-surgery. You decide to give her a dose of milrinone. This results in an increase in her cardiac output. How does this medication work?

(A) It is a cholinergic agonist
(B) It reduces left ventricular filling pressure
(C) It potentiates cardiac phosphodiesterase type 3
(D) It decreases cyclic AMP (cAMP)
(E) It decreases intracellular calcium

12. You are taking care of a 64-year-old man who had just undergone a right hemicolectomy for colon cancer. His blood pressure has been low, and you want to find out whether the shock that this patient is experiencing is related to a possible intraabdominal infection as a consequence of his surgery or is due to his preexisting congestive heart failure (CHF). After analyzing the Swan-Ganz catheter measurements, you deduce that the picture is most compatible with cardiogenic shock. You recall from your pharmacology class that dobutamine can be used successfully for such patients. Which of the following is true regarding dobutamine?

(A) It acts on dopamine receptors
(B) It activates α-receptors
(C) It activates cyclic AMP (cAMP)-related pathways
(D) It increases peripheral resistance
(E) It produces bradycardia

13. A 75-year-old woman, who is admitted for the management of her recent stroke, develops increased blood pressure, up to 195/105, with a heart rate of 95. Her physician is worried about the possibility of cerebral hemorrhage into the preexisting infarct and decides to administer a fast-acting vasodilating agent, which is also commonly used for severe decompensated congestive heart failure (CHF). Which medication did the doctor use?

(A) Nitroprusside
(B) Furosemide
(C) Dobutamine
(D) Losartan
(E) Digoxin

(A) Digoxin
(B) Propranolol
(C) Flecainide
(D) Verapamil
(E) Quinidine

14. While doing your medicine clerkship, you hear an announcement that a CPR team should immediately report to the room of one of the patients. Being an inquisitive student, you decide to observe how the code team manages this unfortunate patient's CPR. The rhythm monitor displays ventricular fibrillation that is quickly converted to atrial fibrillation with rapid ventricular response. The senior resident orders amiodarone to be administered to this patient. Since you forgot how this agent works, you ask one of the residents to explain how this medication works. The resident replies that he is busy, but tells you it is a class III antiarrhythmic agent. What is the mechanism of action of this agent?

(A) It is a β-receptor antagonist
(B) It blocks fast sodium channels
(C) It decreases refractoriness
(D) It interferes with outward potassium current
(E) It has a relatively short half-life

15. Although the rhythm is now under control in the patient described in the question 14, his rate is still rather high, into the 140s–150s. The rhythm strip is consistent with supraventricular tachycardia. The resident that was testing you before is now less busy and asks you what medication he should use next, given that he has in mind an agent that can also be used as an antimalarial. Which agent is it?

16. A 56-year-old retired school teacher with a treated blood pressure of 125/82 mmHg comes in for a semi-annual exam. You have a set of blood chemistries run and his low-density lipoprotein cholesterol (LDLc) is 230 and his high-density lipoprotein cholesterol (HDLc) is 54. You place him on a drug and ask him to return in 1 month. On his return, his LDLc is reduced to 189 but he complains of a cramping pain in his gastrocnemius in both the legs. The drug most likely to have caused this adverse effect is which of the following?

(A) Ezetimibe
(B) Rosuvastatin
(C) Hydrochlorothiazide
(D) Niacin
(E) Gemfibrozil

17. A female patient with a history of bronchospasm complains she felt some shortness of breath that was accompanied with feeling of nausea when playing in a softball game. During her history, she admits that she has felt like that before when walking up a few flights of stairs. You schedule a stress test and the results confirm stable angina. Which of the following drugs would be the best choice for long-term management of this patient?

(A) Nitroprusside
(B) Sildenafil
(C) Metolazone
(D) amilodipine
(E) Propranolol

Answers and Explanations

1. **The answer is A.** Quinidine is associated with QT interval prolongation and torsade de point arrhythmias. Propranolol can cause heart block. Dobutamine rarely causes ventricular arrhythmias.

2. **The answer is D.** Lidocaine is the best agent for the management of ventricular tachycardia associated with acute myocardial infarction (MI). Dobutamine, digitalis, quinidine, and atropine can all induce tachyarrhythmias. Lidocaine does not slow conduction and has little effect on atrial function.

3. **The answer is B.** Hyperthyroidism apparently increases β-adrenoceptors. β-Adrenoceptor antagonists such as propranolol can actually decrease symptoms of hyperthyroidism.

4. **The answer is A.** Quinidine acts to prolong refractoriness and slow conduction rather than as a negative inotropic agent. The ability of digitalis to decrease conduction through the atrioventricular (AV) node makes its effects compatible with quinidine to reduce atrial flutter. Lidocaine must be administered parenterally. The effects of procainamide are synergistic with quinidine, increasing the risk of toxicity; nifedipine has little antiarrhythmic effect.

5. **The answer is A.** The toxicity of nitroprusside is caused by the release of cyanide and the accumulation of thiocyanate. Hydroxocobalamin is used to reduce the toxicity of nitroprusside through the formation of the less toxic cyanocobalamin.

6. **The answer is A.** Angiotensin-converting enzyme (ACE) inhibitors commonly cause dry nonproductive cough. Nitroglycerin can cause headaches. Lovastatin commonly causes liver dysfunction. Digoxin can cause arrhythmias, and quinidine is known to cause muscle weakness.

7. **The answer is C.** Losartan is an angiotensin receptor blocker (ARB) that produces effects similar to those of angiotensin-converting enzyme (ACE) inhibitors while causing less cough and angioedema. Furosemide is a loop diuretic that is used in congestive heart failure. Captopril is an example of another ACE inhibitor. Esmolol is an antiarrhythmic agent. Ezetimibe is a lipid-lowering drug.

8. **The answer is D.** Angiotensin-converting enzyme (ACE) inhibitors cause venodilation and induce natriuresis, thereby reducing preload. A high affinity for angiotensin II receptors represents the mechanism of action of angiotensin-receptor blockers. ACE inhibitors counteract increased peripheral resistance, increase cardiac output, and decrease afterload.

9. **The answer is E.** Digoxin, a cardiac glycoside, increases vagal activity, resulting in inhibition of the sinoatrial (SA) node and delayed conduction through the atrioventricular (AV) node. It also decreases sympathetic tone. Cardiac glycosides increase intracellular sodium while decreasing intracellular potassium; increase intracellular calcium; and increase stroke volume and therefore cardiac output. Cardiac glycosides enhance elimination of sodium and water.

10. **The answer is B.** Hydrochlorothiazide, a diuretic, is known to cause hypokalemia, a state in which the actions of digoxin can be potentiated to a dangerous level. Valsartan is generally not used as a sole agent for hypertension. Hydralazine lowers blood pressure, but it does not generally cause marked electrolyte disturbances. Tadalafil is an agent used for erectile dysfunction. Lovastatin is an HMG-CoA inhibitor, used for hypercholesterolemia.

11. **The answer is B.** Milrinone reduces left ventricular filling pressure and thus enhances cardiac output. It is related to the anticholinergic agent biperiden. Milrinone inhibits cardiac phosphodiesterase type 3. It increases cyclic AMP (cAMP), and therefore intracellular calcium.

12. **The answer is C.** Dobutamine increases cyclic AMP (cAMP)-mediated phosphorylation and the activity of calcium channels. It does not act on dopamine receptors or α-receptors; it only acts on β_1-receptors. Dobutamine does not substantially affect peripheral resistance. This agent produces mild tachycardia.

13. **The answer is A.** Nitroprusside is a vasodilating agent that can be used in hypertensive emergencies. Furosemide is used for long-term treatment of congestive heart failure (CHF). Dobutamine does not significantly affect the vessels to produce vasodilation. Losartan is an angiotensin-converting enzyme (ACE) inhibitor that is used in long-term care of CHF. Digoxin is another long-term agent used in CHF and certain arrhythmias.

14. **The answer is D.** Amiodarone is a class III antiarrhythmic agent that interferes with outward potassium current. β-Receptor antagonists are considered class II antiarrhythmics. Class I antiarrhythmics block fast sodium channels. Amiodarone prolongs the effective refractory period. It has a rather long half-life, up to 100 days.

15. **The answer is E.** Quinidine is used for supraventricular tachycardia and is used to maintain sinus rhythm after conversion of atrial fibrillation. It also has antimalarial properties. Digoxin can be used in long-term management of atrial fibrillation. Propranolol is a class II antiarrhythmic agent. Flecainide is a class IC agent that can be used for ventricular tachyarrhythmias. Verapamil is a class IV antiarrhythmic agent.

16. **The answer is B.** A common adverse effect of statins like rosuvastatin is muscle pain and cramping. Ezetimibe reduces LDLc by interfering with absorption of dietary cholesterol. Hydrochlorothiazide can increase both plasma cholesterol and triglycerides. Niacin can also reduce LDLc and elevated HDLc. The major action of gemfibrozil is to reduce serum triglycerides.

17. **The answer is D.** The calcium-channel blocker amlodipine. Nitroprusside must be given by IV infusion. Sildenafil is useful for erectile dysfunction and pulmonary hypertension. The thiazide-like metolazone would not be of particular benefit. Propranolol is an appropriate choice for treating angina in some patients, but not in the presence of a lung disorder.

chapter 5 Drugs Acting on the Central Nervous System

I. SEDATIVE–HYPNOTIC DRUGS

Drugs that cause sedation and at the same time relieve anxiety (anxiolytics) or can induce sleep. They are used primarily to treat anxiety and insomnia.

A. Benzodiazepines (Table 5.1)
1. **General properties**
   a. Benzodiazepines have a **great margin of safety** over previously available sedative–hypnotic agents (e.g., barbiturates; see Fig. 5.1) that produce a dose-dependent continuum of central nervous system (CNS) depression, leading ultimately to coma and death (Fig. 5.1).
   b. Most benzodiazepines have qualitatively similar therapeutic actions but differ in their relative lipid solubility, biotransformation, and elimination half-life.
2. **Mechanism of action** (Fig. 5.2)
   a. Benzodiazepines facilitate the opening of γ-aminobutyric acid (GABA)-activated chloride channels.
   b. **They bind to a regulatory site,** also referred to as the benzodiazepine receptor, **on the GABA$_A$-receptor,** the major CNS mediator of inhibitory neurotransmission. This site is distinct from the pentameric GABA$_A$-receptor binding site for GABA. Both sites are components of a chloride channel complex that consists of at least four distinct subunits (α, β, γ and their multiple isoforms) in different proportions. A benzodiazepine receptor subtype with α1subunits (BZ$_1$) appears to mediate the sedative effect of benzodiazepines; a receptor subtype (BZ$_2$) with α2 and α3 subunits appears to mediate the anxiolytic effect of the benzodiazepines.
   c. Benzodiazepines **allosterically increase the affinity of the GABA$_A$-receptor for GABA with an increase in the frequency of GABA-stimulated chloride conductance.** This increase in chloride conductance results in neuronal hyperpolarization that leads to inhibition of synaptic transmission in the CNS and inhibition of neuronal depolarization by excitatory neurotransmitters. These drugs have no action in the absence of GABA.
3. **Pharmacological properties**
   a. Generally, benzodiazepines are administered orally to treat anxiety and sleep disorders. The onset of benzodiazepine action is related to the relative degree of lipid solubility, which can vary 50-fold or more. Some can be given parenterally (e.g., **diazepam, midazolam**). Benzodiazepines that are highly lipid soluble (e.g., **midazolam, triazolam, diazepam**) have a more rapid onset of action than benzodiazepines that are relatively less lipid soluble.
   b. The duration of action of benzodiazepines varies considerably. They are classified as either short-, intermediate-, or long-acting. Shorter acting compounds are generally more useful for insomnia without "hangover" on awakening. Longer acting benzodiazepines are generally more useful for anxiety.

table 5.1 Benzodiazepine Indications	
Drug (Half-Life)	**Primary Indications**
Short acting ($t_{1/2} < 5$ h)	
Midazolam	Preanesthetic
Triazolam	Insomnia, preanesthetic
Intermediate acting ($t_{1/2}$ 5–24 h)	
Alprazolam[a]	Anxiety, antidepressant
Clonazepam	Seizures
Estazolam	Insomnia
Lorazepam	Anxiety, insomnia, seizures, preanesthetic
Oxazepam	Anxiety
Temazepam	Insomnia
Long-lasting ($t_{1/2} > 24$ h)	
Chlordiazepoxide[b,d]	Anxiety, preanesthetic, withdrawal states
Clorazepate[b,c]	Anxiety, seizures
Diazepam[b,d]	Anxiety, preanesthetic, seizures, withdrawal states
Flurazepam	Insomnia
Prazepam[b,c]	Anxiety
Quazepam	Insomnia

[a]For panic disorders.
[b]Converted to the long-acting, active metabolite.
[c]Prodrug.
[d]For withdrawal from ethanol and other sedative–hypnotics.

    c. Biotransformation to active metabolites, particularly **desmethyldiazepam,** result from phase I hepatic microsomal oxidation by the cytochrome P450 isozyme CYP3A4, or by acid hydrolysis in the stomach (e.g., the pro-drug clorazepate), and extend the plasma half-life of some benzodiazepines to as long as 60 hours or more (e.g., **chlordiazepoxide, diazepam, flurazepam**) accounting for the hangover and other cumulative effects when administered repeatedly.

    d. Short-medium acting benzodiazepines are those that are biotransformed by ring hydroxylation (e.g., **estazolam**) and/or direct glucuronidation (e.g., **lorazepam, oxazepam, temazepam**=LOT) to inactive metabolites followed by renal clearance.

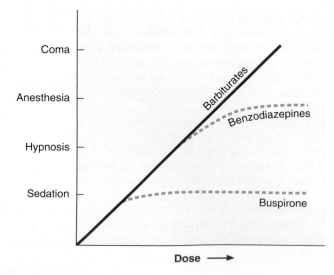

FIGURE 5.1. Theoretical dose–response relationships for sedative–hypnotic drugs and buspirone.

FIGURE 5.2. Representation of GABA-receptor–chloride channel receptor complex. Binding of GABA to its receptor causes the closed chloride channel to open. Binding of benzodiazepine to its receptor allosterically enhances binding of GABA. This causes increased chloride conductance and further hyperpolarization of the cell, making it less excitable.

  e. Clearance of long-acting benzodiazepines is decreased in the elderly who are particularly sensitive to their effects, and in patients with liver disease. In these patients, doses should be reduced or the drug avoided altogether.
4. *Therapeutic uses* (see Table 5.1)
  a. Anxiety disorders. Benzodiazepines (e.g., **clonazepam**, **lorazepam**, **diazepam**) are effective for the short-term management (<6 weeks) of the following anxiety disorders (*selective serotonin-reuptake inhibitors [SSRIs; see III E below] are now considered to be first-line choices for the long-term management of these and other anxiety disorders. Their delayed onset of action limits their effectiveness for acute anxiety states.*):
    (1) Acute anxiety.
    (2) Generalized anxiety disorders (GAD).
    (3) Situational anxiety disorders.
    (4) Panic disorders (PDs) with or without agoraphobia. **Alprazolam and clonazepam**, because of their apparent greater specificity, are widely used for urgent care.
    (5) Social phobia (SP; social anxiety disorder).
  b. Insomnia. Although benzodiazepines that have a rapid onset and sufficient duration with minimal "hangover" are still widely used (e.g., **temazepam**, **flurazepam**, **triazolam**), the nonbenzodiazepine agents zolpidem, zaleplon, and eszopiclone are now preferred for the management of sleep disorders (see below).
  c. Seizures
    (1) Benzodiazepines elevate the seizure threshold.
    (2) Lorazepam (and **diazepam**), given by intravenous (IV) infusion may be used for initial treatment of status epilepticus and drug- or toxin-induced seizures.
    (3) The development of tolerance precludes their long-term use.
  d. Preanesthetic and short medical/surgical procedures. Shorter acting benzodiazepines (e.g., **midazolam**) are preferred for their anxiolytic, sedative, and amnestic actions before and during surgery, endoscopy, or bronchoscopy.
  e. Muscle relaxation. Diazepam is used to treat spontaneous muscle spasms, spasms associated with endoscopy, and the spasticity of cerebral palsy.
  f. Acute mania of bipolar disorder for the initial management of agitation.
  g. Physical dependence. Long-acting benzodiazepines, such as **diazepam** and **chlordiazepoxide**, are used to reduce the withdrawal symptoms of physical dependence associated with the long-term use of shorter acting benzodiazepines and other sedative–hypnotic drugs, including alcohol and the barbiturates.

5. *Adverse effects, contraindications, and drug interactions*

   a. Benzodiazepines commonly produce **daytime drowsiness, sedation, and ataxia** that may impair judgment and interfere with motor skills, particularly in the elderly. In the treatment of insomnia, these adverse effects are more likely to occur with longer acting benzodiazepines.

   b. These drugs may cause **rebound insomnia** on discontinuation.

   c. **In the elderly, overuse of benzodiazepines is the most common cause of reversible confusion and amnesia** as well as a cause of blurred vision, hypotension, tremor, and constipation.

   d. These drugs may **depress respiration** at higher than hypnotic doses, an effect that can be exaggerated in patients with chronic obstructive pulmonary disease or obstructive sleep apnea.

   e. Benzodiazepines, particularly when given intravenously, may decrease blood pressure and decrease heart rate in patients with impaired cardiovascular function.

   f. These drugs cause rare paradoxical excitement.

   g. Benzodiazepines **enhance CNS depression when taken in combination with other drugs that depress the CNS,** most notably alcohol.

   h. Drugs and grapefruit juice that inhibit CYP3A4 can extend the duration of benzodiazepine action.

6. *Tolerance, abuse, and dependence*

   a. Tolerance develops to the sedative, hypnotic, and anticonvulsant actions of benzodiazepines but apparently less so to their anxiolytic action. **Cross-tolerance** occurs with other sedative–hypnotic agents, including **alcohol** and **barbiturates.**

   b. The abuse potential of benzodiazepines is low compared with that of other classes of sedative–hypnotic drugs except when there is already a history of substance abuse.

   c. Signs of withdrawal after long-term benzodiazepine use may include severe anxiety, insomnia, and also gastrointestinal (GI) disturbances, headache, and tremor. Perceptual distortions, delusions, and seizures have also been reported.

   d. Withdrawal occurs sooner and is more severe after abrupt discontinuation of shorter acting benzodiazepines.

   e. The effects associated with withdrawal can be minimized by tapering the dose reduction or substituting longer acting benzodiazepines such as diazepam.

B. Flumazenil

   1. Flumazenil is a **competitive antagonist** at benzodiazepine receptors.

   2. Flumazenil is used to prevent or reverse the CNS effects from benzodiazepine overdose or to speed recovery from the effects of benzodiazepines used in anesthetic and diagnostic procedures; it may precipitate withdrawal. Its short duration of action often necessitates multiple dosing.

C. Zolpidem, zaleplon, and eszopiclone

   1. Zolpidem, zaleplon, and eszopiclone are widely used for **short-term treatment of insomnia.** Due to their relatively high lipid solubility, they have a rapid onset of action. Their duration of action varies between 1 hour (Zolpidem) and 6 hours (eszopiclone). Zolpidem undergoes hepatic metabolism; its half-life may be decreased or increased by other drugs that, respectively, induce the CYP450 system or inhibit CYP3A4 isozymes. Dosage of these drugs should be reduced in the elderly and in patients with hepatic impairment.

   2. These drugs, which act on a specific subtype of the benzodiazepine receptor, BZ_1, to reduce chloride conductance, have a similar mechanism of action but are structurally unrelated to the benzodiazepines.

   3. These drugs have only **weak muscle-relaxing or anticonvulsant activity,** with **reduced potential compared with the benzodiazepines for tolerance, abuse, physical dependence, or rebound insomnia.**

   4. Their actions are blocked or reversed by flumazenil.

   5. Adverse effects include modest daytime sedation, headache, and GI upset. Eszopiclone is reported to also produce dry mouth, some sedation, and an unpleasant taste.

D. Buspirone

1. Buspirone is a **nonbenzodiazepine partial agonist** at serotonin (5-HT1$_A$)-receptors, which selectively relieves anxiety without the sedation, hypnosis, general CNS depression, or drug abuse liability of the benzodiazepines (see Fig. 5.1). It has no other benzodiazepine-like activities.
2. Because a week or more of administration may be required to achieve the therapeutic effects of buspirone, it is **used primarily to treat generalized anxiety disorder**.
3. Buspirone may cause **nervousness, restlessness, dysphoria, tachycardia, or GI distress**. It causes **pupillary constriction.**

E. Ramelteon.
Ramelteon is prescribed for patients who have difficulty falling asleep. It is a selective agonist at melatonin **MT1 and MT2 receptors** that are involved in the promotion of sleep and that maintain the normal circadian rhythm. Adverse effects of ramelteon include dizziness and fatigue.

F. Other sedative–hypnotics.
Barbiturates, chloral hydrate, and meprobamate have been largely supplanted by benzodiazepines, the newer nonbenzodiazepine sedative–hypnotic agents, and the SSRIs, for the treatment of anxiety and sleep disorders.

1. *Barbiturates* (Table 5.2; see also VII C 1 and X C 3)
    a. **Phenobarbital is used as an anticonvulsant; thiopental is used as an IV general anesthetic.**
    b. Barbiturates **interact with a binding site on the GABA$_A$-receptor-chloride channel complex** that is separate from the benzodiazepine-binding site. At low doses, barbiturates **allosterically prolong the GABA-induced opening of chloride channels** and enhance GABA-inhibitory neurotransmission; at higher doses, these drugs have GABA-mimetic activity (they open chloride channels independently of GABA).
    c. **Redistribution from highly vascular (e.g., brain) to less-vascular tissues (e.g., muscle, fat) is responsible for the short duration of the highly lipid-soluble barbiturate thiopental.**
    d. Phenobarbital use is limited by its strong sedation effects, rapid tolerance, drug interactions, abuse potential, and **lethality in overdose due to dose-related respiratory depression** with cerebral hypoxia; this effect results from abuse or suicide attempt. Treatment includes ventilation, gastric lavage, hemodialysis, osmotic diuretics, and, because it is a weak organic base, alkalinization of urine.
    e. With long-term use, **phenobarbital may induce the synthesis of hepatic microsomal enzymes** and may increase its own metabolism and the metabolism of numerous other drugs.
    f. **Phenobarbital may increase porphyrin synthesis** by the induction of hepatic δ-aminolevulinic acid synthase. It **can precipitate the symptoms** of **acute intermittent porphyria.**
    g. Hepatic and renal disease may prolong barbiturate action.
    h. Phenobarbital (and pentobarbital) is occasionally used to treat the physical dependence associated with long-term use of sedative–hypnotic drugs.

t a b l e **5.2**	Classification and Indications of Barbiturates
Drug and Classification	**Indications**

Ultra-short acting
  Thiopental (Pentothal)
  Methohexital (Brevital)
  Thiamylal (Surital)
	Intravenous general anesthesia

Intermediate acting
  Amobarbital (Amytal)
  Pentobarbital (Nembutal)
  Secobarbital (Seconal)
	Preanesthetic medication and regional anesthesia; sedation and hypnosis (largely supplanted by benzodiazepines)

Long acting
  Phenobarbital (Luminal)
  Mephobarbital (Mebaral)
	Seizure disorders; withdrawal syndrome from sedative–hypnotics

II. ANTIPSYCHOTIC (NEUROLEPTIC) DRUGS

A. Classification
1. Antipsychotic drugs may be classified as either **typical** or **atypical.**
2. *Typical antipsychotic drugs* are often sub-classified according to their oral milligram potency (high potency or low potency).
    a. **High-potency** drugs (**piperazine phenothiazines, e.g., fluphenazine,** and **haloperidol**) are more likely to produce extrapyramidal reactions.
    b. **Low-potency** drugs (**aliphatic phenothiazines, e.g., triflupromazine; piperidine phenothiazines, e.g., thioridazine**) are less likely to produce acute extrapyramidal reactions and more likely to produce sedation and postural hypotension.
3. *Atypical antipsychotic agents* (**e.g., risperidone, olanzapine**) have generally replaced the typical drugs for the initial treatment of first-episode patients. **Clozapine** is reserved for treatment-resistant patients.
4. Other **heterocyclic antipsychotic drugs** such as **loxapine** and **molindone,** with intermediate potency, have no clear advantage over other typical drugs.

B. Therapeutic action
1. The therapeutic action of the **typical antipsychotic drugs** not certain, but is correlated best with **antagonist activity** at **postjunctional dopamine (DA) D_2-receptors** in the mesolimbic and mesocortical areas of the CNS where DA normally inhibits adenylyl cyclase activity.
2. The therapeutic action of the **atypical antipsychotic drugs** not certain, but is also correlated with **antagonist activity at 5-HT_{2A} receptors**.

C. Pharmacological properties
1. Most antipsychotic drugs are highly lipophilic and have long half-lives (10–20 h). They show little correlation between plasma levels and therapeutic action. Plasma levels are monitored primarily for compliance and toxicity.
2. Esterification of fluphenazine and haloperidol (fluphenazine decanoate, haloperidol decanoate) results in long-acting depot forms (2- to 3-week duration of action) that can be used to manage compliance issues. **Plasma esterases** convert the parent compound to the active drug.

D. Therapeutic uses
1. *Schizophrenia*
    a. Antipsychotic drugs produce an **immediate quieting action.** However, their antipsychotic effects typically take longer to occur (a week or more). Atypical antipsychotic drugs, particularly **clozapine,** have a seemingly greater effect on negative symptoms than the typical agents.
    b. These drugs **curb acute psychotic attacks** and delay subsequent relapses.
2. *Other selected therapeutic uses*
    a. **Manic phase in bipolar disorder.**
    b. **Schizoaffective disorders.**
    c. **Atypical psychotic disorders.**
    d. **Depression with psychotic manifestations.**
    e. **Tourette syndrome (haloperidol, pimozide** [Orap] or **risperidone**).
    f. Severe nausea or vomiting associated with, e.g., radiation treatment and cancer chemotherapy, as well as postoperative nausea and vomiting. With the exception of thioridazine, typical antipsychotic agents have strong antiemetic activity due to DA D_2-receptor blockade in the chemoreceptor trigger zone (CTZ) of the medulla. The most commonly used are the phenothiazines **prochlorperazine** and **promethazine**.

E. Adverse effects and contraindications. Selection of a specific antipsychotic agent for therapeutic use is often based on its associated adverse effects rather than therapeutic efficacy.

table 5.3 Potency and Selected Adverse Effects of Representative Conventional Antipsychotic Drugs

Drugs	Oral Dose (mg)	Extrapyramidal Effects[a]	Autonomic Effects	Sedation
Conventional drugs				
Aliphatic phenothiazines				
Chlorpromazine	100	++	+++	+++
Triflupromazine	50	++	+++	+++
Piperidine phenothiazines				
Thioridazine[b]	100	+	+++	+++
Mesoridazine	50	+	+++	+++
Piperazine phenothiazines				
Trifluoperazine	10	+++	++	++
Fluphenazine[c]	5	+++	++	++
Butyrophenones				
Haloperidol	2	+++	+	
Other related drugs				
Molindone	20–200	+++	++	++
Loxapine	20–250	+++	++	++

[a]Excluding tardive dyskinesia.
[b]Cardiotoxicity.
[c]Esterification (enanthate or decanoate) results in depot form.

The adverse effects of antipsychotic agents are due to their antagonist actions at DA D_2- and histamine H_1-receptors (and possibly serotonin receptors) in the CNS and to their antagonist actions at muscarinic cholinoceptors and α-adrenoceptors in the periphery.

1. **CNS**
   a. **Extrapyramidal syndromes** (see Tables 5.3 and 5.4)
      (1) These adverse effects are related to a DA-**receptor blockade** in the basal ganglia (and elsewhere in the CNS) that leads to an imbalance in DA and acetylcholine (ACh) actions in the nigrostriatal pathway.
      (2) These effects are a major cause of **noncompliance.**
      (3) Extrapyramidal effects are **most likely to occur with high-potency typical antipsychotic drugs** that have a high affinity for postjunctional DA D_2-receptors in the basal ganglia. They are less likely to occur with low-potency typical antipsychotic drugs such as **thioridazine** and, with the exception of **risperidone,** they are also unlikely to occur with atypical antipsychotic drugs such as **clozapine** and **olanzapine.**
      (4) These effects can sometimes spontaneously remit.

table 5.4 Selected Adverse Effects of Atypical Antipsychotic Drugs

Atypical Drugs	Extrapyramidal Effects[a]	Hypotensive Activity	Sedation	Weight Gain	Increased Prolactin
Aripiprazole	+/−	+	+/−	+/−	+/−
Clozapine[b]	+/−	++	+	+++	+/−
Olanzapine	+/−	+	++	+++	+/−
Quetiapine	+/−	++	++	++	+/−
Risperidone[c]	++	+	+	+	++
Ziprasidone[d]	+/−	+/−	+	+/−	+/−

[a]Excluding tardive dyskinesia.
[b]Agranulocytosis.
[c]Little extrapyramidal effects at low doses.
[d]QTc prolongation.

(5) Extrapyramidal syndromes include the following:

(a) Acute dystonia (often elicited during the first week of therapy). Acute dystonia can be controlled with more-centrally acting antimuscarinic drugs such as **benztropine** and **biperiden,** and the antihistamine **diphenhydramine (Benadryl)** which has central anticholinergic activity, and by reducing the antipsychotic drug dose which, however, may lead to an increase in psychotic symptoms.

(b) Akathisia (can develop as early as the first 2 weeks of treatment or as late as 60 days into therapy). Akathisia can be controlled by drugs with antimuscarinic activity and by the β-receptor antagonist **propranolol.**

(c) Parkinsonian-like syndrome (can develop from 5 days to weeks into treatment). Parkinsonian-like syndrome can be controlled with antimuscarinic drugs (e.g., **benztropine, biperiden**) or by reducing the antipsychotic drug dose.

b. Tardive dyskinesia (generally occurs after months to years of drug exposure).

(1) Tardive dyskinesia is much more likely with typical antipsychotic agents than atypical agents. It does not occur with **clozapine.**

(2) It may be the result of a developing supersensitivity of the postjunctional DA receptors in the CNS, perhaps in the basal ganglia, that results in a relative decrease in cholinergic activity.

(3) Tardive dyskinesia is **often irreversible.**

(4) Tardive dyskinesia has an estimated incidence of 10%–20%; it is more likely to occur in the elderly or in institutionalized patients who receive long-term, high-dose therapy.

(5) The only effective treatment for antipsychotic drug-induced tardive dyskinesia is the discontinuation of drug therapy.

c. Neuroleptic malignant syndrome

(1) Neuroleptic malignant syndrome is most likely in patients sensitive to the extrapyramidal effects of the typical high-potency antipsychotic agents.

(2) This syndrome is characterized by autonomic instability, muscle rigidity, diaphoresis, profound hyperthermia, and myoglobinemia.

(3) This condition occurs, often explosively, in 1% of patients untreated; it is **associated with a 20% mortality rate.**

(4) This condition is treated by discontinuing drug therapy and initiating supportive measures, including the use of **bromocriptine** to overcome the DA receptor blockade and the use of muscle relaxants such as **diazepam** and perhaps **dantrolene** to reduce muscle rigidity.

d. Sedation (see Tables 5.3 and 5.4)

(1) The sedation effects, **more likely with low-potency antipsychotic agents** and with the atypical agents, are due to a central histamine H_1-receptor blockade.

(2) These effects may be mild to severe. The elderly are particularly at risk.

(3) The effects may be temporary.

e. Confusional state with memory impairment. This effect is likely with antipsychotic agents with pronounced antimuscarinic activity.

f. Seizures

(1) Seizures are especially more common with **chlorpromazine and clozapine.**

(2) This effect is due to a lowering of the seizure threshold; antipsychotic drugs may precipitate or unmask epilepsy.

2. *Autonomic nervous system* (see Tables 5.3 and 5.4)

a. α-Adrenoceptor blockade

(1) Blockade of α-adrenoceptors, **more likely to occur with typical low-potency and atypical antipsychotic agents,** causes **orthostatic hypotension** and possibly syncope, as a result of peripheral vasodilation; central depression of the vasomotor center may also contribute. This effect may be severe and may result in reflex tachycardia. Elderly patients and those with heart disease are more at risk. The effect may be temporary.

(2) This blockade also causes **impotence** and **inhibition of ejaculation.**

    b. Muscarinic cholinoceptor blockade

      (1) Blockade of muscarinic cholinoceptors, more common with typical low-potency antipsychotic agents and with the atypical agent clozapine, produces an atropine-like effect, resulting in dry mouth and blurred vision.

      (2) This blockade may also produce constipation, tachycardia, and difficulty in urination leading to urine retention. The effect may be temporary.

      (3) Muscarinic cholinoceptor blockade more rarely causes paralytic ileus and severe bladder infections.

      (4) Elderly patients are more at risk.

  3. *Endocrine and metabolic disturbances,* likely with most typical antipsychotic agents and the atypical agent **risperidone,** are due to DA D_2-receptor antagonist activity in the pituitary, resulting in **hyperprolactinemia** (see Table 5.4).

    a. In **women,** these disturbances include spontaneous or induced **galactorrhea, loss of libido,** and delayed ovulation and menstruation or amenorrhea.

    b. In **men,** these disturbances include **gynecomastia** and **impotence.**

    c. Weight gain is likely with most typical antipsychotic agents and the atypical antipsychotic agents **clozapine** and **olanzapine.** (see Table 5.4). **Hyperglycemia** and **dyslipidemia** have been reported for atypical agents. These drugs may exacerbate or precipitate **diabetes mellitus** or **hyperlipidemia.**

  4. *Other adverse effects*

    a. Withdrawal-like syndrome

      (1) This syndrome is characterized by **nausea, vomiting, insomnia,** and **headache** in 30% of patients, especially those receiving low-potency antipsychotic drugs.

      (2) These symptoms may persist for up to 2 weeks.

      (3) The symptoms can be minimized with a tapered reduction of drug dosage.

    b. Cardiac arrhythmias

      (1) Cardiac arrhythmias result from a quinidine-like effect in which there is local anesthetic activity with an increased likelihood of heart block.

      (2) Cardiac arrhythmias are more likely with **thioridazine** and **ziprasidone,** which can prolong the Q–T interval and lead to conduction block and sudden death.

    c. Blood dyscrasias are rare, except in the case of **clozapine,** which may induce agranulocytosis in up to 3% of patients and, therefore, is used only when other drug groups prove ineffective.

    d. Cholestatic jaundice, which is caused primarily by **chlorpromazine.**

    e. Photosensitivity

      (1) The effect is specific to **chlorpromazine;** it includes dermatitis (5%), rash, sunburn, and pigmentation, and it may be irreversible.

      (2) Chlorpromazine and high-dose **thioridazine** also produce retinitis pigmentosa.

F. Overdose. Overdose with antipsychotics is rarely fatal, except when caused by thioridazine or mesoridazine (and possibly ziprasidone), which may result in drowsiness, agitation, coma, ventricular arrhythmias, heart block, or sudden death.

G. Drug interactions

  1. Antipsychotics have potentiated sedative effects in the presence of **CNS depressants** (e.g., sedative–hypnotics, opioids, antihistamines).

  2. Certain antipsychotic drugs produce additive anticholinergic effects with tricyclic antidepressants, antiparkinsonian drugs, and other drugs with anticholinergic activity.

III. ANTIDEPRESSANT DRUGS

A. Classification (Table 5.5). Antidepressant drugs are classified into five groups: 1) **Selective serotonin reuptake inhibitors (SSRIs);** 2) **drugs that inhibit serotonin and norepinephrine transporters (SNRIs and TCAs);** 3) **serotonin 5HT$_2$-receptor antagonists;** 4) **atypical heterocyclic antidepressants;** and 5) **monoamine oxidase inhibitors (MAOIs).**

| t a b l e   **5.5** | Relative Activity of Selected Antidepressant Drugs on Norepinephrine and Serotonin Prejunctional Neuronal Uptake | |

Drug and Classification	Inhibition of Norepinephrine Uptake	Inhibition of Serotonin Uptake
Tricyclic antidepressants		
Tertiary amines		
Amitriptyline	++	+++
Imipramine	++	+++
Trimipramine	+	0
Doxepin	+	++
Clomipramine	+++	+++
Secondary amines		
Desipramine	+++	0
Nortriptyline	++	+++
Protriptyline	+++	0
Dibenzoxazepine		
Amoxapine[a]	++	+
Selective serotonin reuptake inhibitors		
Fluoxetine	0/+	+++
Paroxetine	0	+++
Sertraline	0	+++
Citalopram	0	+++
Escitalopram	0	+++
Fluvoxamine	0	+++
Other antidepressants		
Trazodone[b]	0	++
Maprotiline	+++	0
Bupropion	0/+	0/+
Venlafaxine	++	+++
Nefazodone[b]	0	0/+
Mirtazapine[c]	0	0
Duloxetine	+++	+++

[a]Has dopamine-receptor antagonist activity.
[b]Has serotonin 5-HT$_1$–receptor antagonist activity at prejunctional receptors.
[c]Has serotonin 5-HT$_2$–receptor and α_2-adrenoceptor antagonist activity.

B. **Mechanism of action** (see Table 5.5)
1. *SSRIs* **(fluoxetine, sertraline, paroxetine, citalopram, escitalopram).** SSRIs are selective inhibitors of serotonin uptake. They allosterically inhibit the prejunctional neuronal serotonin transporter (SERT) to potentiate the action of serotonin.
2. *SNRIs and TCAs*
   a. **SNRIs** are the newer drugs in this drug class **(venlafaxine, desvenlafaxine, duloxetine, milnacipran).** The older drugs are referred to as **TCAs** (e.g., **amitriptyline, desipramine, imipramine, nortriptyline).** Compared with SSRIs and SNRIs, these are now considered second-line drugs for the treatment of depression.
   b. These drugs inhibit SERT and the norepinephrine transporter (NET) to, respectively, potentiate the action of serotonin and norepinephrine. However, individual drugs vary considerably in their inhibition of SERT and NET.
   c. SNRIs are less likely to block α-adrenoceptors, or to have anticholinergic or antihistaminic actions, and thus have fewer adverse effects than the TCAs.
3. *Serotonin (5HT$_2$)-receptor antagonists* **(trazodone, nefazodone).** These drugs block primarily the serotonin 5HT$_2$A-receptor. Trazodone is also an histamine H$_1$-receptor antagonist.
4. *Atypical heterocyclic antidepressants*
   a. **Maprotiline** and **amoxapine** inhibit NET and **have anticholinergic properties. Amoxapine** also inhibits postjunctional DA D$_2$-receptors.

    b. Mirtazapine inhibits 5-HT$_2$-receptors, α_2 auto receptors, and histamine H$_1$-receptors.

    c. Bupropion has a poorly understood mechanism of action.

5. *MAOIs* (phenelzine, tranylcypromine)

    a. MAOIs rapidly, nonselectively, and irreversibly **inhibit the activity of enzymes MAO-A and MAO-B.** Inhibition of MAO-A, which preferentially degrades norepinephrine, epinephrine, and serotonin, is responsible for the therapeutic efficacy of phenelzine and tranylcypromine as antidepressants.

    b. MAO inhibition continues for up to 2–3 weeks after their elimination from the body.

6. *Therapeutic efficacy*

    a. All antidepressant drugs have similar therapeutic efficacy, although individual patients may respond better to one drug than another. Selection is often based on associated adverse effects.

    b. Although the initial effects of the antidepressants on monoamine transmission occur early, their **therapeutic effect occurs only after several weeks of drug administration** and is more closely associated with adaptive changes in neuronal receptors and second messenger activity and over the same time period. Adaptive desensitization of prejunctional norepinephrine and serotonin autoreceptors may also be factors.

    c. Adaptive changes in neurotropic factors such as **brain-derived neurotrophic factor (BDNF)** have also been implicated.

C. Therapeutic uses

  1. *Major depressive disorder*

    a. These drugs are effective in 70% of patients.

    b. SSRIs and SNRIs are preferred over TCAs because of their more limited toxicity.

    c. MAOIs are used rarely, usually only when other antidepressants have proved ineffective or for "atypical" depression.

  2. *Bipolar affective disorder.* The depressed phase of bipolar affective disorder is often treated with antidepressants given in combination with lithium or other drugs used to control mania.

  3. *Anxiety disorders* (SSRIs and SNRIs, although their full efficacy may not be seen for weeks).

    a. Generalized anxiety disorder (GAD) and **Panic disorder (PD).**

    b. Obsessive–compulsive disorder (OCD). Clomipramine and **fluvoxamine** are FDA approved only for the treatment of OCD.

    c. Social phobia (SP), situational anxiety disorder, and **post-traumatic stress disorder (PTSD).**

  4. *Chronic pain disorders*

    a. TCAs and SNRIs are often used for conditions associated with neuropathic pain and other chronic pain conditions.

    b. These drugs may work directly on pain pathways, but the exact mechanism of action is unknown.

  5. Other indications

    a. Bulimia.

    b. Premenstrual dysphoric disorder (fluoxetine, sertraline).

    c. Smoking cessation (bupropion).

    d. Enuresis. TCAs like **imipramine** are used infrequently to suppress enuresis in children (over age 6) and adults.

D. SSRIs

  1. *Pharmacological properties.* Fluoxetine has the longest half-life of all the SSRIs due to its metabolism to a long-acting active agent, **norfluoxetine.**

  2. *Adverse effects* (see Table 5.6). Overall, SSRIs produce fewer serious adverse effects than TCAs, including little sedation, postural hypotension, anticholinergic activity, and cardiovascular toxicity.

    a. Headache that is generally temporary.

    b. Sexual dysfunction in up to 40% of all patients, which is a leading cause of noncompliance.

t a b l e **5.6**	Relationship between Blockade of Neurotransmitter Receptors and Antidepressant-Induced Adverse Effects
Receptor Subtype	**Adverse Effects**
Histamine H$_1$-receptors	Sedation Weight gain Hypotension Potentiation of CNS depressants
Muscarinic receptors	Dry mouth Blurred vision Urinary retention Constipation Memory dysfunction Tachycardia
α_1-Adrenoceptors	Postural hypotension Reflex tachycardia
α_2-Adrenoceptors	Blockade of antihypertensive effects of clonidine, α-methyldopa
Serotonin 5-HT$_2$-receptors	Ejaculatory dysfunction

Reprinted and adapted with permission from Charney DS, et al. Treatment of depression. In: Schatzberg AF, Nemeroff CB, eds. Textbook of Psychopharmacology. Washington, DC: American Psychiatric Press, 1995:578. (Adapted from Richelson, EJ: Side effects of old and new generation antidepressants: a pharmacologic framework. Clin Psychiatry 1991;9:13–19.)

    c. Gastric irritation that is generally transient and includes nausea and heartburn.

    d. Weight loss initially followed in some patients by weight gain (paroxetine).

    e. Stimulation that is mild and often transient may be experienced as dysphoria, and is marked by agitation, anxiety, increased motor activity, insomnia, tremor, and excitement.

    f. Apathy (flattened affect) occurs in some patients.

    g. Rebound/discontinuation syndrome (paroxetine, sertraline). Common effects include flu-like symptoms (dizziness, nausea, headache, and fatigue) and cholinergic rebound. The effects may persist for up to 2 months. Tapered withdrawal minimizes effects.

  3. *Overdose and toxicity.* With only a few reported seizures in overdose, SSRIs are remarkably safe in comparison to other antidepressants. This accounts for their relative popularity. However, SSRIs (and all other antidepressants) may increase suicidal ideation for children, adolescents, and young adults; **"blackbox" warning.**

  4. *Drug interactions*

    a. Fluoxetine and **paroxetine** inhibit liver microsomal enzymes (CYP2D6) and thus can rarely potentiate the actions of other drugs metabolized by the same enzymes.

    b. SSRIs have a rare and potentially fatal interaction with other drugs that increase serotonin activity called **"serotonin syndrome"** that includes tremor, hyperthermia, muscle rigidity, and cardiovascular collapse.

E. SNRIs (venlafaxine, desvenlafaxine, duloxetine, milnacipran)

  1. Duloxetine metabolism is significantly affected by hepatic impairment.

  2. *Adverse effects*

    a. Adverse effects, including rebound/discontinuation effects, are similar to SSRIs.

    b. Additional noradrenergic-related effects include increased blood pressure and heart rate, insomnia, and anxiety.

    c. Duloxetine use is associated with rare hepatotoxicity.

F. TCAs

  1. *Pharmacological properties*

    a. TCAs are generally highly lipid-soluble and have relatively long half-lives.

    b. Monodemethylation of the tertiary amines **imipramine** and **amitriptyline** results in the active secondary amine metabolites **desipramine** and **nortriptyline,** respectively.

    c. Plasma levels are used primarily to monitor compliance and toxicity.

2. *Adverse effects* (Table 5.6). The adverse effects of TCAs are often accounted for by their antagonist activity at α-adrenoceptors, muscarinic cholinoceptors, histamine H_1-receptors, and others.
   a. **CNS**
      (1) **Sedation** is common and probably due to antagonist activity at CNS histamine H_1-receptors.
      (2) **Confusion and memory dysfunction** are central anticholinergic effects and are more common in the elderly.
      (3) **Mania** occasionally occurs in patients with an underlying bipolar affective disorder ("switch" reaction).
      (4) **Agitation** and **psychosis** may worsen in psychotic patients.
      (5) **Tremor** occurs in 10% of patients and is managed with **propranolol.**
      (6) **Seizures** occur occasionally because of lowered seizure threshold; they are more common with tertiary amines.
      (7) **Movement disorders** are occasionally produced by **amoxapine;** these effects are due to DA-receptor antagonist activity.
   b. **Cardiovascular system**
      (1) **Postural hypotension,** which may be severe and may be temporary, is probably due to peripheral α_1-adrenoceptor blockade; it may result in reflex tachycardia.
      (2) Tachycardia, conduction defects, and arrhythmias
         (a) These effects are particularly common with overdose, particularly with **imipramine.**
         (b) Patients with preexisting heart block or compensated cardiac output are at risk.
   c. **Autonomic nervous system**
      (1) Autonomic nervous system effects reflect the very common **muscarinic cholinoceptor antagonist activity** of TCAs. The effects may be temporary.
      (2) TCA use commonly produces dry mouth, blurred vision, difficulty in urination, and constipation.
      (3) TCAs more rarely may precipitate narrow-angle glaucoma or paralytic ileus or cause urine retention.
      (4) These effects are more common in the elderly.
   d. **Rebound/discontinuation effects** (see SSRIs).
   e. **Other adverse effects**
      (1) TCAs often produce **weight gain** that can be extensive.
      (2) TCAs can cause **sexual dysfunction.**
      (3) **TCAs (and all other antidepressants)** may increase **suicidal ideation** for children, adolescents, and young adults; **"blackbox" warning.**
      (4) These drugs produce rare but serious hematologic changes, including hemolytic anemia and agranulocytosis.
      (5) TCAs infrequently cause allergic reactions and obstructive jaundice.
      (6) **Atomoxetine** may increase suicidal thoughts in children and adolescents.
3. *Overdose and toxicity.* Overdose of TCAs produces severe anticholinergic and antiadrenergic signs, respiratory depression, arrhythmias, shock, seizures, coma, and death. Treatment is supportive and includes sodium bicarbonate for cardiac toxicity, benzodiazepines for seizures, and IV fluids and norepinephrine for hypotension.
4. *Drug interactions*
   a. TCAs potentiate the CNS depressant effects of **alcohol** and other drugs with similar activity.
   b. TCAs potentiate the pressor activity of **norepinephrine.**
   c. TCAs have additive anticholinergic effects with **antiparkinsonian drugs, antipsychotic drugs,** and other drugs with anticholinergic activity.
   d. TCAs block α-adrenoceptors and thus reduce the antihypertensive action of **clonidine** and α-**methyldopa.**
   e. Interaction with **other drugs that increase serotonin activity** can cause excitement, hyperpyrexia, and a hypertensive episode. This **"serotonin syndrome"** (see III E 3 c) also may occur with TCAs that more selectively block serotonin reuptake.

G. *Serotonin 5HT$_2$–receptor antagonists*
   1. Trazodone and nefazodone
      a. These drugs are **highly sedating**, particularly trazodone; they cause drowsiness and dizziness, and insomnia.
      b. These drugs cause gastrointestinal disturbances.
      c. These drugs may cause **postural hypotension** in the elderly.
      d. Sexual effects are limited except that trazodone may cause a rare **priapism** in men.
      e. Nefazodone has been associated with a rare **hepatotoxicity** resulting in hepatic failure and death.

H. Atypical heterocyclic antidepressant agents. The pharmacological properties of atypical heterocyclic antidepressant agents are similar to those of TCAs.
   1. *Mirtazapine, maprotiline, amoxapine, and bupropion*
      a. Mirtazepine causes marked **weight gain.**
      b. Maprotiline is highly sedating. The **seizure** risk with maprotiline may be 4% at high therapeutic doses. Also, **cardiotoxicity** in overdose.
      c. Amoxapine causes **movement disorders** similar to those caused by antipsychotic agents, including tardive dyskinesia; these effects are due to DA-receptor antagonist activity. Overdose of amoxapine causes **seizures**.
      d. Bupropion has no significant anticholinergic activity or hypotensive activity; it causes little sexual dysfunction. It is more likely than TCAs to cause **seizures,** particularly at high therapeutic doses. Bupropion causes stimulation, insomnia, and weight loss. Bupropion is also marketed as Zyban, a sustained-release aid for smoking cessation.

I. MAOIs
   1. *Pharmacological properties*
      a. Tranylcypromine and **phenelzine** are used infrequently because of their potential for serious drug interactions.
      b. Phencyclidine is inactivated by acetylation; genetically slow acetylators may show exaggerated effects.
   2. *Adverse effects* include postural hypotension, headache, dry mouth, sexual dysfunction (phenelzine), weight gain, and sleep disturbances.
   3. *Overdose and toxicity.* Uncommon results of overdose of MAOIs include agitation, hyperthermia, seizures, hypotension, or hypertension.
   4. *Drug interactions*
      a. MAOIs may result in headache, nausea, cardiac arrhythmias, hypertensive crisis, and, rarely, **subarachnoid bleeding and stroke** in the presence of indirectly acting sympathomimetics (e.g., **tyramine from certain foods**). These effects are due to the prevention of tyramine metabolism in the GI tract resulting in enhanced noradrenergic activity.
      b. These can potentiate the pressor effect of high doses of directly acting sympathetic amines that are also found in over-the-counter (OTC) preparations.
      c. MAOIs may cause a "**serotonin syndrome**" in the presence of SSRIs, certain TCAs, and opioids such as meperidine that can be fatal.

IV. LITHIUM AND ANTICONVULSANTS USED TO TREAT BIPOLAR DISORDER

A. Mechanism of action (see Fig. 1.1D)
   1. The mechanism of action for lithium is unclear, although it may be directly related to the **inhibition of phospholipid turnover** (lithium inhibits inositol monophosphatase thus decreasing inositol) and, consequently, decreased activity of the second messengers diacylglycerol and inositol 1,4,5-trisphosphate. Effects on protein kinase C, and subsequent neuroplastic alterations, may be important to its therapeutic action.

2. Lithium inhibits glycogen synthase kinase-3 (GSK-3) activity with changes in energy metabolism and gene expression. It also has reported effects on nerve conduction; on the release, synthesis, and action of biogenic amines; and on calcium metabolism.

B. Pharmacological properties
1. The onset of the therapeutic effect takes 2–3 weeks.
2. This drug is eliminated almost entirely by the kidney; 80% is reabsorbed in the proximal renal tubule.
3. Lithium has a low therapeutic index; plasma levels must be monitored continuously.

C. Therapeutic uses
1. *Acute mania or bipolar affective disorder*
   a. Lithium normalizes mood in 70% of patients. Antipsychotic agents and benzodiazepines can be used in the initial stages of the disease to control acute agitation.
   b. The anticonvulsants **carbamazepine, valproic acid,** and **lamotrigene** have been used successfully, and are currently used extensively, either alone or as adjuncts to lithium therapy; the onset of action is sooner than that of lithium. The mechanism of action of these drugs for these conditions is unknown (see VII).
2. *Prophylaxis of bipolar affective disorder,* for which lithium is often administered with a TCA (may precipitate mania).

D. Adverse effects
1. Adverse effects are common at therapeutic doses of 0.5–1.4 mmol/L or slightly higher.
2. These effects include **nausea, vomiting, diarrhea, fine tremor, polydipsia, edema,** and **weight gain.**
3. Lithium administration produces **polydipsia** and **polyuria,** which occurs as the kidney collecting tubule becomes unresponsive to antidiuretic hormone (reversible). More rarely, decreased renal function occurs with long-term treatment, similar to nephrogenic diabetes insipidus.
4. Sodium retention with **edema** is common. **Weight gain** is also common.
5. Adverse effects of lithium also include **benign, reversible thyroid enlargement** caused by reducing tyrosine iodination and the synthesis of thyroxine. Lithium more rarely causes hypothyroidism.
6. Lithium is generally contraindicated during the first trimester of pregnancy because of the possible risk of **fetal congenital abnormalities**. Renal clearance of lithium increases during pregnancy. Breast-feeding is not recommended because lithium is secreted in breast milk with possible neonate dysfunction.
7. Lithium is also contraindicated in patients with **"sick-sinus" syndrome** due to increased depression of the sinus node.

E. Drug interactions
1. Sodium depletion is increased by **low-salt diets, thiazide diuretics, furosemide, ethacrynic acid,** or severe vomiting or diarrhea. This depletion results in increased renal reabsorption of lithium and an **increased chance for toxicity.**
2. Renal clearance of lithium is decreased and the chance of toxicity is enhanced by some nonsteroidal anti-inflammatory drugs (e.g., **indomethacin and phenylbutazone**).

F. Toxicity
1. **Above 2 mmol/L,** confusion (important first sign of toxicity), drowsiness, vomiting, ataxia, dizziness, and severe tremors develop.
2. **Above 2.5 mmol/L,** clonic movements of the limbs, seizures, circulatory collapse, and coma occur.
3. Treatment includes discontinuing lithium administration, hemodialysis, and the use of anticonvulsants.

V. OPIOID ANALGESICS AND ANTAGONISTS

A. Definitions

1. *Opioids* are drugs with morphine-like activity that produce analgesia (i.e., reduce pain) without the loss of consciousness and can induce tolerance and physical dependence.
2. *Opiates* are drugs derived from opium (e.g., morphine, heroin), a powdered, dried exudate of the fruit capsule (poppy) of the plant *Papaver somniferum.*
3. *Opiopeptins* (β-endorphin, *met*-enkephalin, and *leu*-enkephalin, dynorphins A and B, and neoendorphins α and β) are natural substances of the body that are derived from distinct polypeptide precursors and that have opioid-like activity. Opiopeptins are localized in discrete areas of the CNS and in a number of peripheral tissues including the GI tract, kidney, and biliary tract.

B. Mechanism of action

1. Opioids such as morphine are believed to mimic the effects of opiopeptins by interaction with one or more receptors (μ, δ, κ). Each opioid receptor has **distinct subtypes** (e.g., μ_1, μ_2).
   a. Interaction with μ-**receptors** contributes to supraspinal and spinal analgesia, respiratory depression, sedation, euphoria, decreased GI transit, and physical dependence.
   b. Interaction with δ-**receptors** also contributes to supraspinal and spinal analgesia.
   c. The significance of interaction with κ-**receptors** is unclear, but it may contribute to analgesia and also psychomimetic effects of some opioids.
   d. β-Endorphins, enkephalins, and dynorphins have their highest affinity for, respectively, μ-, δ-, and κ-receptors.
2. Opioids produce **analgesia** and some of their other effects by one or more of the following actions:
   a. All opioids activate inhibitory guanine nucleotide binding proteins (G_i; see Fig. 1.1C).
   b. Opioids **inhibit adenylyl cyclase activity,** resulting in a reduction in intracellular cAMP and decreased protein phosphorylation.
   c. Opioids **promote the opening of potassium channels** to increase potassium conductance, which hyperpolarizes and inhibits the activity of postjunctional cells.
   d. Opioids **close voltage-dependent calcium channels** on prejunctional nerve terminals to inhibit release of neurotransmitters (e.g., the release of glutamate and the release of substance P in the spinal cord).
   e. Opioids **raise the threshold** to pain by interrupting pain transmission through ascending pathways (substantia gelatinosa in the dorsal horn of the spinal cord, ventral caudal thalamus) and activating the descending inhibitory pathways (periaqueductal gray area in the midbrain, rostral ventral medulla) in the CNS.
   f. Opioids also raise the threshold to pain by action on peripheral sensory neurons.
   g. Opioids **decrease emotional reactivity to pain** through actions in the limbic areas of the CNS. They dissociate the perception of pain from the sensation. There is significant interpatient variability in this effect.

C. Psychological dependence and compulsive drug use (addiction)

1. The euphoria and other pleasurable activities produced by opioid analgesics, particularly when self-administered intravenously, can result in the development of psychological dependence with compulsive drug use also referred to as addiction. This development may be reinforced by the development of physical dependence (see below).
2. Although physical dependence is not uncommon when opioids are used for therapeutic purposes, addiction is not.

D. Tolerance and physical dependence

1. *Tolerance*
   a. Tolerance occurs gradually with repeated administration; a larger opioid dose is necessary to produce the same initial effect.

t a b l e **5.7**	Relative Development of Tolerance to Opioid Actions
Substantial	**Minimal**
Analgesia	Constipation
Respiratory depression	Seizures
Euphoria and dysphoria	Miosis
Sedation	Antagonist action
Nausea and vomiting	
Cough suppression	

    b. Tolerance is due to a direct neuronal effect of opioids in the CNS (i.e., cellular tolerance).

    c. Tolerance varies in degree (Table 5.7).

    d. Tolerance can be conferred from one opioid agonist to others (cross-tolerance).

  2. *Physical dependence* occurs with the development of tolerance to opioids.

    a. Abstinent withdrawal

      (1) Abstinent withdrawal is a syndrome revealed with discontinuation of opioid administration.

      (2) Abstinent withdrawal is characterized by drug-seeking behavior and physical signs of autonomic hyperexcitability that may include "goose bumps" ("going cold turkey"), muscle spasms ("kicking the habit"), hyperalgesia, lacrimation, rhinorrhea, yawning, sweating, restlessness, dilated pupils, anorexia, irritability, tremor, diarrhea, and flushing.

      (3) Abstinent withdrawal peaks at 48–72 hours.

      (4) This type of withdrawal is generally not life-threatening, except in dependent neonates and the severely debilitated.

      (5) Abstinent withdrawal can be reversed by readministration of opioid.

    b. Precipitated withdrawal

      (1) Precipitated withdrawal is induced by administration of an opioid antagonist such as naloxone.

      (2) Precipitated withdrawal peaks sooner and more explosively than abstinent withdrawal and is more severe.

  3. *Mechanism of morphine tolerance and physical dependence.* Although unclear, persistent morphine activation of μ-receptors has been shown to result in **decreased receptor recycling** and also **receptor uncoupling** with its intracellular targets.

E. Morphine: prototype

  1. *Pharmacological properties*

    a. Morphine is usually given parenterally, but it can be given orally or rectally.

    b. Dosage adjustment of morphine may be necessary in patients with hepatic insufficiency.

    c. Morphine undergoes extensive first-pass metabolism with glucuronide conjugation to morphine-6-glucuronide that possesses analgesic activity and morphine-3-glucuronide that has neuroexcitatory activity, both of which at very high concentrations (e.g., from renal insufficiency) may exert pharmacological actions.

  2. *Therapeutic uses of morphine and other opioids* (Table 5.8)

    a. Analgesia

      (1) Morphine is used for analgesia in severe preoperative and postoperative pain, as well as for the pain of terminal illness; it is used to treat the visceral pain of trauma, burns, cancer, acute myocardial infarction (MI), and renal or biliary colic. Higher doses are necessary for intermittent sharp pain.

      (2) In addition to analgesia, decreased anxiety, sedation that is marked by drowsiness, inability or decreased ability to concentrate, loss of recent memory, and occasional euphoria are useful additional properties of morphine in frightening painful disorders, such as MI and terminal illness.

t a b l e **5.8**	Indications for Morphine and Other Opioids
Indication	**Opioid Used**
Analgesia	Morphine, hydromorphone
Dyspnea	Morphine
Diarrhea	Diphenoxylate, loperamide
Cough	Codeine when not controlled by nonnarcotic cough suppressants
Preanesthesia	Fentanyl often used for its short duration of action (1–2 h)
Regional anesthesia	Morphine, fentanyl
Cardiovascular surgery	High-dose fentanyl as primary anesthetic because it produces minimal cardiac depression
Withdrawal or maintenance therapy	Methadone substitution for treatment of opioid dependence; clonidine, an α-adrenoceptor agonist, is also used for withdrawal because it suppresses autonomic components

b. Diarrhea

(1) Most opioids have strong antidiarrheal action, a pharmacological extension of their constipating effect (see below).

(2) Codeine is popular because of its reduced abuse liability. **Diphenoxylate** and **loperamide** are also used widely.

(3) No significant development of tolerance occurs in humans to the antidiarrheal action of morphine.

c. Acute pulmonary edema

(1) Morphine relieves the dyspnea associated with acute pulmonary edema secondary to left ventricular failure.

(2) This effect may be due to 1) decreased peripheral resistance with a decreased afterload and decreased venous tone with a decreased preload; 2) decreased anxiety of the patient; and/or 3) depression of the respiratory center and the CNS response to hypoxic drive.

d. Myocardial infarction. Vasodilation and the subsequent decreased cardiac preload are of additional therapeutic benefit when morphine is used for the pain of MI. **Pentazocine** and **butorphanol** increase preload and are contraindicated for the treatment of MI.

e. Cough

(1) Opioids directly depress the cough center in the medulla. **Codeine** is widely used for severe cough.

(2) The effect of opioids is unique in that the cough reflex is depressed by L-isomers and also by D-isomers of opioids such as the widely used antitussive, **dextromethorphan** (D-isomers are without analgesic action).

f. Anesthesia applications

(1) Preanesthetic medication or supplement to anesthetic agents during surgery

(a) Opioids are used for analgesic and sedative or anxiolytic effects.

(b) Fentanyl is often used for its short duration of action relative to morphine.

(2) Regional analgesia (epidural or intrathecal administration)

(a) Morphine and **fentanyl** are used to achieve long-lasting analgesia that is mediated through action on the spinal cord.

(b) There is a reduced incidence of adverse effects, but delayed respiratory depression, nausea, vomiting, and pruritus often occur.

(3) High-dose **fentanyl** or congeners (or **morphine**) are used as primary anesthetics in cardiovascular surgery because of their minimal cardiac depression.

g. Physical dependence. Opioids (**methadone, buprenorphine**) are used to mitigate the withdrawal symptoms of physical dependence caused by other opioids, including heroin.

3. *Adverse effects and contraindications of morphine and other opioids*

a. Respiratory depression

(1) Respiratory depression with opioid use is due to the direct inhibition of the respiratory center in the brainstem and to decreased sensitivity of the respiratory center to CO_2 with decreased hypoxic drive; it leads to decreased respiratory rate, minute volume, and tidal exchange.

(2) Opioids are contraindicated if there is a preexisting decrease in respiratory reserve (e.g., emphysema) or excessive respiratory secretions (e.g., obstructive lung disease).

(3) These drugs are contraindicated in patients with head injury. Cerebral vasodilation results from the increased pCO_2 caused by respiratory depression and may result in increased cerebral vascular pressure, which may lead to exaggerated respiratory depression and altered brain function.

(4) Opioids should be used cautiously during pregnancy because they may prolong labor and cause fetal dependence.

(5) Clinical or accidental opioid overdose with respiratory depression may be treated with artificial ventilation. Opioid antagonists can be used to reverse respiratory depression.

b. Constipation

(1) Constipation results from increased tone with decreased coordinated GI motility, increased anal sphincter tone, and inattention to the defecation reflex.

(2) This effect is mediated through actions on the enteric nervous system of the GI tract **to inhibit release of ACh,** and on the CNS.

(3) There is no clinically significant tolerance to this effect.

c. Postural hypotension

(1) Opioids inhibit the vasomotor center in the brainstem, causing peripheral vasodilation; they also inhibit compensatory baroreceptor reflexes and increase histamine release.

(2) Opioids should be used cautiously in patients in shock or with reduced blood volume. The elderly are particularly susceptible.

d. Nausea and vomiting. This common effect of opioids is caused by the direct stimulation of the chemoreceptor trigger zone (CTZ) in the area postrema of the medulla, which leads to activation of the vomiting center; there is also a direct vestibular component.

e. Pneumonia is a potential result of a reduced cough reflex when opioids are used for analgesia, particularly when respiration is compromised.

f. Sedative activity with drowsiness places ambulatory patients at risk for accidents. A paradoxical dysphoria occasionally develops.

g. Pain from biliary or urinary tract spasm

(1) This pain is due to the increased muscle tone of smooth muscle in the biliary tract, the sphincter of Oddi, and the ureters and bladder.

(2) These spasms may result in a paradoxical increase in pain when opioids are used to alleviate the pain associated with the passing of urinary or biliary stones if the dose is insufficient to induce centrally mediated analgesia.

h. Urine retention

(1) This effect, more common in the elderly, is due primarily to decreased renal plasma flow. Other contributing factors include increased tone with decreased coordinated contractility of the ureters and bladder, increased urethral sphincter tone, and inattention to the urinary reflex.

(2) Opioids should be used cautiously in patients with prostatic hypertrophy or urethral stricture.

i. Addiction or physical dependence. The risk for addiction or physical dependence is not a valid excuse to withhold opioids and thereby provide inadequate relief from pain, particularly in the terminally ill.

j. Miosis

(1) Opioid stimulation of the Edinger-Westphal nucleus of the oculomotor nerve results in "pinpoint" pupils even in the dark. This effect is mediated by ACh and blocked by atropine.

(2) No tolerance develops to this effect.

(3) During severe respiratory depression and asphyxia, miosis may revert to mydriasis.

4. *Drug interactions*

a. **Drugs that depress the CNS** add to or potentiate the respiratory depression caused by opioids (e.g., sedative–hypnotic agents).

b. **Antipsychotic and antidepressant agents** with sedative activity potentiate the sedation produced by opioids.

c. In the presence of opioids, particularly meperidine, **MAOIs** produce severe hyperthermia, seizures, and coma.

F. **Other strong opioid agonists**

1. *Hydromorphone, oxymorphone, levorphanol, and heroin*

a. These drugs have actions similar to those of morphine.

b. **Oxymorphone** has little antitussive activity.

c. Heroin (not approved for clinical use) is more lipid-soluble and faster acting than morphine, producing greater euphoria which accounts for its popularity as a drug of abuse.

2. *Fentanyl, sufentanil, alfentanil, and remifentanil*

a. Fentanyl and other synthetic subtypes are administered parenterally. They have a shorter duration of action than morphine.

b. Fentanyl is available as a transdermal patch and lozenge on a stick for breakthrough cancer pain.

c. Fentanyl is administered as a **preanesthetic and intraoperative medication** for its analgesic, anxiolytic, and sedative properties.

d. Fentanyl (or **morphine**) is used in high doses as a **primary anesthetic** for **cardiovascular surgery** because it produces minimal cardiac depression.

e. Fentanyl is used to supplement the analgesia and sedative–hypnotic effects of nitrous oxide and halothane in a "balanced anesthesia" approach. Morphine is also used for this indication.

f. These drugs may cause severe **truncal rigidity** when administered by rapidly at a high dose.

3. *Methadone (also levomethadyl acetate)*

a. Methadone has good analgesic activity. It is administered orally and has a longer duration of action than morphine. It is metabolized by CYP3A4 and CYP2B6 and may accumulate if there is hepatic dysfunction.

b. Methadone is associated with a less severe withdrawal syndrome than morphine; it is often substituted for other opioids as a treatment for physical dependence because it allows a smoother withdrawal with tapered dose reduction. It is also used for maintenance therapy of the heroin-dependent patient.

4. *Meperidine*

a. Although meperidine produces less neonatal respiratory depression than morphine and may have advantages in obstetrics, it is used infrequently.

b. At high doses, it may cause CNS excitation (tremors, delirium, hyperreflexia) and **seizures** due to formation of a metabolite, **normeperidine**. It causes severe restlessness, excitement, and fever ("serotonin syndrome") when administered with MAOIs. It may result in mydriasis and tachycardia due to weak anticholinergic activity.

G. **Weak agonists**

1. *Codeine, oxycodone, and hydrocodone* are partial opioid receptor agonists used for moderate pain.

a. They are orally effective and undergo less first-pass metabolism than morphine.

b. These drugs are usually used in combination with other analgesics such as acetaminophen, aspirin, or ibuprofen (e.g., **codeine**/acetaminophen = Tylenol with codeine; **hydrocodone**/acetaminophen = Vicodin, Lortab; **oxycodone**/aspirin = Percodan; and **oxycodone**/acetaminophen = Percocet).

c. These drugs are associated with less respiratory depression than morphine and have less dependence liability. However, many drug abusers have recently turned to controlled-release tablets that contain high levels of **oxycodone.** Also, overdose with codeine produces seizures.

H. **Mixed agonist–antagonists/partial agonists**
1. ***Buprenorphine, pentazocine, nalbuphine, and butorphanol***
    a. These drugs are used for **moderate pain** and produce modest respiratory depression.
    b. **Buprenorphine** is a partial agonist at opioid μ-receptors and antagonist at κ-receptors.
    c. **Buprenorphine,** because of its slow dissociation from μ-receptors, and long duration of action like methadone, is used for heroin detoxification.
    d. Due to its slow receptor dissociation, and unlike most opioids, its actions are less easily reversed with naloxone.
    e. **Pentazocine, nalbuphine, and butorphanol** are opioid κ-receptor agonists with partial agonist or antagonist activity at opioid μ-receptors.
2. These drugs have less dependence liability than morphine.
3. These drugs, except **nalbuphine,** can increase cardiac preload and should not be used to treat the pain of MI.
4. These drugs can precipitate withdrawal if administered to patients already receiving strong opioid agonists.
5. **Pentazocine** occasionally causes dysphoria, hallucinations, and depersonalization and is not commonly used in clinical practice.

I. **Tramadol and tapentadol**
1. In addition to weak opioid μ-receptor agonist activity, **tramadol** weakly blocks reuptake of serotonin and norepinephrine, whereas **tapentadol** is more specific for the NET—effects that appear to account for their analgesic action.
2. **Tramadol** may have special use for neuropathic pain. **Tapentadol** is used to treat moderate pain.
3. Their actions are only partially reversed by naloxone.
4. **Tramadol** in the presence of MAOIs may precipitate the serotonin syndrome.
5. **Tramadol and tapentadol are** associated with an increased risk of seizures and are contraindicated in patients with epilepsy.

J. **Opioid antagonists**
1. ***Naloxone and naltrexone (also nalmefene)*** are competitive inhibitors of the actions of opioids.
2. These drugs will **precipitate opioid withdrawal.**
3. Naloxone has a relative short duration of action of 1–2 hours. It is used to diagnose opioid dependence and to treat acute opioid overdose. Because of its short duration of action, multiple doses may need to be administered.
4. Naltrexone has a duration of action of up to 48 hours. It is approved for use to help decrease craving for alcohol.

K. **Antidiarrheal agents** (see also Chapter 8 VII B)
1. ***Diphenoxylate/atropine, difenoxin, and loperamide*** are taken orally for the symptomatic treatment of diarrhea.
2. Diphenoxylate is only available combined with atropine to minimize parenteral misuse.
3. Insolubility of diphenoxylate limits its absorption across the GI tract. Loperamide does not penetrate the brain.
4. These drugs have minimal dependence liability or other centrally mediated opioid-like effects at therapeutic doses.

L. **Antitussive agents**
1. ***Dextromethorphan,*** an opioid isomer, is an OTC cough medication that, like codeine, is used for its antitussive activity. However, it has little or no analgesic or addictive properties at therapeutic doses. Some constipation and sedation have been noted.

VI. ANTIPARKINSONIAN DRUGS AND DRUGS USED TO TREAT ALZHEIMER DISEASE

A. **Idiopathic parkinsonian disease**
1. Idiopathic parkinsonian disease is characterized by resting tremor, rigidity, bradykinesia, loss of postural reflexes, and, occasionally, behavioral manifestations.
2. Idiopathic parkinsonian disease is a result of the **progressive degeneration of DA-producing neurons** in the substantia nigra pars compacta that is thought to cause an imbalance in DA and ACh action on neurons of the corpus striatum. The net effect of the reduced output of DA (and relative increase in ACh activity) is a net loss of inhibitory regulation of the neuronal release of GABA in the corpus striatum, which leads to the characteristic movement disorders associated with parkinsonian disease.
3. A parkinsonian-like syndrome may also be induced by antipsychotic drugs, e.g., haloperidol.

B. **Therapeutic goal.** Because it is not yet possible to reverse the degenerative process, drugs are used to increase DA activity or to reduce excitatory interneuron ACh activity, in order to restore their balance in the corpus striatum.

C. **Levodopa (L-dopa), carbidopa, and levodopa/carbidopa**
1. *Mechanism of action* (see Fig. 1.1C). Levodopa is a levorotatory isomer of dopa that is prejunctionally decarboxylated in the CNS to DA in the corpus striatum, where it interacts with postjunctional DA D2- and D_3-receptors to activate inhibitory G proteins, inhibit adenylyl cyclase, decrease cAMP levels, and open potassium channels.
2. *Pharmacological properties*
   a. Absorption is delayed by food and influenced by the rate of gastric emptying and, through competition for absorption sites, by dietary amino acids.
   b. Levodopa is administered with **carbidopa** in a fixed combination (as Sinemet).
      (1) Carbidopa (α-methyldopa hydrazine) is an L-amino acid decarboxylase inhibitor that acts peripherally, does not cross the blood–brain barrier, and has little effect of its own.
      (2) In the presence of carbidopa, less levodopa is decarboxylated by dopa decarboxylase to DA in the periphery; therefore, the therapeutic dose of levodopa can be reduced by up to 80%, substantially minimizing nausea and vomiting and adverse cardiovascular effects.
3. *Therapeutic effects*
   a. Clinical improvement, including major improvement in functional capacity and quality of life, occurs in 70% of patients after several weeks of treatment.
   b. Tremor is more resistant to therapy, and there is little effect on behavioral abnormalities.
   c. The therapeutic effects of L-dopa begin to diminish in about 2–5 years. It is believed that neuronal degeneration progresses to the extent that the remaining functional neurons are unable to process and store (as DA) enough exogenously administered L-dopa to compensate for the decreased endogenous DA levels.
4. *Adverse effects and contraindications*
   a. **Dyskinesias**
      (1) Dyskinesias, characterized by a variety of repetitive involuntary abnormal movements affecting the face, trunk, and limbs, are the major limiting factor in therapy. They occur in 80% of patients.
      (2) Dyskinesias may be relieved by decreasing the dose of levodopa, but the parkinsonian symptoms may then increase.
      (3) **Akinesia paradoxia**, a sudden freezing of movement, may follow an episode of dyskinesia and is often precipitated by stress.
   b. **Akinesias**

(1) End-of-dose akinesia

(a) Each dose of L-dopa improves mobility for a period of time but is followed by the rapid return of muscle rigidity and akinesia before the end of the dosing interval.

(b) Increasing the dose and frequency of L-dopa administration may relieve these symptoms but may also induce dyskinesias.

(2) "On–off" akinesia

(a) "On–off" akinesia is a rapid fluctuation between showing no beneficial effects of L-dopa and showing beneficial effects with dyskinesias.

(b) Clinical improvement can be obtained with continuous IV infusion and, in some instances, with sustained release formulations of **levodopa/carbidopa**.

c. Behavioral effects

(1) Behavioral effects may include anxiety, insomnia, and early-onset psychosis due to exacerbation of a preexisting psychotic problem.

(2) There are also occasional late-onset (2 years) dream alterations, visual hallucinations, and drug-induced psychoses characterized by paranoia and confusional states.

d. Nausea and vomiting

(1) These actions are due to the direct effects of DA on the GI tract and on the CTZ in the CNS. Tolerance to the emetic effect may develop.

(2) Nausea and vomiting are attenuated if levodopa is taken with carbidopa, with food, in divided doses, or with nonphenothiazine antiemetics.

e. Cardiovascular effects

(1) The uncommon cardiovascular effects of levodopa include postural hypotension, occasional hypertension, and (rarely), tachycardia, arrhythmias, and atrial fibrillation due to increased circulating catecholamines.

(2) The incidence of the hypotensive effect of levodopa is reduced with carbidopa.

f. Mydriasis. Mydriasis and precipitation of an attack of acute glaucoma can develop.

5. *Drug interactions and contraindications*

a. The therapeutic action of levodopa is reduced by **antiemetic or antipsychotic drugs** that block DA receptors.

b. Natural aromatic amino acids (tryptophan, histidine, phenylalanine, tyrosine) decrease the absorption of levodopa.

c. Levodopa should not be used with MAO_A **inhibitors.** This combination can cause a severe hypertensive crisis.

d. In the absence of carbidopa, peripheral levels of levodopa are decreased by **pyridoxine** (vitamin B_6), which increases the activity of dopa decarboxylase and increases conversion of levodopa to DA in the periphery.

e. The use of levodopa is **contraindicated in patients with psychosis, narrow-angle glaucoma, and peptic ulcer disease.**

D. DA receptor agonists

1. *Pramipexole* *and* *ropinirole*

a. Characteristics

(1) Pramipexole is a relatively selective DA D_3-receptor agonist; **ropinirole** is a relatively selective DA D_2-receptor agonist.

(2) These drugs are alternative first-line drugs or are given in combination with levodopa for optimal treatment.

(3) Pramipexole is excreted unchanged; dosage adjustments may be necessary in patients with renal insufficiency. **Ropinirole,** which is also approved to treat **restless leg syndrome,** is metabolized by CYP1A2; dosage adjustments may be necessary in the presence of other drugs that are metabolized by the same enzymes.

b. Adverse effects

(1) These drugs have the same adverse effects, cautions, and contraindications as levodopa, although the severity of their effects may differ.

(2) These drugs may induce profound hypotension after an initial dose. Nausea, vomiting, and constipation may be problematic.

(3) Behavioral manifestations are more common and severe than with levodopa.

(4) Rarely, uncontrolled sleep occurs with **pramipexole** and **ropinirole**.

2. *Amantadine*

a. **Characteristics**

(1) Amantadine is an antiviral drug that **increases the release of** DA in the CNS by an unknown mechanism.

(2) Amantadine is useful in the early stages of parkinsonism or as an adjunct to levodopa therapy. The therapeutic effect of this drug may diminish in a few weeks.

b. **Adverse effects**

(1) Amantadine is associated with a reversible occasional headache, insomnia, confusion, hallucinations, and peripheral edema.

(2) Long-term use of amantadine may lead to reversible discoloration of the skin (livedo reticularis) or, more rarely, congestive heart failure.

(3) Overdose may cause a toxic psychosis and seizures.

3. *Selegiline and Rasagilene*

a. **Characteristics**

(1) Selegiline and rasagilene are **selective MAO-B** inhibitors that decrease DA metabolism in the CNS and prolong its action.

(2) These drugs are used as initial therapy or as adjuncts to levodopa therapy.

b. **Adverse effects.** These drugs are well tolerated. Selegiline causes an occasional mild amphetamine-like stimulating action (amphetamine is one of the metabolites).

c. These drugs should be avoided by patients taking SSRIs, TCAs, and meperidine, because of the possibility of precipitating a "**serotonin syndrome.**"

4. *Entacapone and tolcapone*

a. These drugs **inhibit catechol-*o*-methyltransferase,** thereby reducing the peripheral metabolism of levodopa. The decreased clearance of L-dopa increases its CNS bioavailability.

b. **Entacapone, acts only in the periphery.** It decreases the metabolism of levodopa to make more available to the brain; **Tolcapone** acts in the periphery and the brain. In the brain, it inhibits the degradation of DA.

c. **Entacapone** is used to augment the effect of **carbidopa/levodopa** in a combined product (Stalevo) of all three.

d. **Adverse effects** of these drugs include GI disturbances, postural hypotension, sleep disturbances, and an orange discoloration of the urine. **Entacapone** is preferred because tolcapone has been associated (rarely) with acute, fatal hepatic failure.

e. These drugs can exacerbate dysphoria, nausea, and other adverse effects of levodopa; downward dose adjustment of levodopa is necessary.

5. *Benztropine, biperiden, orphenadrine, procyclidine, and trihexyphenidyl*

a. **Characteristics**

(1) These drugs **block muscarinic receptors** and suppress overactivity of cholinergic interneurons in the striatum; they have a somewhat greater ratio of CNS to peripheral activity.

(2) These drugs are often used in the initial stages of mild parkinsonism, often in combination with levodopa. They have a significant effect on tremor and rigidity but little effect on bradykinesia and postural reflexes. These drugs are effective in 25% of patients, many of whom become refractory.

b. **Adverse effects, contraindications, and drug interactions**

(1) These drugs are associated with occasional restlessness, sedation, confusion, mood changes, dry mouth, mydriasis, constipation, tachycardia, and arrhythmias.

(2) These drugs are contraindicated in patients with prostatic hypertrophy, obstructive GI disease (e.g., paralytic ileus) and narrow-angle glaucoma.

(3) To avoid precipitating these conditions, these drugs should not be administered to patients taking other drugs with anticholinergic activity (e.g., TCAs, antihistamines).

E. **Alzheimer disease**
1. *Donepezil, rivastigmine, galantamine, and tacrine* are **acetylcholinesterase inhibitors** (see also Chapter 2 II B) used to treat Alzheimer disease, a disease characterized functionally by a loss of memory and biochemically and cellularly by accumulation of β-amyloid plaques, formation of neurofibrillary tangles, and loss of cortical neurons.
2. *Memantine,* a noncompetitive **inhibitor of *N*-methyl-d-aspartate (NMDA) receptors** that has few side effects, is also used to treat Alzheimer disease.
3. These drugs have only a short-term, modest effect and do nothing to halt the progression of neurodegeneration.
4. *Adverse effects* of the acetylcholinesterase inhibitors include GI dysfunction and muscle cramps. **Tacrine** is associated with liver toxicity.

VII. ANTIEPILEPTIC DRUGS

A. **Drug treatment of seizures**
1. **Epilepsy,** a chronic disease, occurs in approximately 1% of the population. Antiepileptic drugs (AEDs) are effective, at least to some degree, for about 80% of these patients. Lifelong treatment may be necessary.
2. It may take weeks to establish adequate drug plasma levels and to determine the adequacy of therapeutic improvement. **Lack of compliance** is responsible for many treatment failures.
3. AEDs are **most effective** and have the **least adverse effects** when they are used as **monotherapy.** Addition of a second drug to the therapeutic regimen should be gradual, as should discontinuance of the initial drug before the substitution of an alternative drug, because seizures may occur on withdrawal.
4. Some AEDs have **teratogenic potential.** This may call for the reduction or termination of therapy during pregnancy or before planned pregnancy. However, maternal seizures also present a significant risk to the fetus.
5. AEDs may also be used to treat seizures that result from various neurologic disorders, as well as from metabolic disturbances, trauma, and exposure to certain toxins.
6. AEDs may increase the risk of suicidal ideation.

B. **Classification of epilepsies and drug selection.** Epilepsies are characterized by either focal or generalized abnormal neuronal discharges. Drug selection, based on seizure classification, is listed below in the order of general choice.
1. *Partial seizures*
   a. **Simple:** Localized discharge; consciousness unaltered.
   b. **Complex:** Localized discharge that becomes widespread; accompanied by loss of consciousness
      (1) **Phenytoin, carbamazepine, and lamotrigine.**
      (2) Valproic acid and phenobarbital.
2. *Generalized seizures*
   a. **Tonic–clonic** (grand mal): Dramatic bilateral movements with either clonic jerking of the extremities or tonic rigidity of the entire body; accompanied by loss of consciousness.
      (1) **Phenytoin and carbamazepine.**
      (2) Topiramate, other newer AEDs.
   b. **Absence** (petit mal): Sudden onset of altered consciousness that lasts 10–45 seconds, with up to hundreds of seizures per day; begins in childhood or adolescence.
      (1) **Ethosuximide.**
      (2) Valproic acid (when absence seizures coexist with tonic–clonic seizures).
      (3) Clonazepam, lamotrigine and topiramate.

    c. **Myoclonic** syndromes: Lightning-like jerks of one or more extremities occurring singly or in bursts of up to a hundred; accompanied by alteration of consciousness.
      (1) Valproic acid and lamotrigine.
      (2) Other newer AEDs.

3. *Status epilepticus:* Prolonged seizure (>20 min) of any of the types previously described; the most common is life-threatening generalized tonic–clonic status epilepticus. Treatment is **IV diazepam** or **lorazepam** followed by **IV fosphenytoin** (or phenytoin) or **phenobarbital.**

C. Mechanism of action

1. *Phenytoin, carbamazepine, valproic acid, and lamotrigine* block sodium channels and inhibit the generation of action potentials. Their effect is "use dependent," that is, related to their selective binding and prolongation of the inactivated state of the sodium channel (see IX below). They also decrease neurotransmission by actions on prejunctional neurons.
    a. Valproic acid at higher concentrations reduces low-threshold T-type Ca^{2+} current.
    b. Lamotrigine probably has additional therapeutically relevant actions.

2. *Ethosuximide* reduces the low-threshold T-type Ca^{2+} current that provides the pacemaker activity in the thalamus.

3. *Barbiturates* (e.g., phenobarbital) and **benzodiazepines** (e.g., diazepam, lorazepam, clonazepam) facilitate GABA-mediated inhibition of neuronal activity.

D. Phenytoin and fosphenytoin

1. *Pharmacological properties*
    a. Phenytoin is absorbed well after oral administration, but its rate and extent of absorption can be altered considerably by its formulation.
    b. Phenytoin is 90% bound to plasma proteins. Hypoalbuminemia may result in a decrease in total but not free plasma phenytoin. Thus, increasing the dose may be counterproductive and result in toxicity.
    c. Phenytoin is metabolized by microsomal enzymes. Its plasma half-life is approximately 24 hours at therapeutic doses. In some patients, metabolic enzymes become saturated at low doses, and half-life increases dramatically as the dose and plasma concentration increase, resulting in a steady-state mean **plasma concentration that varies disproportionately with dose** (Fig. 5.3).
    d. Phenytoin may interfere with tests of thyroid function.

FIGURE 5.3. Nonlinear accumulation and variable serum levels of phenytoin dosage among different patients. (Modified with permission from Jusko WJ. Bioavailability and disposition kinetics of phenytoin in man. In: Kellaway P, Peterson I. Quantitative Analytic Studies in Epilepsy. New York: Raven Press, 1976:128.)

   e. A steep dose response and **low therapeutic index** require that **phenytoin** plasma levels be carefully monitored.

   f. **Fosphenytoin** is available for parenteral administration as a replacement for phenytoin. Fosphenytoin allows more rapid loading, intramuscular (IM) administration (phenytoin precipitates by the IM route), and IV administration, with minimal vascular erosion.

2. *Adverse effects and toxicity*

   a. Common: Nystagmus (occurs early), diplopia and ataxia (most common), slurred speech, blurred vision, mental confusion, hirsutism (an issue, particularly for females), gingival hyperplasia (can be minimized with good dental hygiene).

   b. Rare: With long-term use, coarsening of facial features, with mild peripheral neuropathy, and osteomalacia due to alteration of vitamin D metabolism; idiosyncratic reactions requiring drug discontinuance (e.g., exfoliative dermatitis; blood dyscrasias, including agranulocytosis).

   c. Fetal malformation ("fetal hydantoin syndrome") includes growth retardation, microencephaly, and craniofacial abnormalities (e.g., cleft palate) and is possibly due to an epoxide metabolite of phenytoin.

3. *Drug interactions*

   a. Phenytoin stimulates hepatic metabolism by microsomal enzyme induction and thereby reduces plasma concentrations of numerous drugs, including other AEDs such as **carbamazepine** and **valproic acid,** and some **antibiotics, oral anticoagulants, and oral contraceptives.**

   b. The plasma concentration of phenytoin is increased by drugs that inhibit its hepatic metabolism (e.g., **cimetidine, isoniazid**).

   c. The plasma concentration of phenytoin is decreased by drugs that stimulate hepatic metabolism (e.g., **carbamazepine, valproic acid**).

E. Carbamazepine and oxcarbazepine

1. *Pharmacological properties*

   a. Carbamazepine has good oral absorption but there is significant interpatient variability in its rate of absorption. An extended-release preparation is available.

   b. Carbamazepine induces microsomal enzymes (autoinduction) and **increases its own hepatic clearance**, thus reducing its half-life from >30 hours to <15 hours. Gradual dosage adjustment is required early in therapy.

   c. Carbamazepine is a drug of choice to treat **trigeminal neuralgia**; it is also used to treat bipolar affective disorder.

   d. Oxcarbazepine is a prodrug whose actions are similar to those of carbamazepine. Its activity is due to a 10-hydroxy metabolite with a half-life of 10 hours. It is a less potent inducer of hepatic microsomal enzymes than carbamazepine.

2. *Adverse effects and toxicity*

   a. Common: Diplopia and ataxia (most common), GI disturbances; sedation at high doses.

   b. Occasional: Retention of water and hyponatremia; rash, agitation in children.

   c. Rare: Idiosyncratic blood dyscrasias and severe rashes.

3. *Drug interactions*

   a. Carbamazepine induces microsomal enzymes and increases the hepatic clearance of numerous drugs including phenytoin, valproic acid, and ethosuximide.

   b. Phenytoin may decrease the steady-state of carbamazepine through microsomal enzyme induction.

   c. Plasma concentration of carbamazepine is increased by drugs that inhibit its metabolism (e.g., valproic acid).

F. Valproic acid

1. *Pharmacological properties*

   a. Valproic acid is also used to treat bipolar affective disorder and is used for **migraine prophylaxis**.

  b. Valproic acid inhibits the metabolism of other drugs including **phenytoin, carbamaze-pine, and ethosuximide.**

  c. Divalproex sodium (Depakote) is a 1:1 enteric formulation of valproic acid and valproate sodium that is absorbed more slowly than valproic acid.

 2. *Adverse effects and toxicity*

  a. Common: GI disturbances and hair loss.

  b. Uncommon: Weight gain, sedation, ataxia, and a fine tremor at high doses.

  c. Rare: Idiosyncratic hepatotoxicity may be fatal in infants and in patients using multiple anticonvulsants.

  d. Fetal malformations: Spina bifida; orofacial and cardiovascular anomalies have been reported.

G. Ethosuximide

 1. *Pharmacological properties*

  a. Although it is effective in fewer patients with absence seizures than valproic acid, ethosuximide is often the drug of choice because of its greater safety.

  b. Valproic acid inhibits its metabolism.

 2. *Adverse effects and toxicity*

  a. Common: GI disturbances, fatigue, and dizziness.

  b. Rare: Idiosyncratic rashes and blood dyscrasias.

H. Phenobarbital at less than hypnotic doses is used most often as a first-line drug for neonatal seizures and for maintenance control of status epilepticus. On occasion, it is used for short-term treatment of febrile seizures in children (see also I E).

I. **Benzodiazepines: diazepam, lorazepam, clonazepam, and clorazepate** (see also I B)

 1. Diazepam and lorazepam are highly effective in short-term treatment of status epilepticus.

 2. Clonazepam is effective for the treatment of absence seizures. Clorazepate is used to treat complex partial seizures. Sedation is their major adverse effect.

J. **Other anticonvulsant agents**

 1. *Lamotrigine* acts like phenytoin and carbamazepine. It is used as **monotherapy for partial seizures**. It is also used for absence seizures, myoclonic seizures, and the Lennox-Gastaut syndrome. Its half-life is reduced by phenytoin and carbamazepine and is increased by valproic acid. Adverse effects include headache, ataxia, dizziness, and (rarely) a rash that may be life-threatening, particularly in children.

 2. *Gabapentin and Pregabalin.* Gabapentin, among other activities, increases GABA levels in the brain. Gabapentin is used as adjunctive therapy for partial and generalized tonic–clonic seizures. Its adverse effects include dizziness, ataxia, and tremor. Pregabalin, an analog of gabapentin, is used as adjunctive therapy for partial seizures. It binds to voltage-gated calcium channels and reduces release of excitatory neurotransmitters. Its major adverse effects are dizziness, dry mouth, blurred vision, and weight gain. Both are also used to treat postherpetic neuralgia, diabetic peripheral neuropathy. Pregabalin is used to treat fibromyalgia.

 3. *Topiramate* acts like phenytoin and carbamazepine and may also act to facilitate the inhibitory action of GABA among other actions. It is used as monotherapy and as adjunctive therapy for partial and generalized tonic–clonic seizures. It is also used for Lennox-Gastaut syndrome. It is FDA approved for migraine headache prophylaxis. It suppresses weight loss and has been used to treat patients with eating disorders. Adverse effects include fatigue, nervousness, and memory dysfunction. Acute myopia and glaucoma may limit its use. Nephrolithiasis has been reported.

 4. *Tiagabine* is used as adjunctive therapy for partial seizures. It inhibits GABA uptake by interaction with its transporter. Dizziness is the most common adverse effect. Confusion and ataxia may limit its use.

 5. *Levetiracetam* acts by an unknown mechanism. It is used as adjunctive therapy to treat partial and generalized tonic–clonic seizures and for myoclonic seizures. Its adverse actions include dizziness. It may cause behavioral changes.

6. **Lacosamide** acts by an undetermined mechanism. It is used as adjunctive therapy to treat partial seizures. Adverse effects include diplopia, dizziness, GI disturbances, and headache.

7. **Ezogabine** increases potassium channel opening. It is used as adjunctive therapy to treat partial seizures. Its adverse effects include blurred vision, confusion, and bladder dysfunction.

8. **Rufinamide** acts like phenytoin and carbamazepine. It is used as adjunctive therapy to treat Lennox-Gastaut syndrome. Its adverse effects include vomiting, diarrhea, and sedation.

9. **Felbamate** use is very limited due to development of aplastic anemia (1:3,000) and severe hepatitis with liver failure (1:10,000).

10. **Zonisamide** acts at the sodium channel and possibly the voltage-dependent calcium channel. Adverse effects include drowsiness, confusion, and rashes.

VIII. GENERAL ANESTHETICS

A. **An overview of general anesthetics**
   1. **General anesthesia** is characterized by a loss of consciousness, analgesia, amnesia, skeletal muscle relaxation, and inhibition of autonomic and sensory reflexes.
   2. **Balanced anesthesia**
      a. Balanced anesthesia refers to a combination of drugs used to take advantage of individual drug properties while attempting to minimize their adverse actions.
      b. In addition to inhalation anesthetics and neuromuscular junction (NMJ)-blocking drugs, other drugs are administered preoperatively, intraoperatively, and postoperatively to ensure smooth induction, analgesia, sedation, and smooth recovery (e.g., benzodiazepines, opioids).
   3. **Stages and planes of anesthesia.** The stages and planes of anesthesia identify the progression of physical signs that indicate the depth of anesthesia. Newer, more potent agents progress through these stages rapidly, and therefore, the stages are often obscured. Mechanical ventilation and the use of adjunct drugs also obscure the signs indicating the depth of anesthesia.
      a. Stage I: Analgesia and amnesia.
      b. Stage II: Excitation.
      c. Stage III: Surgical anesthesia: loss of consciousness.
         (1) Four planes have been described relating to increased depth of anesthesia. Plane IV includes maximal pupil dilation, apnea, and circulatory depression.
         (2) The loss of the eyelash reflex and a pattern of respiration that is regular in rate and depth are the most reliable signs of stage III anesthesia.
      d. Stage IV: Medullary depression: respiratory and cardiovascular failure.

B. **Inhalation anesthetics**
   1. **Nitrous oxide, isoflurane, desflurane, sevoflurane, halothane, and enflurane**
      a. These agents are nonflammable and nonexplosive gases. They are "complete anesthetics" in that they all can produce loss of consciousness, immobility, amnesia, and analgesia to a greater or lesser degree.
      b. These anesthetics are all respiratory depressants; consequently, assisted or controlled ventilation is usually necessary during surgical anesthesia.
      c. Concentrations of halogenated inhalation anesthetics that produce good skeletal muscle relaxation generally produce unacceptable dose-related cardiovascular depression; consequently, NMJ-blocking drugs are commonly used for surgical muscle relaxation. Also, they are generally administered with nitrous oxide, which decreases the extent of cardiovascular and respiratory depression at equivalent anesthetic depths.

2. *Mechanism of anesthetic action.* Inhalation and IV anesthetic agent interaction with **discrete protein binding sites in nerve endings to activate ligand-gated ion channels** best explains their mechanism of action. These channels include the following (see also Fig. 1.1A):

   a. **$GABA_A$-receptor chloride channels,** where these anesthetic agents directly and indirectly facilitate a GABA-mediated increase in chloride (Cl^-) conductance to hyperpolarize and inhibit neuronal membrane activity.

   b. **Ligand-gated potassium (K^+) channels,** where these anesthetic agents increase potassium conductance to hyperpolarize and inhibit neuronal membrane activity.

   c. **NMDA receptors,** where certain anesthetics (e.g., nitrous oxide, ketamine) inhibit excitatory glutamate gated ion channels.

3. *Potency* (Table 5.9)

   a. **Minimum alveolar concentration (MAC)** is a relative term defined as the MAC at steady state (measured in volume/volume percent) that results in immobility in 50% of patients when exposed to a noxious stimulus, such as a surgical incision. Inhalant anesthetics have a steep dose–response relationship.

   b. The lower the MAC value, the more potent the agent; for example, **nitrous oxide** has a MAC of more than 100, indicating that immobility can generally only be achieved under hyperbaric conditions, whereas **isoflurane** has a MAC of 1.2, indicating immobility can be achieved at a relatively low concentration.

   c. MAC is an additive function for inhaled anesthetic agents.

   d. MAC will decrease with increasing age, pregnancy, hypothermia, and hypotension; MAC decreases in the presence of adjuvant drugs such as other general anesthetics, opioids, sedative–hypnotics, or other CNS depressants. It is independent of gender and weight.

4. *Solubility* (see Table 5.9)

   a. The rate at which the partial pressure of an inhalation anesthetic reaches equilibrium between various tissues, notably the CNS, and inspired air depends primarily on the solubility of the drug in blood.

   b. The relative solubility of an inhalation anesthetic in blood relative to air is defined by its blood–gas partition coefficient, lambda (λ), which is directly related to the pharmacokinetics of an anesthetic (see Table 5.9):

$$\lambda = [\text{anesthetic}] \text{ in blood}/[\text{anesthetic}] \text{ in gas}$$

   Relatively few molecules of an anesthetic with low solubility in blood are necessary to increase its partial pressure in blood. This results in its rapid equilibrium in the CNS and a rapid onset of action (e.g., **nitrous oxide, desflurane, and sevoflurane**).

   (1) Increasing the anesthetic concentration in inspired air will increase the rate of induction (Fick's law). For anesthetic agents of moderate solubility (e.g., **halothane**), a higher concentration can be used initially to more rapidly achieve adequate anesthesia.

   (2) Increased rate and depth of ventilation, such as that produced by mechanical hyperventilation or CO_2 stimulation, will increase the partial pressure more rapidly for anesthetics with intermediate or high blood solubility.

t a b l e 5.9	Properties of Inhalation Anesthetics		
Anesthetic	Blood–Gas Partition Coefficient (λ)	Oil–Gas Partition Coefficient	Minimum Alveolar Concentration (%) (MAC)
Nitrous Oxide	0.47	1.4	>100
Halothane	2.3	224	0.75
Enflurane	1.8	95	1.7
Isoflurane	1.5	98	1.4
Desflurane	0.42	??	2.0

(3) Changes in the rate of pulmonary blood flow to and from the lungs will change the rate of rise of arterial tension, particularly for anesthetic agents with intermediate-to-low solubility. Increased pulmonary flow from, for example, increased cardiac output, decreases the rate of rise in partial pressure by presenting a larger volume of blood into which the anesthetic can dissolve. Conversely, decreased pulmonary flow, such as occurs during shock, increases the rate of induction of anesthesia.

(4) The less soluble an anesthetic (low blood:gas partition coefficient), the more rapid its elimination and the more rapid the patient's recovery from anesthesia (e.g., **nitrous oxide, desflurane, sevoflurane**). For soluble anesthetics, the longer the exposure, the longer the time to recovery, because of accumulation of anesthetic in various tissues. Other factors that affect recovery include pulmonary ventilation and pulmonary blood flow.

5. *Pharmacology of commonly used inhalation anesthetics*
   a. **Cardiovascular actions**
      (1) All inhalation anesthetics **depress mean arterial pressure**, halothane and enflurane more than the others.
      (2) **Isoflurane, desflurane,** and **sevoflurane** preserve cardiac output better than **halothane** and **enflurane**. These agents also decrease preload and afterload to a greater degree.
      (3) Nitrous oxide depresses myocardial function that may be offset by its activation of the sympathetic nervous system.
      (4) **Halothane** reduces cardiac output. The result may be a fall in blood pressure. It also sensitizes the heart to endogenous and exogenous catecholamines that may result in arrhythmias.
   b. **Nitrous oxide (N$_2$O)**
      (1) **Advantages**
         (a) Nitrous oxide is an anesthetic gas that has **good analgesic and sedative properties** but no skeletal muscle relaxant properties. It has no odor, results in fast induction and emergence, and produces minimal cardiopulmonary depression.
         (b) Nitrous oxide is often **used in combination with other inhalation anesthetics** to increase their rate of uptake and to add to their analgesic activity while reducing their adverse effects. When given in large volumes, it increases the volume of uptake of a second blood-soluble gas such as **halothane (second-gas effect),** which then speeds the induction of anesthesia.
         (c) This anesthetic is often supplemented in balanced anesthesia with other sedative–hypnotics, analgesics, and skeletal muscle relaxants.
      (2) **Disadvantages**
         (a) Nitrous oxide **lacks sufficient potency to produce surgical anesthesia.**
         (b) Nitrous oxide is commonly associated with **postoperative nausea and vomiting.**
         (c) Nitrous oxide **inactivates methionine synthase** with long-term exposure (e.g., dental personnel, recreational use). This may cause inhibition of DNA and protein synthesis and result in anemia or leukopenia. Chronic exposure can also result in vitamin B$_{12}$ deficiency.
   c. **Isoflurane**
      (1) **Advantages**
         (a) Isoflurane produces more **rapid induction and emergence**.
         (b) Isoflurane undergoes minimal metabolism.
         (c) Isoflurane has **good analgesic** and **sedative–hypnotic** effects.
      (2) **Disadvantages:** Isoflurane has a pungent odor.
   d. **Desflurane**
      (1) **Advantages**
         (a) Desflurane produces more **rapid induction and rapid emergence** than isoflurane and, therefore, is often preferred for outpatient surgical procedures.
         (b) Enflurane undergoes minimal metabolism and, therefore, rarely produces organ toxicity.

(2) Disadvantages

    (a) Desflurane is especially **irritating to the airway** and may cause coughing, laryngospasm, and increased secretions with breath holding.

    (b) Special dispensing equipment for desflurane is necessary because of its low boiling point (23.5°C).

e. Sevoflurane

(1) Advantages

    (a) Sevoflurane produces a very **rapid and smooth induction and rapid recovery** with no respiratory irritation. It is widely used for pediatric anesthesia.

    (b) Sevoflurane causes **bronchodilation,** an effect that is useful for patients with respiratory difficulties.

(2) Disadvantage. Sevoflurane produces fluoride ions during its liver metabolism that potentially could be **nephrotoxic.**

f. Halothane

(1) Advantages

    (a) Halothane has a **pleasant odor** and produces a **smooth and relatively rapid induction.** It is usually administered with nitrous oxide.

    (b) This anesthetic has fair **analgesic** and **skeletal muscle and uterine relaxant** properties; it has excellent **hypnotic properties.**

(2) Disadvantages

    (a) Halothane **decreases cardiac output.** The result may be a fall in blood pressure.

    (b) Halothane may result in an **unpredictable hepatotoxicity,** possibly due to a reactive free radical toxic metabolite, trifluoroacetic acid (on average >40% is metabolized during most anesthetic procedures). However, incidence of this hepatotoxicity is extremely rare (1 in 10,000–30,000).

g. Enflurane

(1) Advantages

    (a) Enflurane produces a **rapid induction and recovery** with little excitation.

    (b) Enflurane produces good **analgesia, muscle relaxation,** and **hypnosis.** It is less likely than halothane to sensitize the heart to catecholamines or cause arrhythmias.

(2) Disadvantages

    (a) Enflurane is **pungent,** which may result in breath holding or coughing; thus, this anesthetic is less well accepted by children.

    (b) At high concentrations, enflurane produces **CNS stimulation** with mild twitching or tonic–clonic movements; hypocapnia exaggerates these effects. It should be avoided in patients with epilepsy or other seizure disorders.

    (c) Enflurane is contraindicated in patients with renal failure because some is **metabolized to fluoride ion** that is excreted by the kidney.

6. *Additional effects of inhalation anesthetics*

a. Inhalation anesthetics are bronchodilators, particularly **halothane** and **sevoflurane,** which allows use in patients with respiratory problems. However, the pungency of **isoflurane** and **desflurane,** which may cause severe irritation of the airway, precludes their use as agents of choice in patients with active bronchospasm.

b. Inhalation anesthetics, except **nitrous oxide,** relax uterine muscle, an advantage during certain obstetrical procedures.

c. Inhalation anesthetics increase cerebral blood flow, which may indirectly result in increased intracranial pressure. Patients with brain tumor or head injury are at risk.

d. Genetically susceptible patients may (rarely) develop potentially lethal **malignant hyperthermia,** which includes tachycardia, hypertension, acid–base and electrolyte abnormalities, muscle rigidity, and hyperthermia. These effects stem from increased free calcium levels in skeletal muscle cells. Treatment is supportive with **dantrolene,** a muscle relaxant that blocks calcium channels.

e. Inhalation anesthetics cause vasodilation and hypothermia by lowering the metabolic rate and lowering the set point for thermoregulatory vasoconstriction.

C. IV anesthetics and preanesthetic drugs

1. *Propofol*

   a. Propofol, which has replaced thiopental as the **agent of choice for rapid sedation and rapid-onset and short-duration anesthesia,** is administered IV. It is rapidly metabolized in the liver. It does not accumulate with continuous infusion.

   b. Propofol is widely used for outpatient surgical procedures, in intensive care settings, and in balanced anesthesia.

   c. Propofol produces no analgesia; it produces minimal postoperative nausea and vomiting.

   d. Propofol produces the following adverse effects: pain at injection site and systemic hypotension from decreased systemic vascular resistance. **Fospropofol** is a water-soluble **prodrug** of propofol that does not cause pain at the site of injection. However, paresthesia is an adverse effect of fospropofol in a majority of patients.

2. *Barbiturates: thiopental* and *methohexital* (*see* also I F 1 and X C 3)

   a. Thiopental, which is highly lipid soluble, is administered IV to induce anesthesia and results in a smooth, pleasant, and rapid induction (~20 s) and minimal postoperative nausea and vomiting, although there may be a "hangover."

   b. Thiopental has a short duration of action (5–10 min) due to redistribution from highly vascular tissue, particularly brain tissue, to less vascular tissue such as muscle and adipose tissue. It accumulates with continuous infusion with an increase in its duration of action.

   c. The action of thiopental in the CNS is similar to that of inhalation anesthetics; it can produce profound respiratory and cardiovascular depression. Thiopental has no analgesic or muscle relaxant properties.

   d. Thiopental is an absolute contraindication for patients with acute intermediate porphyria or variegate porphyria.

3. *Benzodiazepines* (see also I B)

   a. Midazolam may be administered orally or IV and is used preoperatively for sedation and to reduce anxiety. It is used intraoperatively with other drugs as part of balanced anesthesia. It is used as a sole agent for surgical and diagnostic procedures that do not require analgesia (endoscopy, cardiac catheterization, changing burn dressings). **Lorazepam** and **diazepam** may also be used.

   b. Midazolam, produces a clinically useful anterograde amnesia.

   c. Midazolam has a more rapid onset and shorter elimination time than **diazepam** and **lorazepam** and produces less cardiovascular depression.

   d. The actions of the benzodiazepines can be quickly reversed with **flumazenil.**

4. *Opioids: fentanyl, sufentanil, and remifentanil* (see also V)

   a. Opioids are administered preoperatively as adjuncts to inhalation and IV anesthetic to reduce pain.

   b. Remifentanil have a rapid onset of action; **remifentanil** has a short duration of action due to metabolism by nonspecific esterases in the blood and certain tissues.

   c. Fentanyl at high doses is used to achieve general anesthesia during cardiac surgery when circulatory stability is important (may be combined with muscle relaxants and **nitrous oxide** or very small doses of inhalation anesthetic).

   d. Opioids increase the risk of preoperative and postoperative nausea and vomiting.

5. *Etomidate*

   a. Etomidate is a nonbarbiturate anesthetic used as an alternative to propofol and thiopental for rapid-onset, short-duration anesthesia. Unlike thiopental, it causes minimal cardiorespiratory depression, which is useful for the treatment of at-risk patients.

   b. Etomidate has no analgesic effect.

   c. Etomidate produces the following adverse effects: pain at injection site, unpredictable and often severe myoclonus during induction of hypnosis, suppression of adrenocortical function (with continuous use), and postoperative nausea and vomiting.

6. *Ketamine*

   a. Ketamine produces a **dissociative anesthesia,** an effect in which patients feel dissociated from their surroundings; analgesia; and amnesia, with or without loss of consciousness.

    b. This drug is thought to **block the effects of glutamic acid at NMDA receptors.**

    c. Ketamine has a strong analgesic effect. It also has good bronchodilator activity and an amnestic action.

    d. Ketamine is a potent cardiovascular stimulant; it is useful for patients in cardiogenic or septic shock.

    e. At low doses, it is used in infants and children (trauma, minor surgical and diagnostic procedures, changing dressings).

    f. Ketamine's adverse effects include distortions of reality, terrifying dreams, and delirium, particularly in adults.

7. Other agents given in conjunction with general anesthetics

    a. Dexmedetomidine (a selective α_2-adrenoceptor agonist), neuromuscular blocking agents, and antiemetics.

IX. LOCAL ANESTHETICS

A. An overview of local anesthetics

    1. Local anesthetics produce a transient and reversible loss of sensation in a circumscribed region of the body **without loss of consciousness.** As a general rule, smaller nonmyelinated dorsal root type C nerve fibers that carry pain and temperature sensations (and also sympathetic type C unmyelinated postganglionic nerve fibers) are blocked before larger, heavily myelinated type A fibers that transmit sensory proprioception and motor functions.

    2. Most available local anesthetics are classified as either **esters** or **amides** and are usually linked to a lipophilic aromatic group and to a hydrophilic, ionizable tertiary amine. Most are weak bases with pK_a values between 7 and 9 (except benzocaine, $pK_a = 3.5$) and at physiologic pH they are primarily in the charged, cationic form.

    3. The potency of local anesthetics is positively correlated with their lipid solubility, which may vary 16-fold, and negatively correlated with their molecular size.

    4. These anesthetics are selected for use on the basis of the duration of drug action (short, 20 min; intermediate, 1–1.5 h; long, 2–4 h), effectiveness at the administration site, and potential for toxicity.

B. Mechanism of action. Local anesthetics act by blocking sodium channels and the conduction of action potentials along sensory nerves. Blockade is voltage- and time-dependent.

    1. At rest, the voltage-dependent sodium (Na^+) channels of sensory nerves are in the resting (closed) state. Following the action potential, the Na^+ channel becomes active (open) and then converts to an inactive (closed) state that is insensitive to depolarization. During excitation, the cationic charged form of local anesthetics interacts preferentially with the inactivated state of the Na^+ channels on the inner aspect of the sodium channel to **block sodium current** and **increase the threshold for excitation.**

    2. This results in a dose-dependent decrease in impulse conduction and in the rate of rise and amplitude of the action potential. This is more pronounced in rapidly firing axons, suggesting that local anesthetics gain access to the inner axonal membrane by traversing sodium channels while they are more often in an open configuration. Access to the inner axonal membrane may also occur by passage of the more lipophilic anesthetic molecules directly through the plasma membrane.

C. Pharmacological properties

    1. *Administration and absorption*

        a. Local anesthetics are administered topically, by infiltration into tissues to bathe local nerves, by injection directly around nerves and their branches, and by injection into epidural or subarachnoid spaces.

        b. The rate and extent of absorption to and from nerves are important in determining the rate of onset of action and termination of action and also the potential for systemic adverse effects. Their **absorption rate is correlated with the relative lipid**

solubility of the uncharged form and is influenced by the dose and the drug's physico-chemical properties, as well as by tissue blood flow and drug binding.

- **(1) Reduced pH,** as in inflamed tissues, increases the prevalence of the cationic form, which reduces diffusion into nerves and thereby reduces local anesthetic effectiveness.
- **(2) "Carbonation"** of local anesthetic solutions (saturation with carbon dioxide) can decrease intracellular pH, which increases the prevalence and activity of the cationic active form inside the nerve.

c. All local anesthetics, except **cocaine** and **prilocaine,** are vasodilators. Coadministration of a vasoconstrictor like **epinephrine** with a local anesthetic (generally of short or intermediate duration of action) reduces local blood flow, an effect of epinephrine that is mediated through α_1-adrenoceptors. This reduces systemic absorption of the local anesthetic from the site of application, prolongs its action, and reduces its potential for toxicity. **Epinephrine** should not be coadministered for nerve block in areas such as fingers and toes that are supplied with end-arteries because it may cause **ischemia or necrosis,** and it should be used cautiously in patients in labor and in patients with thyrotoxicosis or cardiovascular disease.

2. *Metabolism*
   a. **Ester-type** local anesthetics that enter the blood stream are metabolized by **plasma butyrylcholinesterase** and thus have very short plasma half-lives. The plasma level of these anesthetics may be higher than usual in patients with decreased or genetically atypical cholinesterase.
   b. **Amide-type** local anesthetics are metabolized at varying rates and to varying extents by **hepatic microsomal enzymes**. They are excreted in metabolized and uncharged form by the kidney. The rate of metabolism of these anesthetics is decreased in patients with liver disease or decreased hepatic blood flow, or by drugs that interfere with cytochrome P-450 enzymes.

D. **Specific local anesthetics and their therapeutic uses**
   1. *Amides*
      a. Lidocaine
         (1) Lidocaine is the prototype amide; it has a rapid onset and intermediate duration of action (1–2 h).
         (2) Lidocaine is used for infiltration block, peripheral nerve block, and for epidural and spinal anesthesia.
      b. **Mepivacaine**
         (1) Mepivacaine has a rapid onset and duration of action like lidocaine.
         (2) It is used for peripheral nerve block and spinal anesthesia.
         (3) Mepivacaine has actions similar to those of lidocaine, but it causes less drowsiness and sedation.
      c. **Prilocaine**
         (1) Prilocaine has an intermediate onset and intermediate duration of action like lidocaine. It has vasoconstrictor activity.
         (2) This anesthetic is used for spinal anesthesia; it is widely used but not topically or for obstetrical analgesia.
         (3) Prilocaine has actions similar to those of lidocaine.
         (4) It can cause methemoglobinemia (toluidine metabolites).
      d. **Bupivacaine**
         (1) Bupivacaine has a slow onset and long duration of action.
         (2) It is used for infiltration, regional, epidural, and spinal anesthesia.
         (3) Bupivacaine has actions similar to lidocaine, but greater cardiotoxicity than other amide local anesthetics.
   2. *Esters*
      a. **Procaine**
         (1) Procaine has a medium onset and short duration of action.
         (2) Procaine is used for infiltration anesthesia.
         (3) A metabolite PABA can limit the effectiveness of sulfonamides.

   b. 2-Chloroprocaine
- **(1)** Chloroprocaine has a more rapid onset of action than procaine and a short duration of action. It is very rapidly metabolized by plasma cholinesterase.
- **(2)** It is used for obstetrical anesthesia.
- **(3)** Chloroprocaine has less reported toxicity than procaine.

   c. Cocaine (also see X D)
- **(1)** Cocaine has a medium onset and medium duration of action.
- **(2)** It is used rarely for topical anesthesia of mucous membranes.
- **(3)** It induces intense vasoconstriction.
- **(4)** Euphoria, CNS stimulation, tachycardia, restlessness, tremors, seizures, and arrhythmias limit its clinical use.

   d. Tetracaine
- **(1)** Tetracaine has very slow onset of action (>10 min) and is long acting.
- **(2)** Tetracaine is used primarily for spinal anesthesia and for ophthalmologic use.
- **(3)** Its actions are similar to lidocaine.

E. Adverse effects and toxicity. Adverse effects of local anesthetics are generally an extension of their therapeutic action to block the membrane sodium channel. They are usually the result of overdose or inadvertent injection into the vascular system. Systemic effects are most likely to occur with administration of the amide class.

  1. *CNS*
- **a.** Adverse CNS effects include light-headedness, dizziness, restlessness, tinnitus, tremor, and visual disturbances. Lidocaine and procaine may cause sedation and sleep.
- **b.** At high blood concentrations, local anesthetics produce nystagmus, shivering, tonic–clonic seizures, respiratory depression, coma, and death.
- **c.** Adverse CNS effects are treated by maintenance of airway and assisted ventilation, IV diazepam for seizures (or prophylactically), and succinylcholine to suppress muscular reactions.

  2. *Cardiovascular system*
- **a.** Adverse cardiovascular system effects develop at relatively higher plasma levels than do adverse CNS effects.
- **b.** Bradycardia develops as a result of the block of cardiac sodium channels and the depression of pacemaker activity.
- **c.** Hypotension develops from arteriolar dilation and decreased cardiac contractility.
- **d.** These adverse effects are treated with IV fluids and vasopressor agents.

X. DRUGS OF ABUSE

A. An overview
1. Drugs of abuse generally act on the CNS to modify the user's mental state, although some are used for enhancing physical performance.
2. Long-term use may lead to the development of tolerance and to the development of psychological or physical dependence, or both.
3. Complications related to parenteral drug administration under unsterile conditions or to the coadministration of adulterants are extremely common (e.g., thrombophlebitis, local and systemic abscesses, viral hepatitis, HIV infection).

B. Definitions
1. Drug abuse is the nonmedical, self-administered use of a drug that is harmful to the user. Common abused drugs include opioid analgesics (e.g., heroin), general CNS depressants (e.g., ethanol), inhalants (e.g., toluene, nitrous oxide, amyl nitrate), sedative–hypnotics (e.g., alprazolam, diazepam), CNS stimulants (e.g., cocaine, amphetamines, nicotine), hallucinogens (e.g., LSD, mescaline, phencyclidine, and marijuana).

2. Drug addiction refers to the drug abuser's overwhelming preoccupation with the procurement and use of a drug.

3. Tolerance is the decreased intensity of a response to a drug following its continued administration. A larger dose can often produce the same initial effect.

    a. Metabolic tolerance (pharmacokinetic tolerance): The rate of drug elimination increases with long-term use because of stimulation of its own metabolism (autometabolism).

    b. Cellular tolerance (pharmacodynamic tolerance): Biochemical adaptation or homeostatic adjustment of cells to the continued presence of a drug. The development of cellular tolerance may be due to a compensatory change in the activity of specific neurotransmitters in the CNS caused by a change in their levels, storage, or release or to changes in the number or activity of their receptors, or to changes.

    c. Cross-tolerance. Tolerance to one drug confers at least partial tolerance to other drugs in the same drug class.

    d. Tolerance is often, but not always, associated with the development of physical dependence.

    e. The degree of tolerance varies considerably among different classes of drugs of abuse (e.g., **cocaine>>marijuana**).

4. Dependence refers to the biologic need to continue to take a drug.

    a. Psychological dependence: Overwhelming compulsive need to take a drug (drug-seeking behavior) to maintain a sense of well-being. Psychological dependence may be related to increased DA activity in the "brain reward system" (includes the mesolimbic dopaminergic pathway from the ventral midbrain to the nucleus accumbens and other limbic structures including the prefrontal cortex and limbic and motor systems). Development of psychological dependence generally precedes development of physical dependence but does not necessarily lead to it.

    b. Physical dependence: A latent hyperexcitability that is revealed when administration of a drug of abuse is discontinued after its long-term use ("abstinent withdrawal"). Continued drug use is necessary to avoid the abstinent withdrawal syndrome.

        (1) The **abstinent withdrawal syndrome** is characterized by effects that are often opposite to the short-term effects of the abused drug and that often include activation of the sympathetic nervous system. The severity of the withdrawal syndrome is directly related to the dose of the drug, how long it is used, and its rate of elimination.

        (2) **"Precipitated withdrawal"** that follows administration of an antagonist (e.g., **naloxone**) has a more explosive onset and shorter duration than abstinent withdrawal.

        (3) The development of physical dependence, the mechanism of which is not understood, may involve counter-adaptation of the same systems involved in the development of tolerance, including increased transcription of key enzymes.

        (4) The degree of physical dependence varies considerably among different drugs of abuse (**heroin>>marijuana**).

    c. Cross-dependence: Ability of one drug to substitute for another drug in the same drug class to maintain a dependent state or to prevent withdrawal (e.g., **diazepam** for ethanol; **methadone** for heroin).

C. General CNS depressants

    1. *Ethanol*

        a. Mechanism of action. The precise mechanism of action for ethanol on the CNS is unknown. Among many other actions, ethanol has a direct effect on $GABA_A$-receptors to acutely enhance the inhibitory action of GABA in the CNS. It also has an inhibitory effect on glutamate activation of NMDA-glutamate receptors in the CNS.

        b. Acute effects

            (1) General CNS depression

                (a) At **low-to-moderate levels** in nontolerant individuals (50–100 mg/dL), inhibition of inhibitory CNS pathways (disinhibition) occurs, resulting in decreased anxiety and disinhibited behavior with slurred speech, ataxia, and impaired judgment (drunkenness).

(b) At **moderate-to-toxic levels** (100–300 mg/dL), a dose-dependent general inhibition of the CNS occurs with increasing sedation and respiratory depression and decreasing mental acuity and motor function.

(c) At **toxic levels** (>300 mg/dL), CNS depression can result in coma, profound respiratory depression, and death. **Acute toxicity with respiratory depression** is a serious medical emergency. Respiratory support and avoidance of aspiration of vomitus may be sufficient, but the patient may also require restoration of fluid and electrolyte balance, thiamine to prevent Wernicke-Korsakoff syndrome, and treatment of hypoglycemia.

(2) Depressed myocardial contractility possibly caused by the ethanol metabolite acetaldehyde.

(3) Cutaneous vasodilation

(a) Cutaneous vasodilation is due to probable inhibitory effects on the vasomotor and thermoregulatory centers.

(b) Hypothermia may be significant in cases of severe overdose or in cold environments.

(4) Diuresis develops due to an increase in plasma fluid volume and inhibition of antidiuretic hormone release from the posterior pituitary.

(5) GI effects include increased salivation, decreased GI motility, GI irritation, and occasional nausea and vomiting.

c. Long-term effects

(1) Liver disease

(a) Liver disease, manifested by a progression from reversible fatty liver to alcohol hepatitis, and to irreversible cirrhosis and liver failure, is the most common adverse effect of long-term ethanol consumption.

(b) Other contributing factors to liver disease may include reduced glutathione as a free radical scavenger, damage to mitochondria, and a background of malnutrition.

(2) Peripheral neuropathy with paresthesias of the hands and feet.

(3) Wernicke's encephalopathy with ataxia, confusion, abnormal *eye* movements, and **Korsakoff's psychosis** with impairment of memory that is often irreversible (**Wernicke-Korsakoff syndrome**). This effect is associated with **thiamine deficiency** secondary to malnutrition.

(4) Pancreatitis and gastritis. Chronic alcohol use is a common cause of pancreatitis caused, in part, by direct erosion by ethanol of pancreatic acinar cells. Similarly, the direct action of ethanol may erode the GI epithelium and decrease GI mucosal defense barriers, resulting in GI bleeding, gastritis, esophagitis, and pancreatitis.

(5) Heart disease

(a) Cardiomyopathy may develop due to ethanol-induced membrane disruption with decreased mitochondrial activity, among other effects.

(b) Arrhythmias (and seizures) may develop during "binge" drinking or during the ethanol withdrawal syndrome.

(c) Hypertension, which may be reversible.

(d) Moderate, long-term consumption of ethanol may decrease the risk of coronary heart disease possibly due to an ethanol-induced increase in high-density lipoproteins or to its antioxidant or anti-inflammatory effects.

(6) Fetal alcohol spectrum disorder

(a) Fetal alcohol spectrum disorder results from maternal abuse of ethanol.

(b) Fetal alcohol syndrome is characterized by retarded growth, microencephaly, poorly developed coordination, mental retardation, and congenital heart abnormalities.

(c) Severe behavioral abnormalities can occur in the absence of dysmorphology. There is also an increased rate of spontaneous abortions.

(7) Other long-term effects include mild anemia, hypoglycemia, gynecomastia, testicular atrophy, and cancer of the GI tract.

d. Pharmacological properties
(1) Ethanol is rapidly absorbed from the stomach and small intestine and is rapidly distributed in total body water. Absorption is delayed by food.
(2) Ethanol is oxidized at low plasma concentrations to acetaldehyde by the liver cytosolic enzyme **alcohol dehydrogenase** (ADH), with the generation of reduced nicotinamide adenine dinucleotide (NADH). ADH is also found in the stomach and brain. At higher blood concentrations (>100 mg/dL), ethanol is also oxidized to acetaldehyde by liver microsomal enzymes. Acetaldehyde is further oxidized by mitochondrial **aldehyde dehydrogenase** to acetate, which is further metabolized to CO_2 and H_2O.
(a) Plasma ethanol levels achieved with even one or two alcoholic beverages results in hepatic metabolism that shows **zero-order kinetics** (due to a functional saturation of ADH) so that the rate of ethanol elimination is independent of plasma concentration, with the attendant increased risk of accumulation (in the adult, approximately 6–8 g or 7.5–10 mL of alcohol is metabolized per hour).
(b) **Women** demonstrate less activity of a stomach ADH than men, with resulting higher blood alcohol levels after oral administration of a similar dose. The generally higher fat and blood ratio in women also contributes to the increased effect of ethanol.
(c) Certain **Asian populations** have a genetic alteration in aldehyde dehydrogenase that increases their sensitivity to ethanol because of the relatively greater accumulation of acetaldehyde.
e. Therapeutic uses. Ethanol is used as an antiseptic, as a solvent for other drugs, and as a treatment to prevent methanol-induced toxicity.
f. Drug interactions/contraindications
(1) Ethanol has an additive or potentiative CNS depression and possible respiratory arrest activity with other drugs that also have CNS depressant effects **(benzodiazepines, antihistamines, antipsychotics, antidepressants)**.
(2) Acute ethanol use decreases the metabolism and augments the effects of many drugs because of its inhibitory effects on liver microsomal enzymes.
(3) Long-term ethanol use increases the metabolism and thereby decreases the effect of numerous drugs by induction of liver cytochrome P-450 enzymes (e.g., **phenytoin, warfarin, barbiturates**).
(4) Ethanol use is contraindicated during pregnancy, and in patients with ulcers, liver disease, and seizure disorders.
g. Tolerance and dependence
(1) **Tolerance** to the intoxicating and euphoric effects of ethanol develops with long-term use. Tolerance to ethanol is related to neuronal adaptation and also to some increased autometabolism. A lesser degree of tolerance develops to the potentially lethal action of ethanol. There is cross-tolerance to other CNS depressants, including the benzodiazepines and barbiturates, but not the opioids.
(2) Psychological dependence (see above)
(3) Physical dependence and withdrawal syndrome
(a) **Symptoms** occurring over 1–2 days include anxiety, apprehension, irritability, insomnia, and tremor. More severe cases progress to signs of anorexia, nausea, vomiting, autonomic hyperactivity, hypertension, diaphoresis, and hyperthermia. The most severe cases progress to delirium (agitation, disorientation, modified consciousness, visual and auditory hallucinations, and severe autonomic hyperexcitability also referred to as "**delirium tremens**") and seizures.
(b) The **acute withdrawal syndrome** usually subsides within 3–7 days. This withdrawal syndrome can be life-threatening in debilitated individuals.
(4) **Management of ethanol abuse**
(a) In addition to maintenance and nutritional (e.g., thiamine replacement) and electrolyte therapy and long-term psychological support, treatment may include prevention or reversal of seizures with a benzodiazepine or **phenytoin**, and administration of a long-acting benzodiazepine (e.g., **diazepam**) as a substitute for ethanol, followed by tapered dose reduction over several weeks.

       (b) Disulfiram is used rarely as an adjunct in the supervised treatment of alcoholism, although compliance is low.

          (i) Disulfiram **inhibits aldehyde dehydrogenase,** resulting in the accumulation of toxic levels of acetaldehyde, with nausea, vomiting, flushing, headache, sweating, hypotension, and confusion lasting up to 3 hours.

          (ii) Disulfiram can be toxic in the presence of small amounts of alcohol (e.g., the amount in some OTC preparations). Other drugs with disulfiram-like activity include **metronidazole, sulfonylureas,** and some **cephalosporins**).

          (iii) Disulfiram is absorbed rapidly; its peak effect takes 12 hours. The elimination of disulfiram is slow, so its action may persist for several days.

       (c) Naltrexone, an orally effective opioid-receptor antagonist, **reduces craving for ethanol** and reduces the rate of relapse of alcoholism.

       (d) Acamprosate reduces the incidence of relapse and prolongs abstinence from ethanol. It acts as a competitive inhibitor at the NMDA glutamate receptor.

  2. *Methanol (wood alcohol)*

    a. Methanol is metabolized by ADH to formaldehyde, which is then oxidized to formic acid, which is toxic.

    b. Methanol produces blurred vision and other visual disturbances ("snowstorm") when poisoning has occurred. In severe poisoning, bradycardia, acidosis, coma, and seizures are common.

    c. Treatment of methanol toxicity includes the administration of ethanol to slow the conversion of methanol to formaldehyde (ethanol has a higher affinity for ADH). In addition to other supportive measures, dialysis is used to remove methanol, and bicarbonate is administered to correct acidosis.

    d. Fomepizole, an inhibitor of ADH that reduces the rate of accumulation of formaldehyde, is also used to treat methanol (and ethylene glycol) toxicity.

  3. *Barbiturates (secobarbital, pentobarbital, γ-hydroxybutyric acid [GHB]) and benzodiazepines* (see also I F 1 and VIII C 1)

    a. Adverse effects, drug interactions, and contraindications.

      (1) Barbiturates produce drowsiness at hypnotic doses; they can interfere with motor and mental performance.

      (2) Barbiturates potentiate the depressant effects of other CNS depressants or drugs with CNS depressant activity such as antidepressants.

      (3) Barbiturates produce dose-related respiratory depression with cerebral hypoxia, possibly leading to coma or death. Treatment includes ventilation, gastric lavage, hemodialysis, osmotic diuretics, and (for phenobarbital) alkalinization of urine.

      (4) GHB has been used as a "date rape" drug.

    b. Tolerance and dependence

      (1) Tolerance

        (a) Neuronal adaptation (cellular tolerance) and increased metabolism due to induction of hepatic microsomal enzymes (metabolic tolerance) both contribute to the development of tolerance.

        (b) Abuse and psychological dependence are more likely with the shorter-acting, more rapidly eliminated drugs (e.g., **pentobarbital**).

        (c) Cross-tolerance occurs with other CNS depressants, including the benzodiazepines and **ethanol.**

      (2) Physical dependence

        (a) Withdrawal symptoms include restlessness, anxiety, and insomnia. More severe symptoms of withdrawal include tremor, autonomic hyperactivity, delirium, and potentially life-threatening tonic–clonic seizures.

        (b) For a smoother withdrawal, a longer acting sedative–hypnotic agent (e.g., **chlordiazepoxide** or **phenobarbital**) is substituted for shorter-acting barbiturates.

D. CNS stimulants

  1. *Cocaine and amphetamine/methamphetamine (Desoxyn)* (and dextroamphetamine [Dexedrine]; also methylene-dioxymethamphetamine [MDMA, "Ecstasy"])

a. **Mechanism of action**
   (1) **Cocaine blocks the** DA **transporter** (DAT; also norepinephrine and serotonin transporters, NET and SERT, at higher doses) in the CNS to inhibit the uptake of DA into nerve terminals in the mesolimbic pathway that includes the "brain reward" center. Blockade of NET also leads to increased sympathomimetic activity.
   (2) **Amphetamine increases the release of prejunctional neuronal catecholamines,** including DA and norepinephrine. Amphetamine also exhibits some direct sympathomimetic action and weakly inhibits MAO.
   (3) **MDMA** is more specific for SERT. Serotonin stores are rapidly depleted, perhaps permanently.

b. **Pharmacological properties**
   (1) **Cocaine** is inhaled (snorted) or smoked (free-base form, "**crack cocaine**"); **amphetamine,** usually in the form of **methamphetamine,** is taken orally, IV, or smoked in a form referred to as "**ice.**"
   (2) Short-term, repeated IV administration or smoking (referred to as a **"spree" or "run"**) results in intense euphoria (**"rush"**) as well as increased wakefulness, alertness, self-confidence, and ability to concentrate. Use also increases motor activity and sexual urge and decreases appetite.
   (3) MDMA is usually taken orally.
   (4) Cocaine has a much shorter duration of action (~1 h) than amphetamine.
   (5) **Cocaine** is metabolized by plasma and liver cholinesterase; genetically slow metabolizers are more likely to show severe adverse effects. A nonenzymatic metabolite, **benzoylecgonine,** is measurable for 5 days or more after a spree and is used to detect cocaine use.

c. **Therapeutic uses**
   (1) **Cocaine** is used as a **local anesthetic** for ear, nose, and throat surgery. It is the only one with inherent vasoconstrictor activity (see also IX D 2 c).
   (2) **Methylphenidate** (Ritalin), an amphetamine congener
      (a) **Attention-deficit/hyperactivity disorder**; also **amphetamine.**
      (b) **Narcolepsy.**

d. **Cocaine and amphetamine short-term and adverse effects**
   (1) Short-term, repeated IV administration or smoking results in intense **euphoria** as well as increased wakefulness, alertness, self-confidence, and ability to concentrate. The use also increases motor activity and sexual urge and decreases appetite. Adverse effects may occur during this same time or from overdose and are due to excessive sympathomimetic activity. These adverse effects include the following:
   (2) **Anxiety, inability to sleep, hyperactivity, sexual dysfunction,** and stereotypic and sometimes **dangerous behavior,** often followed by exhaustion ("crash") with increased appetite and increased sleep with disturbed sleep patterns (the withdrawal pattern)
   (3) **Toxic psychosis**
      (a) Toxic psychosis is marked by paranoia and tactile and auditory hallucinations.
      (b) This condition is usually reversible, but it may be permanent.
   (4) **Necrotizing arteritis**
      (a) Necrotizing arteritis is produced by **amphetamine.**
      (b) This effect sometimes results in brain hemorrhage and renal failure.
   (5) **Perforation of the nasal septum** from the vasoconstrictor effects of "snorting" **cocaine.**
   (6) **Cardiac toxicity** caused by **cocaethylene** that forms when cocaine and ethanol are taken together.
   (7) **Fetal abnormalities** and early childhood learning disabilities from the maternal use of **cocaine.**
   (8) **Overdose**
      (a) Overdose results in tachycardia, hypertension, hyperthermia, and tremor.
      (b) Overdose, particularly with **cocaine,** may cause hypertensive crisis with **cerebrovascular hemorrhage and MI.**
      (c) Overdose occasionally produces seizures, coronary vasospasm, cardiac arrhythmias, shock, and death.

   e. Cocaine and amphetamine tolerance and dependence
   (1) Extremely strong psychological dependence to these drugs develops.
   (2) Tolerance can develop.
   (3) The withdrawal-like syndrome includes long periods of sleep, increased appetite, anergia, depression, and drug craving.
   f. MDMA (Ecstasy) short-term and adverse effects
   (1) MDMA increases feelings of "intimacy" and "understanding".
   (2) MDMA causes hyperthermia, seizures, and the "serotonin syndrome".
   (3) Withdrawal is associated with long-term depression and also aggression.
2. *Nicotine* is a constituent of tobacco, along with various gases and particulate matter.
   a. Mechanism of action: Nicotine mimics the action of ACh at cholinergic nicotinic receptors of ganglia, in skeletal muscle, and in the CNS.
   b. Pharmacological properties
   (1) Nicotine is well absorbed from the lung after smoking and is rapidly distributed.
   (2) Nicotine is rapidly metabolized in the liver: it has a plasma half-life $(t_{1/2})$ of approximately 1 hour.
   (3) Nicotine may cause nausea and vomiting in the early stages of smoking. It increases psychomotor activity and cognitive function, increases release of adrenal catecholamines and antidiuretic hormone (ADH), increases blood pressure and heart rate, and increases tone and secretions of the GI tract.
   c. Adverse effects. Nicotine use contributes to cancer of the lungs, oral cavity, bladder, and pancreas; obstructive lung disease; coronary artery disease; and peripheral vascular disease.
   d. Tolerance and dependence
   (1) Tolerance
      (a) Tolerance to the subjective effects of nicotine develops rapidly.
      (b) Tolerance is primarily cellular; there is some metabolic tolerance.
   (2) Dependence
      (a) Nicotine produces strong psychological dependence; it increases the activity of DA in the nucleus accumbens.
      (b) The withdrawal-like syndrome indicative of physical dependence occurs within 24 hours and persists for weeks or months. Dizziness, tremor, increased blood pressure, drug craving, irritability, anxiety, restlessness, difficulty in concentration, drowsiness, headache, sleep disturbances, increased appetite, GI complaints, nausea, and vomiting may occur.
   e. Medications and replacement therapies
   (1) **Nicotine polacrilex** is a **nicotine resin** contained in a chewing gum that, when used as a nicotine replacement, has therapeutic value for diminishing withdrawal symptoms while the patient undergoes behavioral modification to overcome psychologic dependence. It has an objectionable taste and may cause stomach discomfort, mouth sores, and dyspepsia.
   (2) A nicotine **transdermal patch** containing nicotine is also available. Local skin irritation is a common problem. A nicotine nasal spray is also available (which may cause nasal irritation) as is a nicotine inhaler, which may cause local irritation of the mouth and throat. Because of potential nicotine overdose, the gum or nicotine patch should be used with caution in patients who continue to use cigarettes.
   (3) **Varenicline** is a partial agonist at certain nicotine receptors that reduces the actions of nicotine. It may cause drowsiness and has been associated with suicidal ideation.
   (4) **Other available pharmacological therapies** that have been used with some reported success include **clonidine**, **nortriptyline** and **bupropion**, and **selegiline**.

E. Hallucinogens (psychotomimetics)
1. *LSD (d-lysergic acid diethylamide); also mescaline, psilocybin*
   a. LSD is an extremely potent synthetic drug that, when taken orally, causes altered consciousness, euphoria, increased sensory awareness ("mind expansion"), perceptual distortions, and increased introspection.

    b. It acts at neuronal postjunctional serotonin 5-HT$_{2A}$-receptors.

    c. The sympathomimetic activity of LSD includes pupillary dilation, increased blood pressure, and tachycardia.

    d. Adverse effects of LSD include alteration of perception and thoughts with misjudgment, changes in sense of time, visual hallucinations, dysphoria, panic reactions, suicide (bad trips), "flashbacks," and psychosis; treatment includes benzodiazepines for sedation.

    e. A high degree of tolerance to the behavioral effects of LSD develops rapidly.

    f. Dependence and withdrawal do not occur with these hallucinogens.

  2. *Phencyclidine (PCP, "angel dust")*

    a. PCP is a veterinary anesthetic used initially in humans, like ketamine, as a dissociative anesthetic.

    b. PCP is taken orally and IV; it is also "snorted" and smoked. It is considered a "club drug."

    c. The behavioral actions related to PCP are thought to be related to its **antagonist activity at NMDA receptors** for the excitatory amino acid glutamate.

    d. Low doses of PCP produce a state resembling ethanol intoxication. High doses cause euphoria, hallucinations, changed body image, and an increased sense of isolation and loneliness; it also impairs judgment and increases aggressiveness.

    e. Overdose with PCP may result in seizures, respiratory depression, cardiac arrest, and coma. Treatment of PCP overdose includes maintenance of respiration, control of seizures, reduction of sensory input, and therapy directed at behavioral manifestations, possibly including benzodiazepine or antipsychotic drug therapy.

F. Marijuana (cannabis) and dronabinol (marinol)

  1. The active ingredient in marijuana is Δ**-9 tetrahydrocannabinol;** it acts prejunctionally as an agonist to inhibit adenylyl cyclase through G-protein-linked cannabinoid receptors. Through disinhibition of DA neurons it inhibits the activity of GABA neurons in the ventral tegmentum area (VTA).

    a. Cannabinol CB$_1$ receptors, which account for most CNS effects, are localized to cognitive and motor areas of the brain. Cannabinol **CB$_2$-receptors** are found in the immune system among other peripheral organs.

    b. Anandamide and 2-arachidonylglycerol, naturally occurring ligands derived from arachidonic acid that act at prejunctional CB$_1$-receptors to inhibit the release of GABA and glutamate; their normal physiologic function is unclear.

  2. Marijuana is mostly smoked, but can be taken orally. It is very lipid soluble. The effects of smoking are immediate and last up to 2–3 hours.

  3. The **initial phase** of marijuana use (the "high") consists of euphoria, uncontrolled laughter, loss of sense of time, and increased introspection. The **second phase** includes relaxation, a dreamlike state, sleepiness, and difficulty in concentration. At extremely high doses, acute psychosis with depersonalization has been observed.

  4. The physiologic effects of marijuana include increased pulse rate and a characteristic reddening of the conjunctiva.

  5. Marijuana, and its analog **dronabinol**, is used therapeutically to decrease intraocular pressure for the treatment of glaucoma, as an antiemetic in cancer chemotherapy, and to stimulate appetite in patients with AIDS. **Nabilone**, another marijuana analog, is used to treat chronic pain.

  6. Tolerance is difficult to demonstrate in man except among long-term high-dose users, for whom a mild form of psychological and physical dependence has been noted.

  7. Adverse effects of marijuana, some of which are controversial, include the following:

    a. Long-term effects similar to those of cigarette smoking, including periodontal disease.

    b. Exacerbation of preexisting paranoia or psychosis.

    c. "Amotivational syndrome" that may be more related to user's personality type.

    d. Impairment of short-term memory and disturbances of the immune, reproductive, and thermoregulatory systems.

DRUG SUMMARY TABLE

Sedative–Hypnotic Drugs
Benzodiazepines
Alprazolam (Xanax, generic)
Clonazepam (Klonopin, generic)
Clorazepate (Tranxene, generic)
Chlordiazepoxide (Librium, generic)
Diazepam (Valium, generic)
Estazolam (ProSom, generic)
Flurazepam (Dalmane, generic)
Lorazepam (Ativan, generic)
Midazolam (Versed)
Oxazepam (Serax, generic)
Prazepam (Centrax)
Quazepam (Doral)
Temazepam (Restoril, generic)
Triazolam (Halcion, generic)
Nonbenzodiazepines
Buspirone (BuSpar, generic)
Eszopiclone (Lunesta)
Zaleplon (Sonata)
Zolpidem (Ambien, generic)
Melatonin receptor agonists
Ramelteon (Rozerem)
Barbiturates
Amobarbital (Amytal)
Pentobarbital (Nembutal, generic)
Secobarbital (Seconal, generic)
Benzodiazepine receptor antagonists
Flumazenil (Romazicon, generic)

Antipsychotic Drugs
Typical
Chlorpromazine (Thorazine, generic)
Triflupromazine (Vesprin, generic)
Thioridazine (Mellaril, generic)
Loxapine (Loxitane)
Molindone (Moban)
Trifluoperazine (Stelazine, generic)
Fluphenazine (Prolixin, generic)
Perphenazine (Trilafon, generic)
Thiothixene (Navane, generic)
Haloperidol (Haldol, generic)
Atypical
Aripiprazole (Ability)
Asenapine (Saphris)
Clozapine (Clozaril, generic)
Olanzapine (Zyprexa)
Paliperidone (Invega)
Quetiapine (Seroquel)
Risperidone (Risperdal)
Ziprasidone (Geodon)
Other
Pimozide (Orap)
Prochlorperazine (Compazine)

Antidepressant Drugs
Tricyclic Antidepressants
Amitriptyline (Elavil, generic)
Imipramine (Tofranil, generic)
Trimipramine (Surmontil)
Doxepin (Sinequan, generic)
Clomipramine (Anafranil, generic)
Desipramine (Norpramin, generic)
Nortriptyline (Pamelor, generic)
Protriptyline (Vivactil, generic)
Amoxapine (Asendin, generic)

Selective Serotonin Reuptake Inhibitors
Citalopram (Celexa, generic)
Escitalopram (Lexapro)
Fluoxetine (Prozac, generic)
Fluvoxamine (Luvox, generic)
Paroxetine (Paxil, generic)
Sertraline (Zoloft, generic)
Selective Norepinephrine Reuptake Inhibitors
Desvenlafaxine (Pristiq)
Duloxetine (Cymbalta)
Milnacipran (Savella)
Venlafaxine (Effexor)
Serotonin 5-HT$_2$ Antagonists
Nefazodone (Serzone, generic)
Trazodone (Desyrel, generic)
Atypical Heterocyclic Drugs
Bupropion (Wellbutrin, generic)
Maprotiline (Ludiomil, generic)
Mirtazapine (Remeron, generic)
Monoamine Oxidase Inhibitors
Phenelzine (Nardil, generic)
Tranylcypromine (Parnate, generic)

Drugs Used to Treat Bipolar Disorder
Carbamazepine (Tegretol, generic)
Divalproex (Depakote)
Lamotrigine (Lamictal)
Lithium (Eskalith, generic)
Topiramate (Topamax)
Valproic acid (Depakene, generic)

Opioid Analgesics, Antagonists, and Antitussives
Opioid Analgesics
Alfentanil (Alfenta, generic)
Buprenorphine (Buprenex)
Butorphanol (Stadol, generic)
Codeine (Generic)
Fentanyl (Sublimaze, others, generic)
Hydrocodone (Used only in analgesic combinations, e.g., Vicodin)
Hydromorphone (Dilaudid, generic)
Levomethadyl acetate (Orlaam)
Levorphanol (Levo-Dromoran, generic)
Meperidine (Demerol, generic)
Methadone (Dolophine, generic)
Morphine (Generic)
Nalbuphine (Nubain, generic)
Oxycodone (Generic)
Oxymorphone (Numorphan)
Pentazocine (Talwin)
Propoxyphene (Damon, generic)
Remifentanil (Ultiva)
Sufentanil (Sufenta, generic)
Tapentadol (Nucynta)
Tramadol (Ultram, generic)
Opioid Antagonists
Alvimopan (Entereg)
Methylnaltrexone (Relistor)
Nalmefene (Revex)
Naloxone (Narcan, generic)
Naltrexone (ReVia, Depade, generic)

Antidiarrheal Agents
Difenoxin (Motofen)
Diphenoxylate (Lomotil, generic))
Loperamide (Imodium, generic)

Antitussive Agents
Dextromethorphan (Benylin DM, generic)

Antiparkinsonian Drugs
Amantadine (Symmetrel)
Benztropine (Cogentin)
Biperidin (Akineton)
Bromocriptine (Parlodel)
Carbidopa (Lodosyn)
Carbidopa/levodopa/entacapone (Stalevo)
Entacapone (Comtan)
Levodopa (Dopar)
Levodopa/Carbidopa (Sinemet)
Orphenadrine (Norflex)
Pramipexole (Mirapex)
Procyclidine (Kemadrin)
Rasagiline (Azilect)
Ropinirole (Requip)
Selegiline (deprenyl) (Eldepryl, generic)
Tolcapone (Tasmar)
Trihexyphenidyl (Artane)

Drugs Used to Treat Alzheimer Disease
Donepezil (Aricept)
Galantamine (Reminyl)
Memantine (Axura)
Rivastigmine (Exelon)
Tacrine (Cognex)

Antiepileptic Drugs
Carbamazepine (Tegretol, generic)
Clonazepam (Klonopin, generic)
Clorazepate (Tranxene, generic)
Diazepam (Valium, generic)
Ethosuximide (Zarontin, generic)
Ethotoin (Peganone)
Ezogabine (Potiga)
Felbamate (Felbatol)
Fosphenytoin (Cerebyx)
Gabapentin (Neurontin)
Lacosamide (Vimpat)
Lamotrigine (Lamictal, generic)
Levetiracetam (Keppra, generic)
Lorazepam (Ativan, generic)
Mephenytoin (Mesantoin)
Methsuximide (Celontin)
Oxcarbazepine (Trileptal)
Phenobarbital (Luminal, generic)
Phensuximide (Milontin)
Phenytoin (Dilantin, generic)
Pregabalin (Lyrica)
Primidone (Mysoline, generic)
Rufinamide (Banzel)
Stiripentol (Diacomit, imported for compassionate use)
Tiagabine (Gabitril)
Trimethadione (Tridione)

Topiramate (Topamax)
Valproic acid (Depakene, generic)
Vigabetrin (Sabril)
Zonisamide (Zonegran, generic)

Anesthetic Agents
Desflurane (Suprane)
Dexmedetomidine (Precedex)
Diazepam (Valium, generic)
Droperidol (Inapsine, generic)
Enflurane (Enflurane, Ethrane)
Etomidate (Amidate)
Fospropofol (Lusedra)
Halothane (Fluothane, generic)
Isoflurane (Isoflurane, Forane)
Ketamine (Ketalar, generic)
Lorazepam (Ativan, generic)
Methohexital (Brevital)
Midazolam (Versed, generic)
Nitrous oxide
Propofol (Diprivan, generic)
Sevoflurane (Ultane, generic)
Thiopental (Pentothal, generic)

Local Anesthetics
Articaine (Septocaine)
Benzocaine (generic)
Bupivacaine (Marcaine, Sensorcaine, generic)
Butamben picrate
Chloroprocaine (Nesacaine, generic)
Cocaine (Generic)
Dibucaine (Nupercainal, generic)
Dyclonine (Dyclone)
Etidocaine (Duranest)
Lidocaine (Xylocaine, generic)
Mepivacaine (Carbocaine, generic)
Pramoxine (Tronothane, generic)
Prilocaine (Citanest)
Procaine (Novocain, generic)
Proparacaine (Alcaine, generic)
Ropivacaine (Naropin)
Tetracaine (Pontocaine, generic)

Medications (selected) for Drug Abuse
Opioids
Clonidine (Catapres, generic)

L-Acetylmethadol (ORLAAM)
Methadone (Dolophine, generic)
Ethanol
Acamprosate (Campral)
Chlordiazepoxide (Librium, generic)
Diazepam (Valium, generic)
Disulfiram (Antabuse, generic)
Lorazepam (Ativan, generic)
Naltrexone (ReVia, generic)
Oxazepam (Serax, generic)
Thiamine (generic)
Methanol, Ethylene Glycol
Ethanol (generic)
Fomepizole (Antizol, generic)
Nicotine
Bupropion (Zyban)
Nicotine replacements (Nicorette, Nic-oderm, generic)
Varenicline (Chantix)

Review Test

Directions: Each of the numbered items or incomplete statements in this section is followed by answers or by completions of the statement. Select the ONE lettered answer or completion that is BEST in each case.

1. A 42-year-old businessman visits a psychiatrist for what he describes as a very "embarrassing problem." The patient has found it difficult to make it to work on time because he keeps driving back to his house to make sure that the garage door is shut. He has begun waking up 2 hours early to facilitate these obsessions and compulsions. He is otherwise without additional complaints. The psychiatrist is concerned that the patient has developed obsessive-compulsive disorder (OCD) and has him try which of the following?

(A) Imipramine
(B) Clomipramine
(C) Atomoxetine
(D) Propranolol
(E) Desipramine

2. A 56-year-old truck driver is on disability for a back injury he sustained while making a delivery 3 months ago. He has been on several opioid drugs but continues to complain of "nagging back pain." The pain specialist he sees decides to try treating him with an antidepressant approved for the management of chronic pain. Which of the following would he chose?

(A) Fluoxetine
(B) Promethazine
(C) Trazodone
(D) Prochlorperazine
(E) Venlafaxine

3. A 56-year-old man recently suffered a myocardial infarction (MI). He is on numerous medications, many of which are metabolized by the cytochrome P-450 system. He now presents to the psychiatrist with difficulty sleeping and decreased appetite and reports "no longer enjoying golf like I used to." Recognizing that depression is common in patients who have recently had an MI, the psychiatrist decides to start the patient on selective serotonin reuptake inhibitor (SSRI) therapy. Given his multiple medications, which SSRI should be avoided?

(A) Fluoxetine
(B) Tranylcypromine
(C) Sertraline
(D) Escitalopram
(E) Phenylzine

4. The above patient returns for follow-up 6 months later. He has joined a health club and has lost several pounds and notes "feeling better mentally." However, upon questioning he still has not returned to the activities he once enjoyed and is still not sleeping or eating well. The psychiatrist recommends increasing the dose of his selective serotonin reuptake inhibitor (SSRI). The patient reluctantly admits that he has not been taking his medication because of some of the side effects. Which one is likely to be the most bothersome?

(A) Weight gain
(B) Tachycardia
(C) Headache
(D) Sexual dysfunction
(E) Tremor

5. A 36-year-old man has been smoking two packs of cigarettes a day for the last 20 years. He is concerned that his health has deteriorated, and he has a persistent hacking cough. He also states that he doesn't want to "get lung cancer and die, like my father did." He has tried nicotine patches with no success and wants to know if there is any "pill" he could try. What medication could the physician recommend?

(A) Mirtazapine
(B) Citalopram
(C) Phenelzine
(D) Buspirone
(E) Bupropion

6. A 23-year-old man is brought to the emergency room after he was found walking the streets naked while proclaiming himself "the son of God." His urine toxicology screen comes back negative for illicit drugs or alcohol. During the interview with the on-call psychiatrist, the patient displays flight of ideas as he jumps from topic to topic. The physician recommends starting the patient on lithium therapy for acute mania. Which of the following is associated with lithium use?

(A) Urinary retention
(B) Weight loss
(C) Fine tremor
(D) A wide therapeutic margin
(E) Hyperthyroidism

7. A first-year surgery intern has rotated on numerous surgical services during the first year, including general surgery, cardiothoracic surgery, urology, surgical oncology, trauma surgery, and colorectal surgery. He has gotten quite used to liberally ordering morphine for pain control. However, which of the following is an absolute contraindication to opioid use?

(A) Closed head injury
(B) Myocardial infarction
(C) Acute pulmonary edema
(D) Renal colic
(E) Biliary colic

8. A 5-year-old child is admitted to the hospital with a low-grade fever and a persistent cough that has resulted in vomiting episodes following prolonged coughing spells. His throat culture is negative, his fever has resolved, and all that is left is a slight cough. He is discharged from the hospital by the pediatrician who recommends an over-the-counter opioid antitussive. Which of the following does he recommend?

(A) Tramadol
(B) Diphenoxylate
(C) Loperamide
(D) Dextromethorphan
(E) Naloxone

9. An anesthesia resident is on his first case alone. The surgeons are preparing the patient's abdomen for their eventual incision when the attending physician enters the operating room and asks the anesthesia resident if the patient is anesthetized. Which of the following is the most reliable sign that surgical anesthesia has been reached?

(A) Analgesia
(B) Amnesia
(C) Loss of consciousness
(D) Maximum papillary dilation
(E) Loss of eyelash reflex

10. A 16-year-old patient visits his dentist for a routine checkup. He finds that his wisdom teeth are severely impacted and need to be removed. The oral surgeon to whom he is referred plans on using an agent that has good analgesic and sedative properties but does not cause skeletal muscle relaxation. Which agent has these ideal properties?

(A) Enflurane
(B) Nitrous oxide
(C) Thiopental
(D) Halothane
(E) Isoflurane

11. A 6-year-old child was badly burned when his house caught on fire. He sustained full-thickness burns on approximately 40% of his body. He has spent many months enduring multiple skin-grafting procedures. To aid in reducing the pain associated with dressing changes, he is given ketamine IV. This drug has been associated with which of the following adverse reactions?

(A) Irritation to the respiratory airways
(B) Sensitization of the heart to catecholamines
(C) Reduction of cardiac output
(D) Malignant hyperthermia
(E) Distortion of reality and terrifying dreams

12. A patient sees an otolaryngologist with complaints of recurrent sinusitis. The surgeon decides to perform sinus surgery to debride the scarred sinus tissue. During the procedure, the surgeon elects to use an agent that has good local anesthesia as well as vasoconstrictive properties. What agent might he use?

(A) Cocaine
(B) Procaine
(C) Tetracaine
(D) Lidocaine
(E) Mepivacaine

13. A 28-year-old alcoholic woman learns that she is pregnant after missing her last two menstrual periods. She received poor prenatal care, missing many of her appointments. The neonatologist that cared for her child at birth learned that the mother did not refrain from her normal heavy alcohol binges throughout her pregnancy. Which of the following is the most likely consequence of such abuse to the child during pregnancy?

(A) Abruptio placentae and learning difficulties as the child ages
(B) Spina bifida and orofacial defects
(C) Fetal hemorrhage and defects in fetal bone formation
(D) Microcephaly, retarded growth, and congenital heart defects
(E) Growth retardation, microcephaly, and craniofacial abnormalities

14. A 16-year-old boy is brought to the emergency room at 4 am by his friends, who report that the patient was at an all-night rave party and was agitated, hyperactive, and hypersexual. The physician learns that the boy took several pills, which his friends thought were "ecstasy" (methylenedioxymethamphetamine).

Which of the following describes the mechanism of this "party" drug?

(A) Antagonistic activity at the N-methyl-d-aspartate (NMDA) receptor for lutamic acid
(B) Binding to the cannabinol CB1 receptor
(C) Increased release of dopamine and norepinephrine
(D) Mimics the action of acetylcholine
(E) Agonist at postjunctional serotonin receptors

15. A 31-year-old lawyer is transferred to the emergency room after collapsing at a party. He complained of chest pain, and an electrocardiogram demonstrated ventricular fibrillation, for which he received cardioversion. A primary survey of the patient showed little trauma, with the exception of a perforated nasal septum. A close friend accompanied the patient and confides in you that the patient was "doing" an illicit substance at the party. Which of the following is the most likely?

(A) Phencyclidine (PCP)
(B) γ-Hydroxybutyric acid (GHB)
(C) Lysergic acid diethylamide (LSD)
(D) Cocaine
(E) Marijuana

Answers and Explanations

1. **The answer is B.** Clomipramine, a tricyclic antidepressant (TCA) that inhibits serotonin uptake as well as the selective serotonin-reuptake inhibitors (SSRIs), is used for the treatment of obsessive-compulsive disorder (OCD). Imipramine is a tricyclic agent that is used infrequently to suppress enuresis in children and that is metabolized to yet another TCA, desipramine. Atomoxetine is a selective inhibitor of the norepinephrine reuptake transporter that is used in the management of attention-deficit disorders. Propranolol is a β-blocker used to treat hypertension and other cardiovascular conditions.

2. **The answer is E.** Venlafaxine and some tricyclic antidepressants are used in the management of chronic pain. Promethazine and prochlorperazine are two dopamine receptor blockers, without antipsychotic activity, used to treat nausea and vomiting. Trazodone is an atypical antidepressant that is highly sedating and has been associated with orthostatic hypotension and priapism. Fluoxetine is a selective serotonin reuptake inhibitor (SSRI). SSRIs are not effective therapy for chronic pain.

3. **The answer is A.** Fluoxetine and paroxetine inhibit cytochrome P-450 and thus need to be used with caution as they can potentiate the action of other drugs metabolized by this system. Tranylcypromine and phenelzine are monoamine oxidase inhibitors (MAOIs) that, when used with selective serotonin reuptake inhibitors (SSRIs), can cause a potentially fatal "serotonin syndrome." Sertraline and escitalopram are two SSRIs that are not metabolized by the P-450 system and might be good choices for this individual.

4. **The answer is D.** Sexual dysfunction is a common complaint with selective serotonin reuptake inhibitors (SSRIs), occurring in up to 40% of all patients, and a leading cause of noncompliance. Weight loss is usually experienced initially with SSRIs, and some persons may eventually gain weight. Headache is associated with SSRIs, although it is often transient. Tremor and tachycardia are side effects that are more typical with tricyclic antidepressants (TCAs).

5. **The answer is E.** Bupropion is an atypical heterocyclic antidepressant that is useful as an aid in smoking cessation. Mirtazapine is another atypical agent used in the treatment of depression that blocks both serotonin and α-adrenergic receptors. Phenelzine is an MAOI, sometimes used for depression. Citalopram is a selective serotonin reuptake inhibitor (SSRI), which are typically not used for smoking cessation. Buspirone is an antianxiety drug useful in situations where nonsedating agents are favored.

6. **The answer is C.** Lithium use is associated with a fine tremor that can often be successfully managed with β-blockers. Lithium is associated with polydipsia and polyuria, not urinary retention. Likewise, the other choices are opposite what might be expected with lithium use, as patients experience weight gain and hypothyroidism. Lithium has a narrow therapeutic margin, with therapeutic doses not too much lower than toxic doses.

7. **The answer is A.** Opioids are contraindicated in cases of head trauma, as they increase cerebral vascular pressure and may cause hemorrhage and/or herniation. Morphine is used during myocardial infarction, as it decreases cardiac preload and chest pain. Morphine is also used to reduce dyspnea associated with acute pulmonary edema. Renal colic, pain due to a kidney stone passing through the ureter, or biliary colic, which is a similar pain associated with gallstones passing through biliary ducts, are both well managed with morphine.

8. **The answer is D.** Dextromethorphan is an opioid isomer available in over-the-counter cough remedies. It has no analgesic properties and limited abuse potential at recommended doses. Tramadol is a weak μ-opioid-receptor agonist, which also blocks serotonin and norepinephrine uptake and is used for neuropathic pain. Diphenoxylate is an opioid that, combined with atropine, is taken orally to treat diarrhea. Loperamide is an opioid that does not cross

the blood–brain barrier and is also used for the treatment of diarrhea. Naloxone is an opioid antagonist used to reverse opioid overdose.

9. **The answer is E.** Loss of eyelash reflex and a pattern of respiration that is regular and deep are the most reliable indications of stage III, or surgical, anesthesia. Analgesia and amnesia are characteristics of stage I anesthesia, whereas the loss of consciousness is associated with stage II anesthesia. Maximum papillary dilation also occurs during stage III anesthesia, but closer to the progression to stage IV anesthesia, an undesirable stage associated with respiratory and cardiovascular failure.

10. **The answer is B.** Nitrous oxide is an anesthetic gas that has good analgesic and sedative properties without the skeletal muscle-relaxing effects. It can be used along with other inhaled agents decreasing their concentrations and thus their side effects. Enflurane produces anesthesia, hypnosis, and muscle relaxation, as do the others, and is very pungent. Thiopental is a barbiturate that is too short acting for this application. Halothane has a pleasant odor and produces a smooth and relatively rapid induction but decreases cardiac output and can result in an unpredictable hepatotoxicity. Isoflurane is associated with more rapid induction and recovery than halothane and may have some benefits in patients with ischemic heart disease.

11. **The answer is E.** Ketamine is a dissociative anesthetic related to phencyclidine (PCP) and is thought to block glutamic acid *N*-methyl-d-aspartate (NMDA) receptors. Its use is associated with distortions of reality, terrifying dreams, and delirium, more commonly in adults. Malignant hyperthermia may be associated with any of the inhaled anesthetics, such as halothane, in genetically prone individuals. Halothane and isoflurane sensitize the heart to catecholamines. Desflurane is especially irritating to airways, and enflurane can reduce cardiac output.

12. **The answer is A.** Cocaine is ideal for such surgery because of its topical activity; it does not require the addition of epinephrine, as it has intrinsic vasoconstrictive activity that aids in hemostasis. Similar to cocaine, both procaine and tetracaine are ester-type compounds; however, procaine is not topically active and tetracaine is used primarily for spinal anesthesia and ophthalmologic procedures. Lidocaine is an amide anesthetic preferred for infiltrative blocks and epidural anesthesia. Mepivacaine is another amide local anesthetic, although not topically active, which, like all such agents, acts by blocking sodium channels.

13. **The answer is D.** Fetal alcohol syndrome is a leading cause of congenital abnormalities, especially microcephaly, growth retardation, and congenital heart defects. Abruptio placentae and learning difficulties are more typical with maternal use of cocaine during pregnancy. Spina bifida and orofacial defects are associated with valproic acid use during pregnancy, and the anticonvulsant phenytoin is associated with fetal growth retardation, microcephaly, and craniofacial abnormalities. Fetal hemorrhage and bone malformation are a consequence of warfarin use during pregnancy.

14. **The answer is C.** Like other amphetamines, ecstasy increases the release of dopamine and norepinephrine. Its use is often associated with "rave" parties. Phencyclidine (PCP) is an antagonist at the *N*-methyl-d-aspartate (NMDA) receptor for glutamic acid, causing euphoria and hallucinations. Marijuana causes euphoria, uncontrollable laughter, loss of time perception, and increased introspection. It binds to the cannabinol CB-1 receptor. Nicotine is a powerful stimulant in tobacco products and works by mimicking the effects of acetylcholine at cholinergic nicotinic receptors. Lysergic acid diethylamide (LSD) is an agonist of the postjunctional serotonin receptors.

15. **The answer is D.** Cocaine is cardiotoxic and can cause arrhythmias that can be life-threatening. These effects are even more likely when alcohol is also consumed. Cocaine causes vasoconstriction, and snorting the drug causes necrosis and eventual perforation of the nasal septum. γ-Hydroxybutyric acid (GHB) is a barbiturate that is used as a "date rape" drug. Lysergic acid diethylamide (LSD) causes increased sensory awareness, perceptual distortions, and altered consciousness. Phencyclidine (PCP) can cause euphoria, hallucinations, an increased sense of isolation and loneliness, and increased aggression. Marijuana causes euphoria, laughter, a loss of time perception, and increased introspection.

chapter 6

Autocoids, Ergots, Anti-inflammatory Agents, and Immunosuppressive Agents

I. HISTAMINE AND ANTIHISTAMINES

A. **Histamine** (Fig. 6.1). Histamine is a small molecule produced by decarboxylation of the amino acid histidine; it is catalyzed by the enzyme L-histidine decarboxylase in a reaction that requires pyridoxal phosphate.

1. *Synthesis*
   a. Histamine is found in many tissues, including the brain; it is stored and found in the highest amounts in mast cells and basophils. Mast cells, which are especially abundant in the respiratory tract, skin (especially hands and feet), gastrointestinal (GI) tract, and blood vessels, store histamine in a granule bound in a complex with heparin, adenosine triphosphate (ATP), and an acidic protein.
   b. **Release** of histamine can occur by two processes:
      (1) **Energy- and Ca^{2+}-dependent degranulation reaction.** The release of histamine from mast cells is induced by immunoglobulin E (IgE) fixation to mast cells (sensitization) and subsequent exposure to a specific antigen; complement activation (mediated by immunoglobulin G or immunoglobulin M) may also induce degranulation.
      (2) **Energy- and Ca^{2+}-independent release (displacement).** Displacement is induced by drugs such as morphine, tubocurarine, guanethidine, and amine antibiotics. In addition, mast cell damage, which is caused by noxious agents such as venom or by mechanical trauma, can release histamine.

2. *Mechanism of action*
   a. **Histamine (H_1)-receptors**
      (1) H_1-receptors are found in the brain, heart, bronchi, GI tract, vascular smooth muscles, and leukocytes.
      (2) H_1-receptors are membrane bound and coupled to G-proteins, specifically $G_{q/11}$, and their activation causes an increase in phospholipase A_2 and D activity, increases in diacylglycerol and intracellular Ca^{2+}, and increased cyclic guanosine 5′-monophosphate (cGMP).
      (3) Activation of H_1-receptors in the brain increases wakefulness.
      (4) Activation of H_1-receptors in vessels causes vasodilation and an increase in permeability.
      (5) Activation of H_1-receptors typically stimulates nonvascular smooth muscle.
   b. **Histamine (H_2)-receptors**
      (1) H_2-receptors are membrane bound; they are found in the brain, heart, vascular smooth muscles, leukocytes, and parietal cells.
      (2) The response of H_2-receptors is coupled via $G\alpha_s$ to increased cyclic AMP (cAMP) production.

151

$$HN \diagdown N \quad CH_2 - CH_2 - NH_2$$

FIGURE 6.1. Structure of histamine.

(3) Activation of H_2-receptors increases gastric acid production, causes vasodilation, and generally relaxes smooth muscles.

c. Histamine-H_3 and H_4-receptors are located in the brain and hematopoietic cells and thymus. There are no approved drugs that act through these receptors but it is a very active area of research.

B. **Histamine agonists**
1. *Prototypes.* These agents include **histamine, betahistine,** and **impromidine**.
   a. **Betazole** has approximately tenfold greater activity at H_2-receptors than at H_1-receptors.
   b. **Impromidine** is an investigational agent; its ratio of H_2 to H_1 activity is about 10,000:1.
   c. Methimepip is an H_3-specific agonist.
2. *Uses.* The uses of histamine agonists are primarily diagnostic. These agents are used in **allergy testing** to assess histamine sensitivity and in the **test of gastric secretory function** (they have been largely supplanted for this use by **pentagastrin** [Peptavlon], a synthetic peptide analog of gastrin with fewer adverse effects).
3. *Adverse effects.* The adverse effects of these agents can be quite severe; they include flushing, a burning sensation, hypotension, tachycardia, and bronchoconstriction.

C. **Histamine (H_1)-receptor antagonists** are competitive inhibitors at the H_1-receptor (see Table 6.1)
1. *Classification*
   a. **First-generation agents include chlorpheniramine, most often used in cold remedies, diphenhydramine, dimenhydrinate**, used in anti-motion sickness preparations, **doxylamine** is marketed only as a sleeping aid, and meclizine and promethazine used almost exclusively as anti-emetics. As a class, these agents are lipid soluble, readily cross the blood–brain barrier, and have significant CNS actions mediated in large part by their anti-cholinergic activity.

table 6.1 Major Pharmacologic Properties of H_1-Receptor Antagonists

Drug Class	Prototype	Duration of Action (h)	Antihistamine Potency	Anticholinergic Potency	Antiemetic Potency	Sedative Effect
First-generation agents						
Alkylamines	Chlorpheniramine	4–25	+++	++	Marginal	+
Ethanolamines	Diphenhydramine	4–6	++	+++	+++	+++
	Dimenhydrinate	4–8	++	++	+	+++
	Clemastine	10–24	++	++	+	+
Ethylenediamines	Pyrilamine	4–6	+	++	Marginal	+
Piperazines	Cyclizine	4–24	++	++	+++	+
Phenothiazines	Promethazine	4–24	+/+++	+++	++++	+++
Methylpiperidines	Cyproheptadine	6–8	++	++	++	++
Second-generation agents						
Alkylamines	Acrivastine	6–8	++++	Marginal	None	Marginal +
Piperazines	Cetirizine	12–24	++++	+	Marginal	14%
	Levocitirizine	12–24	++++	+	Marginal	6%
Piperidines	Loratadine	24	++	None	None	8%
	Desloratadine	24	++++	None	None	2.1%
	Fexofenadine	12	++++	None	None	1.3%

    b. Second-generation agents include Loratadine (Claritin), desloratadine (Clarinex), and clemastine. These agents were designed to have much reduced lipid solubility and poor CNS penetration. Little or no anticholinergic activity and greatly reduced sedation compared with earlier agents. Desloratadine is the active metabolite of loratadine and has about 15-fold greater affinity for the H_1 receptor than the parent compound.

2. *Pharmacologic properties* (Table 6.1)

    a. Histamine (H_1)-receptor antagonists are well absorbed after oral administration. The effects of these agents are usually seen in 30 minutes (with maximal effects at 1–2 h); the duration of action is 3–8 hours for first-generation compounds and 3–24 hours for second-generation compounds.

    b. H_1-receptor antagonists are lipid soluble; most first-generation agents cross the blood–brain barrier, a property reduced but not eliminated with second-generation agents.

    c. H_1-receptor antagonists are metabolized in the liver; many induce microsomal enzymes and alter their own metabolism and that of other drugs.

3. *Pharmacologic actions*

    a. Many H_1-receptor antagonists, especially diphenhydramine and pyrilamine have muscarinic-cholinergic antagonist activity.

    b. Most of these agents are effective local anesthetics, probably because of a blockade of sodium channels in excitable tissues. **Dimenhydrinate** and **promethazine** are potent local anesthetics.

    c. H_1-receptor antagonists relax histamine-induced contraction of bronchial smooth muscle and have some use in allergic bronchospasm.

    d. These agents block the vasodilator action of histamine.

    e. H_1-receptor antagonists inhibit histamine-induced increases in capillary permeability.

    f. These agents block mucus secretion and sensory nerve stimulation.

    g. H_1-receptor antagonists, especially the first-generation agents, frequently cause CNS depression (marked by sedation, decreased alertness, and decreased appetite). In children and some adults, these agents stimulate the CNS.

4. *Therapeutic uses*

    a. Treatment of allergic rhinitis and conjunctivitis. Clemastine is approved for the treatment of rhinorrhea. Many antihistamines are used to treat the common cold, based on their anticholinergic properties, but they are only marginally effective for this use. Diphenhydramine also has an antitussive effect not mediated by H_1-receptor antagonism.

    b. Treatment of urticaria and **atopic dermatitis,** including hives.

    c. Sedatives. Several (**doxylamine, diphenhydramine**) are marketed as over-the-counter sleep aids.

    d. Prevention of **motion sickness.**

    e. Appetite suppressants.

5. *Adverse effects* (significantly reduced with second-generation agents)

    a. H_1-receptor antagonists produce sedation (synergistic with alcohol and other depressants), dizziness, and loss of appetite.

    b. These agents can cause GI upset, nausea, and constipation or diarrhea.

    c. H_1-receptor antagonists produce anticholinergic effects (dry mouth, blurred vision, and urine retention).

    d. Two second-generation H_1 antagonists, astemizole and terfenadine (a prodrug of fexofenadine) were discontinued or removed from the market because they were associated with Q–T prolongation and ventricular tachycardias.

D. Histamine (H_2)-receptor antagonists (see also Chapter 8 III C 1)

    1. Histamine (H_2)-receptor antagonists include **cimetidine** (Tagamet), **ranitidine** (Zantac), **famotidine** (Pepcid AC), and **nizatidine** (Axid).

    2. These agents are competitive antagonists at the H_2-receptor, which predominates in the gastric parietal cell.

3. H_2-receptor antagonists are used in the treatment of GI disorders, including heartburn and acid-induced indigestion.

4. These agents promote the healing of **gastric and duodenal ulcers** and are used to treat hypersecretory states such as **Zollinger-Ellison** syndrome.

E. The chromones: Cromolyn (Intal) and Nedocromil Sodium (Tilade)
   1. These are poorly absorbed salts; they must be administered by **inhalation.**
   2. They inhibit the release of histamine and other autocoids mast cells.
   3. Each is used **prophylactically in the treatment of asthma; they do not reverse bronchospasm.**
   4. These agents produce **few adverse effects** that are usually confined to the site of application; these effects include **sore throat** and **dry mouth.**
   5. Nedocromil sodium appears to be more effective than cromolyn in reducing **bronchospasm** caused by exercise or cold air.

II. SEROTONIN AND SEROTONIN ANTAGONISTS

A. Serotonin (5-hydroxytryptamine, 5-HT)
   1. *Biosynthesis and distribution*
      a. Serotonin is synthesized from the amino acid L-tryptophan by hydroxylation and decarboxylation.
      b. Approximately 90% of serotonin is found in the enterochromaffin cells of the GI tract. Much of the remaining 10% is found in the platelets; small amounts are found in other tissues, including the brain. Platelets acquire serotonin from the circulation during passage through the intestine by a specific and highly active uptake mechanism.
      c. Serotonin is stored in granules as a complex with ATP.
      d. The major breakdown product of serotonin is **5-hydroxyindoleacetic acid. Serotonin is also the precursor of melatonin.**
   2. *Mechanism of action.* Serotonin acts on several classes of 5-HT receptors, which are located on cell membranes of many tissues:
      a. **5-HT$_1$** (subtypes 5-HT$_{1A}$ through 5-HT$_{1E}$, HT$_{1P}$). 5-HT$_1$ receptors are coupled to an inhibition in cAMP; stimulation contracts arterial smooth muscle, especially in carotid and cranial circulation. At presynaptic sites, neuronal serotonin release is inhibited.
      b. **5-HT$_2$** (subtypes 5-HT$_{2A}$ through 5-HT$_{2C}$). 5-HT$_2$ receptors are coupled to an increase in phospholipase C activity; stimulation causes contraction of vascular and intestinal smooth muscle and increases microcirculation and vascular permeability. Stimulation of this receptor on platelet membranes causes platelet aggregation; in the CNS, this receptor mediates hallucinogenic effects.
      c. **5-HT$_3$** receptors are coupled to a ligand-gated ion channel. Stimulation of this receptor in the area postrema causes nausea and vomiting; stimulation on peripheral sensory neurons causes pain.
      d. **5-HT$_4$** receptors increase cAMP; in the GI tract, these receptors mediate an increase in secretion and peristalsis.
      e. **5-HT$_{5a,b}$** are expressed in the brain and are coupled to a decrease in cAMP.
      f. **5-HT$_6$** and **5-HT$_7$** expressed in the brain are coupled to an increase in cAMP. 5-HT$_6$ receptors appear to be involved in anxiety and cognitive function. 5-HT$_7$ receptors are involved in thermoregulation, learning memory, and nociceptive processing.

B. Serotonin agonists (see Table 6.2)
   1. *Buspirone (BuSpar)*
      a. Buspirone is a relatively specific 5-HT$_{1A}$-receptor agonist, with weak dopamine receptor antagonism.

t a b l e 6.2 Drugs that Interact with Serotonin Receptors

Drug	Receptor	Action
Buspirone	5-HT$_{1a}$ agonist	Anxiolytic
Sumatriptan	5-HT$_{10,1B,1F}$ agonist	Acute migraine
Almotriptan	5-HT$_{10,1B,1F}$ agonist	Acute migraine
Dolasetron (Anzemet)	5-HT$_3$ antagonist	Antiemetic
Granisetron (Kytril)	5-HT$_3$ antagonist	Antiemetic
Ondansetron (Zofran)	5-HT$_3$ antagonist	Antiemetic
Alosetron	5-HT$_3$ antagonist	Severe irritable bowel
Risperidone	5-HT$_{2A,2C}$ antagonist (and D$_2$ antagonist)	Atypical antipsychotic

    b. Buspirone is useful for the management of **anxiety disorders, especially generalized anxiety disorder.**

    c. It may be useful in the treatment of the agitation associated with Alzheimer's and ADHD.

    d. Therapeutic actions can take as long as 2 weeks to appear.

2. *Triptans:* **Sumatriptan, Rizatriptan, Eletriptan, Zolmitriptan, Almotriptan, Frovatriptan, and Naratriptan**

    a. The "triptans" as a class are 5-HT$_{1D}$- and 5-HT$_{1B}$-receptor agonists and have 5-HT$_{1F}$ agonist activity. Activation of 5-HT$_{1D}$ receptors inhibits vasodilation and inflammation of the meninges and pain transmission and the release of vasodilator substances such as calcitonin gene-related peptide (CGRP) in trigeminal neurons. 5-HT$_{1B}$ agonist activity results in vasoconstriction of dilated cerebral vessels.

    b. The major use of the triptans is the treatment of **acute migraine;** about 50%–80% of patients report relief from pain within 2 hours. Triptans may be useful to treat cluster headaches.

    c. 5-HT$_{1B}$ activity can cause coronary vasospasm, and chest pain is an adverse effect of the triptans. They are contraindicated in patients with CAD or angina. Other adverse effects of this class include flushing, hypertension, nausea, and vomiting.

    d. All are available as oral agents. Sumatriptan and zolmitriptan are also available as nasal sprays, and sumatriptan is also available for subcutaneous injection.

3. *Trazodone (Desyrel)*

    a. The parent drug is metabolized to *m*-chlorophenylpiperazine, an activator of 5-HT$_{1B}$ and 5-HT$_2$ receptors. It also blocks the reuptake of serotonin.

    b. Trazodone is used to treat **depression, especially with insomnia.**

    c. Side effects are numerous with headache, dizziness, constipation, chest pain arrhythmias, and priapism seen in multiple patients.

4. *Tegaserod (Zelnorm) and Alosetron (Lotronox)*

    a. Tegaserod is a specific 5-HT$_4$ agonist used to treat irritable bowel syndrome and constipation.

    b. Tegaserod speeds gastric emptying and reduces GI sensitivity.

    c. Alosetron is a 5-HT$_3$ antagonist used for irritable bowel syndrome and can have severe GI side effects; its use is restricted to women.

C. Serotonin antagonists

    1. *Cyproheptadine*

        a. Cyproheptadine is a potent H$_1$-receptor antagonist of the phenothiazine class; it also blocks both 5-HT$_1$ and 5-HT$_2$ receptors.

        b. Cyproheptadine is used most frequently to limit diarrhea and intestinal spasms produced by **serotonin-secreting carcinoid tumors** and postgastrectomy **dumping syndrome.**

        c. Cyproheptadine produces sedation and anticholinergic actions.

2. *Ondansetron, Granisetron, Dolasetron, and Palonosetron*
   a. These drugs are 5-HT$_3$-receptor antagonists.
   b. The 5-HT$_3$-receptor antagonists are highly effective in treating the nausea and vomiting associated with chemotherapy and radiation therapy and have become the primary agents used with these therapies.
   c. Administered intravenously (IV) or orally; IV administration 30 minutes before anticancer treatment is the most effective. Palonosetron is administered IV and has a much longer half-life (40 h) compared with the other agents (3 h).
3. *Clozapine*
   a. While clozapine mainly blocks D$_1$ and D$_4$ receptors, it also blocks 5-HT$_{2A}$ and 5-HT$_{2C}$ receptors and has mixed acetylcholine muscarinic antagonist/agonist activities.
   b. Clozapine is an atypical **antipsychotic** with reduced extrapyramidal effects.
4. *Risperidone (Risperdal)*
   a. Risperidone is an antagonist at 5-HT$_{2A}$, 5-HT$_{2C}$, and dopamine (D$_2$) receptors.
   b. Risperidone is an **atypical antischizophrenic agent** with reduced extrapyramidal activity.

D. Other serotonergic agents. *Fluoxetine (Prozac)* and other SSRIs (see also Chapter 5, Table 5.5). The actions of this class of antidepressants are presumed to be due to decreased serotonin uptake into neurons.

III. ERGOTS

A. Structure. Ergots include a wide variety of compounds sharing the tetracyclic ergoline nucleus that are produced by the fungus *Claviceps purpurea*. These agents have a strong structural similarity to the neurotransmitters norepinephrine, dopamine, and serotonin.
   1. **Amine ergot alkaloids** include **methysergide, lysergic acid** and **LSD,** and **methylergonovine.**
   2. **Peptide ergot alkaloids** include **ergotamine (Ergomar), dihydroergotamine (Migranol), ergocristine, ergonovine, bromocriptine (Parlodel), cabergoline,** and **pergolide (Permax).**

B. Mechanism of action
   1. Ergots display varying degrees of agonist or antagonist activity in three receptor types: α-adrenoceptors, dopamine receptors, and serotonin receptors.
   2. The pharmacologic use of ergots is determined by the relative affinity and efficacy of the individual agents for these receptor systems. Many agents exhibit partial agonist activities and thus can cause either stimulatory or inhibitory effects.

C. Pharmacologic properties (Table 6.3)
   1. Ergots may be administered parenterally, rectally, sublingually, as inhalants, or orally, and vary widely in their absorption. Amine alkaloids are slowly and relatively poorly absorbed; the peptide alkaloids are completely absorbed.
   2. Ergots are extensively metabolized to compounds of varying activity and half-life.

D. Therapeutic uses
   1. *Postpartum hemorrhage*
      a. **Methylergonovine** (methergine) is the most uterine-selective agent; causes prolonged and forceful **contraction of uterine smooth muscle.**
      b. Ergots should not be used to induce labor.
      c. Uterine sensitivity varies with hormonal status; the uterus at term is most sensitive.
   2. *Migraine*
      a. **Ergotamine** (ergomar and ergostat) is widely used for relief of an acute migraine attack.

t a b l e **6.3**	Pharmacologic Properties of Ergots			
Drug	Receptor	Target Tissue and Response	Therapeutic Uses	Toxicity
Methylergonovine	α-Adrenoceptor agonist	Uterine smooth muscle contraction	Postpartum hemorrhage	Hypertension, nausea
Ergotamine	α-Adrenoceptor agonist, 5-HT receptor agonist	Vascular smooth muscle; vasoconstriction	Acute migraine attacks	Nausea, diarrhea
Methysergide	5-HT receptor antagonist	Vascular smooth muscle; prevent initial vasoconstriction	Migraine prophylaxis	Fibroblastic changes
Bromocriptine, pergolide	Dopamine agonists	Breast, uterus, pituitary; suppress lactation and decrease growth hormone levels	Hyperprolactinemia, amenorrhea, acromegaly	Dose-related effects, ranging from nausea to Parkinsonian-like symptoms

(1) The major effect of ergotamine is **cerebral vasoconstriction;** it reverses the rebound vasodilation that is the probable cause of pain.

(2) Ergotamine acts as a central 5-HT receptor and α-adrenoceptor agonist.

(3) Ergotamine is most effective if administered in the early (prodromal) stages of attack to reverse rebound vasodilation. Much less effective if treatment is delayed.

(4) Ergotamine is frequently **combined with caffeine,** which probably increases absorption.

(5) Ergotamine produces long-lasting and cumulative effects; weekly dosage must be strictly limited.

b. Methysergide (Sansert) is used for the **prophylaxis of migraine.**

   (1) Methysergide acts as a serotonin-receptor (5-HT$_{2A,C}$) antagonist, and it inhibits initial vasoconstriction in the early stages of a migraine.

   (2) Methysergide is effective in 60% of patients for the prophylaxis of migraine; it is ineffective after the onset of an attack.

   (3) The cumulative toxicity of methysergide requires drug-free periods of 3–4 weeks every 6 months.

c. Propranolol and other **β-adrenergic antagonists** are also effective agents for the prophylaxis of migraine.

3. *Hyperprolactinemia*

a. Bromocriptine mesylate (Parlodel) and **pergolide** (Permax), **cabergoline,** dopaminergic agonists, cause specific **inhibition of prolactin secretion** (elevated prolactin secretion can induce infertility and amenorrhea in women and galactorrhea in men and women).

b. These agents are used to treat prolactin-secreting tumors of the pituitary, to counteract central dopaminergic antagonists, and to suppress normal lactation.

c. Bromocriptine mesylate and pergolide are used as adjuncts to agents such as **levodopa** in the management of **Parkinson disease** (not a prolactin-lowering effect).

d. These agents reduce growth hormone secretion.

E. Adverse effects

1. The most serious adverse effect is **prolonged vasospasm;** this can lead to gangrene and is most frequently caused by **ergotamine** and **ergonovine.**

2. The most common side effect is **GI disturbance.**

3. Methysergide toxicity includes retroperitoneal fibroplasia and coronary and endocardial fibrosis, as well as CNS stimulation and hallucinations.

IV. EICOSANOIDS

A. An overview

1. Eicosanoids are a large group of autocoids with potent effects on virtually every tissue in the body; these agents are derived from the metabolism of 20-carbon, unsaturated fatty acids (**eicosanoic acids**).
2. The eicosanoids include the prostaglandins, thromboxanes, leukotrienes, hydroperoxye-icosatetraenoic acids (**HPETEs**), and hydroxyeicosatetraenoic acids (**HETEs**).

B. Biosynthesis (Fig. 6.2)

1. **Arachidonic acid,** the most common precursor of the eicosanoids, is formed by two pathways:

   a. **Phospholipase A_2**-mediated production from membrane phospholipids; this pathway is inhibited by glucocorticoids by the action of annexin-A1.

   b. **Phospholipase C** in concert with diglyceride lipase can also produce free arachidonate.

2. **Eicosanoids** are **synthesized** by two pathways:

   a. The **prostaglandin H synthase (COX, cyclooxygenase) pathway** produces **thromboxane,** the primary prostaglandins (**prostaglandin E,** or PGE; **prostaglandin F,** or PGF; and **prostaglandin D,** or PGD), and **prostacyclin (PGI$_2$).**

   (1) There are **two forms** of **COX: COX-1** is located platelets, kidney, GI tract, and many other locations; **COX-2** is found in great abundance in connective tissues, in the kidney, and in the endothelium.

   (2) The **COX-1** enzyme is expressed at fairly constant levels and may provide protective action on gastric mucosa, on endothelium, and in the kidney.

   (3) The **COX-2** enzyme is highly inducible by numerous factors associated with inflammation. Current theories suggest that the COX-2 isoform is predominantly associated with **eicosanoid production** in inflammation.

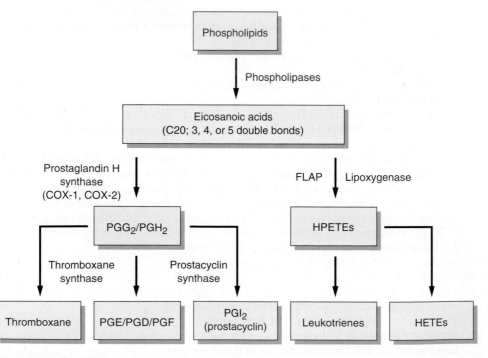

FIGURE 6.2. Biosynthesis of eicosanoids.

b. The **lipoxygenase pathway** produces the HPETEs, HETEs, and the leukotrienes.

   (1) 5-Lipoxygenase in association with 5-LOX activating protein (FLAP) produces 5-HPETEs, which are subsequently converted to 5-HETEs and then to leukotrienes.

   (2) 12-Lipoxygenase and 15-lipoxygenase produce 12-HPETEs and 15-HPETES, respectively, which are converted to corresponding HETEs.

c. Additional metabolites of the HPETEs, hepoxilins and lipoxins, have been identified, but their biologic role is unclear.

3. The eicosanoids all have short plasma half-lives (typically 0.5–5 min). Most catabolism occurs in the lung.

   a. Prostaglandins are metabolized by prostaglandin 15-OH dehydrogenase (PDGH) to 15-keto metabolites, which are excreted in the urine.

   b. **Thromboxane A$_2$ (TXA$_2$)** is rapidly hydrated to the less active TXB$_2$.

   c. **PGI$_2$** is hydrolyzed to 6-keto-PGF$_{1\alpha}$.

4. Various eicosanoids are synthesized throughout the body; synthesis can be very tissue specific:

   a. **PGI$_2$** is synthesized in endothelial and vascular smooth muscle cells.

   b. **Thromboxane** synthesis occurs primarily in platelets.

   c. **HPETEs, HETEs,** and the **leukotrienes** are synthesized predominantly in mast cells, white blood cells, airway epithelium, and platelets.

C. **Actions.** There is no universal mediator of eicosanoid action. A separate cell-surface receptor appears to mediate the activities of each class of metabolite. Virtually all of the known second-messenger systems have been implicated in the action of the eicosanoids, including stimulation or inhibition of cAMP and cGMP, and alterations in Ca^{2+} flux.

1. *Vascular smooth muscle*

   a. **PGE$_2$** and **PGI$_2$** are potent vasodilators in most vascular beds. **PGE$_2$** also antagonizes the effects of vasoconstrictor substances such as norepinephrine.

   b. **PGF$_{2\alpha}$** causes arteriolar vasodilation and constriction of superficial veins.

   c. **Thromboxane** is a potent vasoconstrictor.

2. *Inflammation*

   a. **PGE$_2$** and **PGI$_2$** cause an increase in blood flow and promote, but do not cause, edema. PGE also potentiates the effect of other inflammatory agents such as bradykinin.

   b. **HETEs** (5-HETE, 12-HETE, and 15-HETE) and **leukotrienes**, especially LTB4, cause chemotaxis of neutrophils and eosinophils.

3. *Bronchial smooth muscle*

   a. **PGFs** cause smooth muscle contraction.

   b. **PGEs** cause smooth muscle relaxation.

   c. **Leukotrienes** and **thromboxane** are potent bronchoconstrictors and are the most likely candidates for mediating allergic bronchospasm. The leukotrienes **LTC$_4$** and **LTD$_4$** are the components of **slow-reacting substance of anaphylaxis (SRS-A)** and are secreted in asthma an anaphylaxis.

4. *Uterine smooth muscle.* **PGE$_2$** and **PGF$_{2\alpha}$** cause contraction of uterine smooth muscle in pregnant women. The nonpregnant uterus has a more variable response to prostaglandins; **PGF$_{2\alpha}$** causes contraction, and **PGE2** causes relaxation.

5. *GI tract*

   a. **PGE$_2$** and **PGF$_{2\alpha}$** increase the rate of longitudinal contraction in the gut and decrease transit time.

   b. The **leukotrienes** are potent stimulators of GI smooth muscle.

   c. **PGE$_2$** and **PGI$_2$** inhibit acid and pepsinogen secretion in the stomach. In addition, prostaglandins increase mucus, water, and electrolyte secretion in the stomach and the intestine.

6. *Blood*

   a. **TXA$_2$** is a potent inducer of platelet aggregation.

   b. **PGI$_2$** and **PGE$_2$** inhibit platelet aggregation.

   c. **PGEs** induce erythropoiesis by stimulating the renal release of erythropoietin.

   d. **5-HPETE** stimulates release of histamine; **PGI$_2$** and **PGD** inhibit histamine release.

7. *Neurotransmission*
   a. **PGE2 and PGI2 sensitize peripheral nerve endings by increasing membrane excitability**. They are NOT direct nociceptive neurotransmitters.
   b. **Both COX1 and COX2 are expressed in the spinal cord and prostanoids decrease inhibitory GABA-nergic activity resulting in increased transmission of pain stimuli.**
   c. In the brain, prostaoids contribute to **allodynia**.

D. **Therapeutic uses**
   1. *Induction of labor at term.* Induction of labor is produced by infusion of **PGF$_{2\alpha}$** (carboprost tromethamine) (Hemabate) or **PGE$_2$** (dinoprostone) (Prostin E).
   2. *Therapeutic abortion.* Infusion of **carboprost tromethamine** or administration of vaginal suppositories containing **dinoprostone** is effective in inducing abortion in the second trimester. Currently, these prostaglandins are combined with **mifepristone (RU486)** to induce first-trimester abortion.
   3. *Maintenance of ductus arteriosus* is produced by **PGE$_1$** (Prostin VR) infusion; PGE$_1$ will maintain patency of the ductus arteriosus, which may be desirable before surgery.
   4. *Treatment of peptic ulcer.* **Misoprostol** (Cytotec), a methylated derivative of PGE$_1$, is approved for use in patients taking high doses of nonsteroidal anti-inflammatory drugs (NSAIDs) to reduce gastric ulceration.
   5. *Erectile dysfunction.* Alprostadil (PGE$_1$) can be injected directly into the corpus cavernosum or administered as a transurethral suppository to cause vasodilation and enhance tumescence.
   6. *Glaucoma.* Latanoprost, a PGF$_{2\alpha}$ analog and the similar bimatoprost and travoprost are the first-line agents for glaucoma. They reduce intraocular pressure by increasing the outflow of aqueous humor.
   7. *Pulmonary hypertension.* PGI$_2$ analogs are effective in treating pulmonary hypertension of several etiologies. Epoprostenol (IV infusion) and treprostinil (IV or subcutaneous injection), and iloprost (inhaled 6–9 times per day) are approved for this use.

E. **Adverse effects** of eicosanoids include local pain and irritation, bronchospasm, and GI disturbances, including nausea, vomiting, cramping, and diarrhea.

F. **Pharmacologic inhibition of eicosanoid synthesis**
   1. **Phospholipase A2-mediated** release of eicosanoic precursors, such as arachidonic acid, is inhibited by glucocorticoids, in part by the action of annexin-1 (lipocortin).
   2. **Aspirin** and most **NSAIDs** inhibit synthesis of prostaglandin G (PGG) and prostaglandin H (PGH) by their actions on the **COX pathways.** Aspirin can increase the synthesis of eicosanoids through the lipoxygenase pathway, perhaps by shunting biosynthesis towards the LOX pathway.
   3. **Eicosatetraenoic acid** is an arachidonic acid analog that inhibits both COX and lipoxygenase activity.
   4. Imidazole derivatives such as **dazoxiben** appear to inhibit thromboxane synthase preferentially.

V. NONSTEROIDAL ANTIINFLAMMATORY DRUGS (NSAIDS) (TABLE 6.4)

A. **An overview**
   1. The inflammatory response is complex, involving the immune system and the influence of various endogenous agents, including prostaglandins, bradykinin, histamine, chemotactic factors, and superoxide free radicals formed by the action of lysosomal enzymes.
   2. Aspirin, other salicylates, and newer drugs with diverse structures are referred to as **NSAIDs** to distinguish them from the anti-inflammatory glucocorticoids. NSAIDs are used to **suppress the symptoms of inflammation associated with rheumatic disease.** Some are also used to relieve **pain** (analgesic action) and **fever** (antipyretic action).

t a b l e **6.4**	Nonsteroidal and Analgesic Compounds and Their Therapeutic Effectiveness			
Chemical Class	Prototype	Analgesia	Antipyresis	Anti-inflammatory
Salicylates	Aspirin	+++	+++	+++
Para-aminophenols	Acetaminophen	+++	+++	Marginal
Indoles	Indomethacin	+++	++++	++++
Pyrrole acetic acids	Tolmetin, mefenamic acid	+++	+++	+++
Propionic acids	Ibuprofen, naproxen	++++	+++	++++
Enolic acids	Phenylbutazone, piroxicam	+++	+++	++++
Alkanones	Nabumetone	++	++	+++
Sulfonamide	Celecoxib	++++	+++	++++

B. Mechanism of action
  1. *Anti-inflammatory effect*
     a. The anti-inflammatory effect of NSAIDs is due to the inhibition of the enzymes that produce prostaglandin H (COX-1 and COX-2), in the conversion of arachidonic acid to **prostaglandins**, and to **TXA$_2$** and **prostacyclin**.
     b. Aspirin irreversibly inactivates COX-1 and COX-2 by acetylation of a specific serine residue. This distinguishes it from other NSAIDs, which reversibly inhibit COX-1 and COX-2.
     c. NSAIDs have no effect on lipoxygenase and therefore do not inhibit the production of leukotrienes.
     d. Additional anti-inflammatory mechanisms may include interference with the potentiative action of other mediators of inflammation (bradykinin, histamine, serotonin), modulation of T- cell function, stabilization of lysosomal membranes, and inhibition of chemotaxis.
  2. *Analgesic effect*
     a. PGE$_2$ and PGI$_2$ are the most important prostaglandins involved in pain. Inhibition of their synthesis is a primary mechanism of NSAID-mediated analgesia.
        (1) Prostaglandins sensitize pain receptors and processing; peripheral input via C and Aδ fibers and TRPV-1 Ca^{2+} channels
           – prostaglandin primary hyperalgesia
        (2) Afferent input processed in dorsal horn (prostaglandins inhibit GABA and glycine inhibitory interneurons)
           – prostaglandin secondary hyperalgesia
        (3) Prostaglandins produce changes in central pain processing that leads to **allodynia**: painful sensation caused by normally innocuous stimuli.
     b. NSAIDs prevent the potentiating action of prostaglandins on endogenous mediators of peripheral nerve stimulation (e.g., bradykinin).
  3. *Antipyretic effect.* The antipyretic effect of NSAIDs is believed to be related to inhibition of production of prostaglandins induced by interleukin-1 (IL-1) and interleukin-6 (IL-6) in the hypothalamus and the "resetting" of the thermoregulatory system, leading to vasodilatation and increased heat loss.

C. Therapeutic uses
  1. *Inflammation*
     a. NSAIDs are first-line drugs used to arrest inflammation and the accompanying pain of rheumatic and nonrheumatic diseases, including **rheumatoid arthritis, juvenile arthritis, osteoarthritis, psoriatic arthritis, ankylosing spondylitis, Reiter syndrome,** and **dysmenorrhea.** Pain and inflammation of bursitis and tendonitis also respond to NSAIDs.
     b. NSAIDs do not significantly reverse the progress of rheumatic disease; rather they slow destruction of cartilage and bone and allow patients increased mobility and use of their joints.

    c. Treatment of chronic inflammation requires the use of these agents at doses well above those used for analgesia and antipyresis; consequently, the incidence of adverse drug effects is increased. Drug selection is generally dictated by the patient's ability to tolerate the adverse effects, and the cost of the drugs.

    d. Anti-inflammatory effects may develop only after several weeks of treatment.

2. *Analgesia.* NSAIDs **alleviate mild-to-moderate pain** by decreasing PGE_2- and PGI_2, which are hyperalgesic in the periphery and centrally. They are less effective than opioids, and they are more effective against pain associated with integumental structures (pain of muscular and vascular origin, arthritis, and bursitis) than with pain associated with the viscera.

3. *Antipyresis.* NSAIDs **reduce elevated body temperature** with little effect on normal body temperature.

4. *Miscellaneous uses.* Aspirin **reduces** the **formation of thrombi** and is used prophylactically to reduce recurrent transient ischemia, unstable angina, and the incidence of thrombosis after coronary artery bypass grafts.

D. Aspirin (acetylsalicylic acid) and nonacetylated salicylates include sodium salicylate, magnesium salicylate, choline salicylate, sodium thiosalicylate, sulfasalazine (Azulfidine), mesalamine (Asacol), and salsalate.

1. *Pharmacologic properties*

    a. Salicylates are weak organic acids; **aspirin** has a pK_a of 3.5.

    b. These agents are rapidly absorbed from the intestine as well as from the stomach, where the low pH favors absorption. The rate of absorption is increased with rapidly dissolving (buffered) or predissolved (effervescent) dosage forms.

    c. Salicylates are hydrolyzed rapidly by plasma and tissue esterases to acetic acid and the active metabolite **salicylic acid.** Salicylic acid is more slowly oxidized to gentisic acid and conjugated with glycine to **salicyluric acid** and to ether and ester glucuronides.

    d. Salicylates have a $t_{1/2}$ of 3–6 hours after short-term administration. Long-term administration of high doses (to treat arthritis) or toxic overdose increases the $t_{1/2}$ to 15–30 hours because the enzymes for glycine and glucuronide conjugation become saturated.

    e. Unmetabolized salicylates are excreted by the kidney. If the urine pH increases to above 8, clearance is increased approximately fourfold as a result of decreased reabsorption of the ionized salicylate from the tubules.

2. *Therapeutic uses*

    a. Salicylates are used to treat **rheumatoid arthritis, juvenile arthritis,** and **osteoarthritis,** as well as other inflammatory disorders. 5-Amino salicylates (mesalamine, sulfasalazine) can be used to treat **Crohn's disease.**

    b. Salicylic acid is used **topically** to treat **plantar warts, fungal infections,** and **corns; its** use is based on the destruction of keratinocytes and dermal epithelia by the free acid.

    c. Aspirin has significantly greater antithrombotic activity than other NSAIDs and is useful in preventing or reducing the risk of myocardial infarction in patients with a history of myocardial infarction, angina, cardiac surgery, and cerebral or peripheral vascular disease.

3. *Adverse effects*

    a. GI effects

        (1) GI effects are the most common adverse effects of high-dose **aspirin** use (70% of patients); these effects may include nausea, vomiting, diarrhea, constipation, dyspepsia, epigastric pain, bleeding, and ulceration of stomach, duodenum, and small intestine.

        (2) These GI effects are thought to be due to a direct chemical effect on gastric cells and a decrease in the production and cytoprotective activity of prostaglandins, which leads to gastric tissue susceptibility to damage by hydrochloric acid.

        (3) The GI effects may contraindicate **aspirin** use in patients with an active ulcer. Aspirin may be taken with prostaglandins to reduce gastric damage.

(4) Substitution of enteric-coated or timed-release preparations, or the use of **nonacetylated salicylates,** may decrease gastric irritation. Gastric irritation is not prevented by using buffered tablets.

b. Hypersensitivity (intolerance)

(1) Hypersensitivity is relatively **uncommon with the use of aspirin** (0.3% of patients); hypersensitivity results in rash, bronchospasm, rhinitis, edema, or an anaphylactic reaction with shock, which may be life-threatening. The incidence of intolerance is highest in patients with asthma, nasal polyps, recurrent rhinitis, or urticaria. Aspirin should be avoided in such patients.

(2) **Cross-hypersensitivity** may exist to other **NSAIDs** and to the yellow dye tartrazine, which is used in many pharmaceutical preparations.

(3) Hypersensitivity is not associated with **sodium salicylate** or **magnesium salicylate.**

(4) The use of **aspirin** and other **salicylates** to control fever during viral infections (influenza and chickenpox) in children and adolescents is associated with an increased incidence of **Reye syndrome,** an illness characterized by vomiting, hepatic disturbances, and encephalopathy that has a 35% mortality rate. **Acetaminophen** is recommended as a substitute for children with **fever of unknown etiology.**

c. Miscellaneous adverse effects and contraindications

(1) Salicylates occasionally **decrease** the **glomerular filtration rate,** particularly in patients with renal insufficiency.

(2) Salicylates occasionally produce **mild hepatitis,** usually asymptomatic, particularly in patients with systemic lupus erythematosus, juvenile or adult rheumatoid arthritis, or rheumatic fever.

(3) These agents **prolong bleeding time. Aspirin** irreversibly inhibits platelet COX-1 and COX-2 and, thereby, **TXA$_2$** production, suppressing platelet adhesion and aggregation. The use of salicylates is contraindicated in patients with bleeding disorders, such as hypothrombinemia, hemophilia, hepatic disease, and vitamin K deficiency, and use should be avoided in patients receiving anticoagulants such as coumarin and **heparin.**

(4) Salicylates are not recommended during pregnancy; they may induce **postpartum hemorrhage** and lead to **premature closure** of the **fetal ductus arteriosus.**

4. Drug interactions

a. The **action of anticoagulants** may be enhanced by their displacement by aspirin from binding sites on serum albumin. Aspirin also displaces **tolbutamide, phenytoin,** and other drugs from their plasma protein-binding sites.

b. The hypoglycemic action of **sulfonylureas** may be enhanced by displacement from their binding sites on serum albumin or by inhibition of their renal tubular secretion by aspirin.

c. Usual analgesic doses of **aspirin** (<2 g/day) decrease renal excretion of **sodium urate** and antagonize the uricosuric effect of **sulfinpyrazone** and **probenecid; aspirin** is contraindicated in patients with gout who are taking uricosuric agents.

d. Antacids may alter the absorption of **aspirin.**

e. Aspirin competes for tubular secretion with **penicillin G** and prolongs its half-life.

f. Corticosteroids increase renal clearance of **salicylates.**

g. Alcohol may increase GI bleeding when taken with aspirin.

5. Toxicity

a. Aspirin toxicity is dose-dependent and effects are determined by plasma drug levels.

b. In adults, **salicylism** (tinnitus, hearing loss, vertigo) occurs as initial sign of toxicity after **aspirin** or **salicylate overdose** or poisoning.

c. In children, the common signs of toxicity include **hyperventilation** and **acidosis,** with accompanying lethargy and hyperpnea.

d. Disturbance of acid–base balance results in **metabolic acidosis** in infants and young children and in **compensated respiratory alkalosis** in older children and adults. **Salicylate toxicity** initially increases the medullary response to carbon dioxide, with resulting hyperventilation and respiratory alkalosis. In infants and young children, increases in lactic acid and ketone body production result in metabolic acidosis. With increased severity of toxicity, respiratory depression occurs, with accompanying respiratory acidosis.

   e. The uncoupling of oxidative phosphorylation by **aspirin** results in **hyperthermia** and **hypoglycemia,** particularly in infants and young children. Nausea, vomiting, tachycardia, hyperpnea, dehydration, and coma may develop.

   f. **Treatment** includes correction of acid–base disturbances, replacement of electrolytes and fluids, cooling, alkalinization of urine with bicarbonate to reduce salicylate reabsorption, forced diuresis, and gastric lavage or emesis.

E. Other NSAIDs
   1. An o*verview*
      a. Like aspirin, these agents are used for the treatment of **inflammation** associated with rheumatic and nonrheumatic diseases.
      b. NSAIDs are absorbed rapidly after oral administration. These agents are extensively bound to plasma proteins, especially albumin. They cause drug interactions due to the displacement of other agents, particularly anticoagulants, from serum albumin; these interactions are similar to those seen with **aspirin.**
      c. NSAIDs are metabolized in the liver and excreted by the kidney; the half-lives of these agents vary greatly (from 1 to 45 h, with most between 10 and 20 h). The required frequency of administration may influence drug choice because of possible problems with compliance.
      d. These agents commonly produce **GI disturbances;** they demonstrate **cross-sensitivity with aspirin** and with each other. Other adverse effects, such as hypersensitivity, are generally the same as for aspirin; the cautions and contraindications are also similar to those for aspirin.
      e. NSAIDs are associated with nondose-related instances of acute renal failure and nephrotic syndrome, and they may lead to renal toxicity in combination with angiotensin-converting enzyme inhibitors. **Indomethacin, meclofenamate, tolmetin,** and **phenylbutazone** are generally more toxic than other NSAIDs.
   2. *Ibuprofen, naproxen (Naprosyn, Aleve), fenoprofen (Nalfon), and ketoprofen (Orudis)*
      a. These agents are propionic acid derivatives; ibuprofen can be administered IV.
      b. There is no reported interaction of **ibuprofen** or **ketoprofen** with anticoagulants. **Fenoprofen** has been reported to induce **nephrotoxic syndrome.**
      c. Long-term use of ibuprofen is associated with an increased incidence of hypertension in women.
   3. *Sulindac (clinoril), tolmetin (tolectin), and ketorolac (toradol)*
      a. Sulindac and tolmetin are pyrrole acetic acid derivatives. **Sulindac** is a prodrug that is oxidized to a sulfone and then to the active sulfide, which has a relatively long $t_{1/2}$ (16 h) because of enterohepatic cycling.
      b. **Tolmetin** has minimal effect on platelet aggregation; it is associated with a higher incidence of anaphylaxis than other NSAIDs. Tolmetin has a relatively short $t_{1/2}$ (1 h).
      c. **Ketorolac** is a potent analgesic with moderate anti-inflammatory activity that can be administered IV or topically in an ophthalmic solution.
   4. *Indomethacin (indocin)*
      a. Indomethacin is the drug of choice for treatment of **ankylosing spondylitis** and **Reiter syndrome;** it is also used for acute gouty arthritis.
      b. Indomethacin is also used to speed the closure of **patent ductus arteriosus** in premature infants (otherwise it is not used in children); it inhibits the production of prostaglandins which prevent closure of the ductus.
      c. Indomethacin is not recommended as a simple analgesic or antipyretic because of the potential for severe adverse effects.
      d. Bleeding, ulceration, and other adverse effects are more likely with **indomethacin** than with most other NSAIDs. Headache is a common adverse effect; tinnitus, dizziness, or confusion also occasionally occurs.

5. *Piroxicam (Feldene)*
   a. Piroxicam is an oxicam derivative of enolic acid.
   b. Piroxicam has $t_{1/2}$ of 45 hours.
   c. Like **aspirin** and **indomethacin, bleeding** and **ulceration** are more likely with piroxicam than with other NSAIDs.
6. *Meclofenamate (Meclomen) and mefenamic acid (Ponstel)*
   a. Meclofenamate and mefenamic acid have $t_{1/2}$ of 2 hours.
   b. A relatively high incidence of GI disturbances is associated with these agents.
7. *Nabumetone (Relafen)*
   a. Nabumetone is another chemical class of **NSAIDs,** but it has **similar effects.**
   b. Compared with NSAIDs, nabumetone is associated with **reduced inhibition of platelet function** and **reduced incidence of GI bleeding.**
   c. Nabumetone inhibits COX-2 more than COX-1.
8. *Other NSAIDs* include flurbiprofen (Ansaid), diclofenac (Voltaren), and etodolac (Lodine). Flurbiprofen is also available for topical ophthalmic use.
9. *COX-2 selective agents*
   a. Several agents, celecoxib (Celebrex), rofecoxib (Vioxx), valdecoxib (Bextra), that inhibit COX-2 more than COX-1 have been developed and approved for use. The relative COX-2/COX-1 specificity of these agents is about 10, 35, and 30, respectively. Rofecoxib and valdecoxib are no longer marketed.
   b. The rationale behind the development of these drugs was that inhibition of COX-2 would reduce the inflammatory response and pain but not inhibit the cytoprotective action of prostaglandins in the stomach, which is largely mediated by COX-1.
   c. Concern has arisen due to a doubling in the incidence of heart attack and stroke in patients taking rofecoxib and valdecoxib. This appears to be class-wide adverse effect, but only rofecoxib and valdecoxib have been removed from the market. Valdecoxib has also been associated with serious adverse skin reactions. One possible explanation, as illustrated in Figure 6.3, is that inhibition of COX-2-mediated production of the vasodilator PGI_2 by endothelial cells, while not affecting the prothrombotic actions of COX-1 in platelets, increases the chance of blood clots.
   d. While the incidence of GI adverse effects is reduced with COX-2 selective inhibitors (especially the frequency of endoscopically detected microerosions), there have still been occurrences of serious GI adverse effects with these agents.
   e. Celecoxib remains on the market and is approved for osteoarthritis and rheumatoid arthritis; pain including bone pain, dental pain, and headache; and ankylosing spondylitis.

F. **Other anti-inflammatory drugs** are used in the more advanced stages of some rheumatoid diseases.
   1. *Aurothioglucose (Solganal), gold sodium thiomalate (Myochrysine), and auranofin (Ridaura)*
      a. Aurothioglucose, gold sodium thiomalate, and auranofin are gold compounds that may **retard** the **destruction of bone and joints** by an unknown mechanism.
      b. These agents have long latency.
      c. **Aurothioglucose** and **gold sodium thiomalate** are administered intramuscularly (IM). **Auranofin** is administered orally and is 95% bound to plasma proteins.
      d. These agents can produce **serious GI disturbances, dermatitis,** and **mucous membrane lesions.** Less common effects include hematologic disorders such as aplastic anemia and proteinuria, with occasional nephrotic syndrome.
   2. *Penicillamine (Cuprimine, Depen)*
      a. Penicillamine is a chelating drug (will chelate gold) that is a metabolite of **penicillin.**
      b. Penicillamine has **Immunosuppressant activity,** but its mechanism of action is unknown.
      c. This agent has long latency.
      d. The incidence of severe adverse effects is high; these effects are similar to those of the gold compounds.

FIGURE 6.3. COX-2 inhibition and increased risk of cardiovascular accident.

3. *Methotrexate*
   a. Methotrexate is an antineoplastic drug used for **rheumatoid arthritis** in patients who do not respond well to NSAIDs or glucocorticoids.
   b. Methotrexate commonly produces **hepatotoxicity.**
4. *Chloroquine and hydrochloroquine (Plaquenil)*
   a. Chloroquine and hydrochloroquine are **antimalarial drugs.**
   b. These agents have immunosuppressant activity, but their mechanism of action is unknown.
   c. Used to treat joint pain associated with lupus and arthritis.
5. *Adrenocorticosteroids*

G. **Nonopioid analgesics and antipyretics**
   1. *An overview*
      a. **Aspirin, NSAIDs,** and **acetaminophen** are useful for the treatment of mild-to-moderate pain associated with integumental structures, including **pain of muscles and joints, postpartum pain,** and **headache.**
      b. These agents have **antipyretic activity** and, **except for acetaminophen,** have anti-inflammatory activity at higher doses.
      c. These agents act by an unknown mechanism to reduce pain and temperature. Their peripherally mediated analgesic activity and centrally mediated antipyretic activity are correlated with the inhibition of prostaglandin synthesis.

2. *Acetaminophen*
   a. Unlike aspirin and other NSAIDs, acetaminophen does not displace other drugs from plasma proteins; it causes minimal gastric irritation, has little effect on platelet adhesion and aggregation, and does not block the effect of uricosuric drugs on uric acid secretion.
   b. Acetaminophen has no significant anti-inflammatory or antiuricosuric activity.
   c. Acetaminophen is administered orally and is rapidly absorbed. It is metabolized by hepatic microsomal enzymes to sulfate and glucuronide.
   d. Acetaminophen is a **substitute for aspirin** to treat mild-to-moderate pain for selected patients who are intolerant to aspirin, have a history of peptic ulcer or hemophilia, are using anticoagulants or a uricosuric drug to manage gout, or are at risk for Reye syndrome. Acetaminophen can be administered in pregnancy with greater safety than aspirin.
   e. Overdose with acetaminophen results in accumulation of a minor metabolite, N-acetyl-p-benzoquinone, which is responsible for hepatotoxicity. When the enzymes for glucuronide and sulfate conjugation of acetaminophen and the reactive metabolite become saturated, an alternative glutathione conjugation pathway (cytochrome P-450 dependent) becomes more important. If hepatic glutathione is depleted, such as may occur with alcohol consumption, the reactive metabolite accumulates and may cause hepatic damage by interaction with cellular macromolecules, such as DNA and RNA. Overdose is treated by emesis or gastric lavage and oral administration of **N-acetylcysteine** within 1 day to neutralize the metabolite and increase biosynthesis of glutathione.
   f. Long-term use of acetaminophen has been associated with a threefold increase in kidney disease; and women taking more than 500 mg/day had a doubling in the incidence of hypertension.

H. **Disease-modifying antiarthritic drugs**
   1. *Tumor necrosis factor (TNF)* plays an important causative role in rheumatoid arthritis, and this has led to development of drugs that specifically target this ligand or its receptor to treat the disease. TNF-α is responsible for inducing IL-1 and IL-6 and other cytokines that further the disease.
   2. *Anti-TNF-α drugs* (Table 6.5)

t a b l e **6.5** Selected Disease-Modifying Anti-Rheumatic Drugs

Drug	Characteristic	Molecular Target	Use
Adalimumab	Anti-TNF-α antibody	Plasma and tissue TNF-α	Rheumatoid arthritis
Infliximab	Anti-TNF-α antibody	Plasma and tissue TNF-α	Rheumatoid arthritis, Crohn's disease, uveitis, psoriasis
Certolizumab	Pegolated Anti-TNF-α antibody	Plasma and tissue TNF-α	Crohn's disease, rheumatoid arthritis
Golimumab	Anti-TNF-α antibody	Plasma and tissue TNF-α	RA, AS, psoriatic arthritis
Etanercept	TNF-receptor fusion protein	Plasma and tissue TNF-α	Rheumatoid arthritis, psoriasis
Anakinra	Recombinant IL-1a	Interleukin-1	Rheumatoid arthritis
Abatacept	CTLA4 (CD152) fusion protein	T cells	Rheumatoid arthritis
Rituximab	Anti CD20 antibody	B cells	Rheumatoid arthritis, leukemia, lymphoma
Tocilizumab	Anti IL-6 receptor antibody	Leukocyte and mesenchymal IL-6R	Rheumatoid arthritis
Natalizumab	Anti-α4 integrin	Intestinal and endothelial Adherence junctions	Multiple sclerosis, Crohn's disease

a. **Infliximab** (Remicade) is a recombinant antibody with human constant and murine variable regions that specifically binds TNF-α, thereby blocking its action.

   (1) Approved for use for rheumatoid arthritis, Crohn's disease, psoriasis, and other autoimmune diseases.

   (2) Administered by IV infusion at 2-week intervals initially and repeated at 6 and 8 weeks.

b. **Adalimumab** (Humira) is approved for the treatment of rheumatoid arthritis. It is a humanized (no murine components) anti-TNF-α antibody administered subcutaneously every other week.

c. **Etanercept** (Enbrel) is a fusion protein composed of the ligand-binding pocket of a TNF-α receptor fused to an IgG1 Fc fragment. The fusion protein has two TNF-binding sites per IgG molecule and is administered subcutaneously weekly.

d. The most serious adverse effect with these drugs is **infection** including tuberculosis, immunogenicity, and lymphoma. Injection site infections are common.

3. *Anti IL-1 drugs.* **Anakinra** (Kineret) is a recombinant protein essentially identical to IL-1a, a soluble antagonist of IL-1 that binds to the IL-1 receptor but does not trigger a biologic response. Anakinra is a competitive antagonist of the IL-1 receptor. It is approved for use for the treatment of rheumatoid arthritis. It has a relatively short half-life and must be administered subcutaneously daily.

I. Other immunosuppressive biologicals

1. Alefacept (Amevive)

   a. Alefacept is a recombinant fusion protein composed of the extracellular domain of LFA-3 and a portion of human IgG heavy chain. This protein acts as an antagonist of the LFA-3/CD2 interaction and causes a marked decrease in the number of CD2 T cells.

   b. Alefacept is administered IV or IM.

   c. Treatment with alefacept has demonstrated a rapid improvement and lessening of the severity of **psoriasis,** a disease with an autoimmune component.

2. Rituximab (Rituxan)

   a. Rituximab is an engineered monoclonal antibody to **CD20,** a B-lymphocyte differentiation antigen on pre-B and mature B-lymphocytes. Rituximab binding to the surface of B-cells results in their destruction.

   b. Rituximab, in combination with methotrexate, is approved for use in rheumatoid arthritis unresponsive to other therapies. It is also approved for treating refractory or large B-cell non-Hodgkin lymphoma.

3. Abatacept (Orencia)

   a. T-cell activation requires co-stimulation by an antigen presenting cell. **Abatacept blocks the co-stimulatory signal**. It is a fusion protein consisting of a portion of human CTLA4 and a fragment of the Fc domain of human IgG1. Abatacept mimics endogenous CTLA4 and competes with CD28 for CD80 and CD86 binding. This prevents complete T-cell activation, reduces T-cell proliferation, and reduces plasma cytokine levels.

   b. **Abatacept** is approved for use in rheumatoid arthritis.

   c. The most common side effect with its use is **infection.**

4. Efalizumab (Raptiva)

   a. **Efalizumab** is a monoclonal antibody that binds to CD11a of T cells. A component of T-cell activation is an interaction of CD-11a with ICAM-1. Efalizumab binding to T cells prevents their activation without their destruction.

   b. Efalizumab has proven effective in treating psoriasis. Its most adverse effects are nausea, headache, chills, and fever.

5. Tocilizumab (Actemra)

   a. Tocilizumab is a monoclonal antibody against the human IL-6 receptor. IL-6 is a potent inflammatory cytokine involved in the pathogenesis of several autoimmune diseases including rheumatoid arthritis, multiple myeloma, and prostate cancer.

   b. **Tocilizumab** is approved for use in juvenile idiopathic arthritis.

    c. Most common adverse effect is upper respiratory tract infection (10%).

  6. Natalizumab (Tysabri)

    a. Tysabri is a monoclonal antibody against $\alpha4$-integrin, a cell adhesion molecule that participates in cell–cell and cell–ECM interactions. It is infused every 4 weeks and is thought to reduce the penetration of immune cells through the cells lining the intestine and through the blood–brain barrier.

    b. The drug is useful in multiple sclerosis and Crohn's disease.

    c. It has been associated in several patients with the development of the neurological disorder progressive multifocal leukoencephalopathy (PML), especially when co-administered with α-interferon.

VI. DRUGS USED FOR GOUT

A. Gout

  1. Gout is a familial disease characterized by recurrent hyperuricemia and arthritis with severe pain; it is caused by **deposits of uric acid** (the end-product of purine metabolism) in joints, cartilage, and the kidney. Serum urate in excess of 6 mg/dL is associated with gout.

  2. Acute gout is treated with nonsalicylate NSAIDs, particularly **indomethacin,** or with **colchicine.**

  3. Chronic gout is treated with the uricosuric agent **probenecid** or **sulfinpyrazone,** which increases the elimination of uric acid, or **febuxostat** or **allopurinol,** which inhibit uric acid production.

  4. Serious gout refractory to the above treatments can be treated with **pegloticase**, a recombinant uricase that is administered by infusion.

B. Colchicine

  1. Colchicine is an alkaloid with anti-inflammatory properties; it is used for relief of inflammation and pain in **acute gouty arthritis.** Reduction of inflammation and relief from pain occur 12–24 hours after oral administration.

  2. The mechanism of action in acute gout is unclear. Colchicine prevents polymerization of tubulin into microtubules and inhibits leukocyte migration and phagocytosis. Colchicine also inhibits cell mitosis.

  3. The adverse effects after oral administration, which occur in 80% of patients at a dose near that necessary to relieve gout, include **nausea, vomiting, abdominal pain,** and particularly **diarrhea.** IV administration reduces the risk of GI disturbances and provides faster relief (6–12 hours) but increases the risk of sloughing skin and subcutaneous tissue. Higher doses may (rarely) result in liver damage and blood dyscrasias.

C. NSAIDs

  1. Historically, **indomethacin** has been the NSAID most often used to treat **acute gout** attacks; however, because they have fewer adverse effects, the use of **naproxen** and **sulindac** is increasing.

  2. NSAIDs are preferred to the more disease-specific colchicine because of the diarrhea associated with the use of colchicine.

D. Probenecid

  1. Probenecid is an organic acid that reduces urate levels by acting at the anionic transport site in the renal tubule **to prevent reabsorption of uric acid.**

  2. These agents are used for **chronic gout,** often in combination with **colchicine.**

  3. Probenecid and sulfinpyrazone undergo rapid oral absorption.

  4. These agents inhibit the excretion of other drugs that are actively secreted by renal tubules, including **penicillin,** NSAIDs, cephalosporins, and **methotrexate.** Dose reduction of these drugs may be warranted.

5. Increased urinary concentration of uric acid may result in the formation of urate stones (**urolithiasis**). This risk is decreased with the ingestion of large volumes of fluid or alkalinization of urine with potassium citrate.

6. Low doses of uricosuric agents and salicylates inhibit uric acid secretion. Aspirin is contraindicated in gout.

7. Common adverse effects include **GI disturbances** and **dermatitis;** rarely, these agents cause blood dyscrasias.

E. **Allopurinol (Lopurin, Zyloprim) and Febuxostat (Uloric)**

1. Allopurinol is used prophylactically to treat **chronic, tophaceous gout** because it reduces the size of the established tophi; **colchicine** is administered concomitantly during the first week of therapy to prevent gouty arthritis.

2. Allopurinol inhibits the synthesis of uric acid by inhibiting **xanthine oxidase,** an enzyme that converts hypoxanthine to xanthine and xanthine to uric acid. Allopurinol is metabolized by xanthine oxidase to alloxanthine, which also inhibits xanthine oxidase. Allopurinol also inhibits de novo purine synthesis.

3. Allopurinol commonly produces **GI disturbances** and **dermatitis.** This agent more rarely causes hypersensitivity, including fever, hepatic dysfunction, and blood dyscrasias. Allopurinol should be used with caution in patients with liver disease or bone marrow depression.

4. **Febuxostat also inhibits xanthine oxidase** but is more specific in its action.

F. **Pegloticase (Krystexxa)**

1. Humans (and great apes) do not have functional uricase as do other mammals. Uricase converts uric acid to the water-soluble allantoin. **Pegloticase** is a recombinant form of porcine uricase that is also pegylated to slow its degradation.

2. **Pegloticase** can reduce serum urate in a matter of hours. It is approved for use in patients with gout who have been unresponsive to other drug therapies.

3. The most serious side effect with pegloticase s serious allergic reactions.

VII. IMMUNOSUPPRESSIVE AGENTS

A. **Inhibition of immune response**

1. *Nonspecific inhibition.* **Azathioprine, cyclophosphamide,** and **methotrexate** suppress immune function by their cytotoxic action achieved through a variety of mechanisms, particularly by inhibition of DNA synthesis. Generally, immunosuppressive activity is achieved at nearly toxic doses.

2. *Specific inhibition* (Fig. 6.4). **Glucocorticoids, cyclosporine, tacrolimus** (Prograf), and **sirolimus** (rapamycin) (Rapamune) inhibit the activation or actions of specific cells of the immune system and are generally less toxic than the nonspecific agents.

3. *Suppression* of the immune system increases the risk of opportunistic viral, bacterial, and fungal infections.

4. *Development of tolerance.* To overcome an allergic reaction, small quantities of antigen are administered gradually to develop tolerance, most probably as a result of the induction of IgG antibodies to neutralize a subsequent IgE reaction with the allergen.

B. **Use of immunosuppressive agents**

1. Immunosuppressive agents are used to treat syndromes or diseases that reflect **imbalances in the immune system,** including rheumatoid arthritis, systemic lupus erythematosus, inflammatory bowel disease, chronic active hepatitis, lipoid nephrosis, Goodpasture syndrome, and autoimmune hemolytic anemia.

2. Immunosuppressive agents are also used to **prevent allograft rejection,** which results when cytotoxic T lymphocytes develop in response to incompatible transplanted organs.

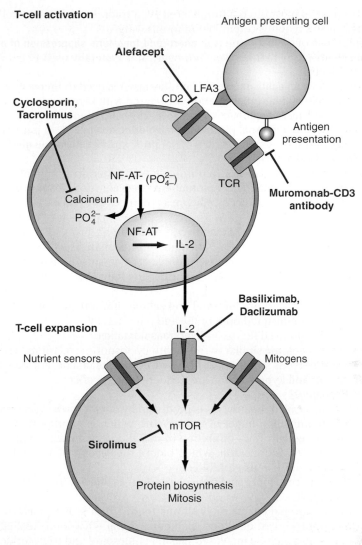

FIGURE 6.4. Sites of action of immunomodulators.

C. Individual agents

1. Glucocorticoids

a. Glucocorticoids are thought to interfere with the cell cycle of activated lymphoid cells and stimulate apoptosis in some lymphoid lineages. Glucocorticoids mainly affect T-cells but chronic use causes a reduction in antibody production as well.

b. Glucocorticoids are used for a wide variety of immunologically mediated diseases.

c. Glucocorticoids are important agents in suppressing allograft rejection; they are often used in **combination** with either **cyclosporine** or a cytotoxic agent.

2. Cyclosporine (Sandimmune, Neoral)

a. **Cyclosporine** is a potent immunosuppressive cyclic polypeptide that binds to **cyclophilin** and inhibits T-helper cell activation, mostly by the nuclear translocation of the transcription factor NF-AT and subsequently by the production of interleukin-2 and the first phase of T-cell activation.

b. Cyclosporine has variable absorption from the GI tract (20–50%). Doses must be established by monitoring the blood levels. Cyclosporine has a biphasic $t_{1/2}$, with a terminal phase of 10–25 hours; it is metabolized in the liver and eliminated primarily in bile.

    c. Cyclosporine is most often administered IV; a microemulsion (Neoral) permits oral dosing but still requires careful blood monitoring.

    d. The main use of cyclosporine is in **short- and long-term suppression of organ rejection in transplants** of the kidney, liver, and heart. It is generally used in combination with glucocorticoids.

    e. **Cyclosporine as an ophthalmic emulsion** (Restasis) is used to increase tear production in patients with ocular inflammation associated with keratoconjunctivitis sicca.

    f. Cyclosporine causes **nephrotoxicity** in 25%–75% of patients, with a reduction in glomerular filtration and renal plasma flow; **hypertension** in 30% of patients; neurotoxicity (tremor and seizures) in 5%–50% of patients; and **hirsutism** and **gingival hyperplasia** in 10%–30% of patients.

    g. Cyclosporine is synergistically nephrotoxic with other drugs that affect kidney function. Inhibition of hepatic microsomal enzymes elevates plasma concentration; the induction of drug-metabolizing enzymes enhances clearance.

3. *Tacrolimus (FK-506) (Prograf)*

    a. Tacrolimus is produced by *Streptomyces tsukubaensis*. Like cyclosporine, it decreases the activity of **calcineurin,** a Ca^{2+}-dependent phosphatase, which leads to a decrease in nuclear NF-AT and the transcription of T-cell-specific lymphokines and early T-cell activation. Inhibition of calcineurin is mediated by tacrolimus binding to **FKBP** (FK-binding protein).

    b. Tacrolimus decreases both humoral and cellular immune responses.

    c. This agent is administered both orally and parenterally.

    d. Tacrolimus is approved for use in **liver transplantation.**

    e. The adverse effects are similar to those with cyclosporine; tacrolimus can damage the kidneys and nervous system, manifest by tremors, headache, and renal impairment. Hypertension and hyperkalemia are frequent adverse effects.

4. *Sirolimus (Rapamune)*

    a. Sirolimus (also called rapamycin) is produced by *Streptomyces hygroscopius*. It inhibits mTOR (mammalian target of rapamycin), which is an important component of several signaling pathways. Inhibition of mTOR interferes with protein biosynthesis and delays the G_1–S transition, which blocks the second phase of T-cell activation; B-cell differentiation is also inhibited.

    b. Sirolimus is approved for renal transplantation; its efficacy in liver transplant has not been determined.

    c. Many of the adverse effects of sirolimus follow from growth factor inhibition and include suppression of all blood elements, impaired wound healing, and rashes; metabolic effects include increased plasma cholesterol and triglycerides.

5. *Azathioprine (Imuran)*

    a. Azathioprine is a cytotoxic agent that suppresses T-cell activity to a greater degree than B-cell activity. Azathioprine also inhibits the proliferation of promyelocytes in the marrow. It is S-phase specific.

    b. Azathioprine is metabolized to **mercaptopurine,** which is also immunosuppressive.

    c. Azathioprine is most effective when given just after an immunologic challenge. This agent may enhance antibody response if given before a challenge. Azathioprine is not effective on established responses.

    d. Azathioprine can be administered orally. It is eliminated mainly by metabolic degradation by **xanthine oxidase.** Dose reduction is necessary when azathioprine is administered with **allopurinol or febuxostat,** which inhibit xanthine oxidase activity.

    e. Azathioprine is used with **prednisone** in **transplantation procedures** and in some diseases of the immune system, including **systemic lupus erythematosus** and **rheumatoid arthritis.**

    f. The major adverse effect associated with this agent is bone marrow suppression. At higher doses, occasional nausea and vomiting, GI disturbances, and hepatic dysfunction occur.

6. *Cyclophosphamide (Cytoxan, Neosar)*

    a. Cyclophosphamide is an alkylating agent developed as an anticancer drug.

    b. Cyclophosphamide suppresses B lymphocytes to a greater degree than T cells.

    c. This agent is the drug of choice in the treatment of **Wegener granulomatosis;** it is also used in severe cases of **rheumatoid arthritis** and other autoimmune disorders.

    d. Cyclophosphamide causes adverse effects that include cystitis and cardiomyopathy.

7. *Methotrexate (Folex, Mexate)*

    a. Methotrexate is an anticancer agent that has immunosuppressive action.

    b. Methotrexate inhibits replication and function of T cells and possibly B cells.

    c. Methotrexate has been used for **graft rejection** and for autoimmune and inflammatory diseases.

    d. This agent has also proved beneficial in the treatment of **severe psoriasis** that is refractory to other agents.

    e. Hepatotoxicity is the major adverse effect.

8. *Mycophenolate mofetil*

    a. Mycophenolate mofetil is hydrolyzed to mycophenolic acid, which inhibits T- and B-cell responses by inhibiting the synthesis of purines.

    b. It is useful in organ transplant patients, especially those intolerant of cyclosporine or tacrolimus. It has also been used in lupus, rheumatoid arthritis, and inflammatory bowel disease.

    c. Toxicities are mostly GI disturbances, headache, and reversible neutropenia.

9. *Thalidomide*

    a. Thalidomide was used as a sedative in the 1960s and removed from the market due to horrible teratogenic effects if administered during pregnancy. **Thalidomide does have significant immunomodulatory actions.**

    b. Thalidomide increases IL-10, decreases TNF-α activity, decreases cellular adhesion molecules, and enhances cell-mediated immunity.

    c. Thalidomide is used for multiple myeloma, myelogenous leukemia, solid tumors such as colon and prostate cancer.

10. *Immunosuppressive antibody reagents*

    a. *Antithymocyte globulin (Atgam)*

        (1) Polygonal antibodies raised against human thymic lymphocytes.

        (2) Following intravenous administration, T lymphocytes are removed from the circulation, resulting in decreased T-cell-mediated immune response.

        (3) Used to treat allograft rejection and to prevent rejection.

        (4) Adverse effects include serum sickness and nephritis.

    b. *Muromonab-CD3 antibody (Orthoclone OKT3)*

        (1) Monoclonal antibodies that recognize the CD3 surface glycoprotein on T lymphocytes.

        (2) Attachment of antibodies to CD3 impairs antigen recognition by T cells.

        (3) Following IV administration, T-cell levels fall rapidly and immune responses are impaired.

        (4) Used to prevent acute allograft rejection.

        (5) Adverse effects include cytokine release syndrome, anaphylactoid reactions, and CNS toxicity.

    c. *Basiliximab (Simulect) and daclizumab (Zenapax)*

        (1) Both are monoclonal antibodies against CD25, one of the subunits of the IL-2 receptor.

        (2) Both reduce the incidence and the severity of renal transplant rejection, but they cannot be used to treat acute rejection.

        (3) Side effects include shortness of breath, hypersensitivity reactions including itching and rash, and infections.

    d. *Ustekinumab (Stelara)*

        (1) Ustekinumab is a human monoclonal antibody against IL-12 and IL-23 and blocks binding of those cytokines to their receptors. This decreases activation of T-cells.

        (2) Administered by subcutaneous injection.

        (3) Adverse reactions are upper airway infections and allergic responses.

DRUG SUMMARY TABLE

Histamine H₁-receptor Antagonists
Chlorpheniramine (generic)
Brompheniramine (generic)
Diphenhydramine (Benadryl, Compose, generic)
Doxylamine (Unisom, generic)
Clemastine (Tavist, Contact-D, others)
Dimenhydrinate (Dramamine, others)
Pyrilamine (generic)
Antazoline (Vasocon-A)
Meclizine (Antivert, others)
Cyclizine (Marezine)
Promethazine (Phenergan, others)
Cyproheptadine (Periactin)
Loratadine (Claritin)
Desloratadine (Clarinex)
Fexophenadine (Allegra)
Acrivastine (Semprex-D)
Cetirizine (Zyrtec)
Levocitirizine (Xyzal)

Chromones
Cromolyn (Intal)
Nedocromil sodium (Tilade)

Ergots
Methysergide (Sansert)
Methylergonovine (Methergine)
Ergotamine (Ergomar, Ergostat)
Dihydroergotamine (Migranol)
Bromocriptine (Parlodel)
Pergolide (Permax)

Eicosanoids
Carboprost tromethamine (Hemabate)
Dinoprostone (Prostin E)
Misoprostol (Cytotec)
Prostaglandin E₁ (Caverject)
Epoprostenol (Veletri)

Nonsteroidal Analgesics
Acetaminophen (generic)

Gold Salts
Aurothioglucose (Solganal)
Gold sodium thiomalate (Myochrysine)
Auranofin (Ridaura)

Other Anti-RA Drugs
Penicillamine (Cuprimine, Depen)
Methotrexate (Rheumatrex)
Chloroquine (Aralen)

DMARDs
Infliximab (Remicade)
Adalimumab (Humira)
Etanercept (Enbrel)
Anakinra (Kineret)
Alefacept (Amevive)
Abatacept (Orencia)

Antigout Drugs
Probenecid (Benemid)
Allopurinol (Lopurin, Zyloprim)
Febuxistat (Uloric)
Colchicine (generic)
Pegloticase (Krystexxa)

Histamine H₂-receptor Antagonists
Cimetidine (Tagamet)
Ranitidine (Zantac)
Famotidine (Pepcid AC)
Nizatidine (Axid)

Serotonin Receptor Agonists
Buspirone (BuSpar)
Sumatriptan (Imitrex)
Rizatriptan (Maxalt)
Eletriptan (Relpax)
Zolmitriptan (Zomig)
Almotriptan (Axert)
Frovatriptan (Frova)
Naratriptan (Amerge)
Trazodone (Desyrel)
Tegaserod (Zelnorm)

Serotonin-Receptor Antagonists
Cyproheptadine (Periactin)
Ondansetron (Zofran)
Granisetron (Kytril)
Dolasetron (Anzemet)
Palonosetron (Aloxi)
Clozapine (Clozaril)
Risperidone (Risperdal)

NSAIDs
Acetylsalicylic acid
Magnesium salicylate (Tricosal)
Sulfasalazine (Azulfidine)
Mesalamine (Asacol)
Salsalate (Amigesic, generic)
Ibuprofen (Advil, Motrin, generic)
Naproxen (Aleve, generic)
Fenoprofen (Nalfon)
Ketoprofen (Orudis)
Sulindac (Clinoril)
Tolmetin (Tolectin)
Ketoralac (Toradol)
Indomethacin (Indocin)
Piroxicam (Feldene)
Meclofenamate (Meclomen)
Mefenamic acid (Ponstel)
Nabumetone (Relafen)
Flurbiprofen (generic)
Diclofenac (Voltaren)
Etodolac (Lodine)
Celecoxib (Celebrex)

Immunosuppressive Drugs
Azathioprine (Imuran)
Cyclophosphamide (Cytoxan, Neosar)
Methotrexate (Folex, Mexate)
Cyclosporine (Sandimmune, Neoral)
Tacrolimus (FK-506) (Prograf)
Sirolimus (Rapamune)
Antithymocyte globulin (Atgam)
Muromonab-CD3 antibody (Orthoclone OKT3)
Basiliximab (Simulect)
Daclizumab (Zenapax)
Thalidomide (Thalomid)
Mycophenolate Mofetil (CellCept)

Review Test

Directions: Each of the numbered items or incomplete statements in this section is followed by answers or by completions of the statement. Select the ONE lettered answer or completion that is BEST in each case.

1. A long-haul truck driver comes into your asthma clinic complaining that he is sneezing constantly and has burning and watery eyes. He indicates that he seems to have a month or so of these symptoms every spring. Which of the following drugs would be most appropriate to treat this patient?

(A) Dimenhydrinate
(B) Scopolamine
(C) Fexofenadine
(D) Cetirizine

2. Following a prolonged first labor, an alert nurse notices persistent bleeding in the postpartum patient with no vaginal or cervical laceration, and her uterine fundus feels very soft. The patient's heart rate is mildly elevated, and her blood pressure is 105/55 mmHg. Which of the following would be the best choice in this circumstance?

(A) Acetaminophen
(B) Buspirone
(C) Methylergonovine
(D) Methysergide

3. A 24-year-old woman has a history of migraine headaches with accompanying aura. During her last attack, ergotamine was much less effective, and you decide to try an alternative to treat her current attack. Agonist activity at which of the following receptors would be the best target for your new treatment?

(A) Histamine H_1
(B) α-Adrenoreceptors
(C) Serotonin 5-HT_{1B}
(D) Prostaglandin FP

4. An elderly patient has a history of taking both prescription medications and over-the-counter (OTC) "pain killers" for her rheumatoid arthritis. She is not diabetic and has no history of kidney disease. She is admitted into your clinic in acute renal failure and comments that the pain in her hands has become much worse in the last week. Which of the following drugs is most likely responsible for the adverse renal effect?

(A) Ibuprofen
(B) Prednisone
(C) Colchicine
(D) Probenecid

5. A neonate is identified as having atrial septal defect of congenital origin that will require surgical repair. Adequate systemic perfusion requires that the patency of the ductus arteriosus be maintained. Which of the following agents would best accomplish this goal?

(A) Indomethacin
(B) PGE_1
(C) PGI_2
(D) Celecoxib

6. A 24-year-old student has been taking over-the-counter (OTC) diphenhydramine for her allergy symptoms most of her life. Lately, however, she has had more frequent symptoms, so she increased the dose of the medication. She now asks her friend, who is a medical student, to explain to her how exactly this agent makes her more sleepy lately. What is the most likely answer regarding diphenhydramine?

(A) It blocks H_1-receptors in the brain
(B) It modulates the release of dopamine and serotonin
(C) It acts peripherally, since it does not cross the blood–brain barrier
(D) It exerts its effects via muscarinic-cholinergic agonist activity
(E) It contains tryptophan, which produces sedation

7. A 35-year-old man presents to his doctor with complaints of epigastric pain. He explains that he has been taking aspirin for many years for pain related to his low back injury. The doctor suspects gastritis and prescribes a trial of medication that might be helpful to this patient. What medication did the physician most likely prescribe?

(A) Doxylamine
(B) Desloratadine
(C) Cetrizine
(D) Famotidine
(E) Buspirone

8. A 30-year-old woman has suffered from cyclical migraines for many years. She now presents to her physician asking for a medication designated specifically for migraines, not just a general pain reliever. Her physician decided to prescribe sumatriptan as a trial medication. The patient, who is a biochemist, would like to know how this medication works.

(A) It is a 5-HT$_{1A}$ agonist
(B) It is a 5-HT$_{1D}$ agonist
(C) It blocks reuptake of serotonin
(D) It is a 5-HT$_3$ antagonist
(E) It is a 5-HT$_{2A}$ antagonist

9. A 35-year-old woman presents to her physician with a chief complaint of headaches. She states that her symptoms started several months ago and most recently have been associated with occasional vomiting. She also complains of milky discharge from her breasts and lack of menstruation in the last 3 months. Her physician orders a magnetic resonance imaging (MRI) scan of brain, and the patient is diagnosed with a large pituitary adenoma. Which medication would most likely benefit this patient if she is deemed not a good operative candidate?

(A) Methysergide
(B) Bromocriptine
(C) Ergotamine
(D) Aprotinin
(E) Allopurinol

10. A 24-year-old woman who is 42 weeks pregnant is admitted to the labor and delivery ward for induction of labor. A fetal heart monitor shows that the fetus is currently in no acute distress. Sterile examination shows the patient to be minimally dilated without significant effacement. She is given carboprost. Which eicosanoid does this medication represent?

(A) PGG
(B) TXA$_2$
(C) PGF$_{2a}$
(D) PGE$_1$
(E) PGH

11. A 70-year-old man suffers a myocardial infarction (MI). He is admitted to the cardiac intensive care unit and is given aspirin and a β-blocker. A catheterization procedure is scheduled. The patient's wife, who is a pharmacy technician, wants to know why the patient is being given aspirin and not another nonsteroidal anti-inflammatory drug (NSAID). What is the best answer to this question?

(A) Aspirin inhibits both COX-1 and COX-2
(B) Aspirin irreversibly binds to COX-1 and COX-2
(C) Aspirin is a weak acid
(D) Aspirin is excreted by the kidneys
(E) Aspirin has much greater antithrombotic activity

12. Following a kidney transplant, a 24-year-old male patient is placed on cyclosporine but after 48 hours complains of serious nausea and diarrhea and has a sudden increase in transaminases. You switch him to tacrolimus but the nausea persists and he complains of getting dizzy and has dyspnea. Which of the following immunosuppressive agents would be an alternate drug in this scenario?

(A) Mycophenolate mofetil
(B) Etanercept
(C) Tocilizumab
(D) Colchicine
(E) Basiliximab

13. You have been treating a 42-year-old woman with mild rheumatoid arthritis for 4 years with ibuprofen. She has returned to your office and complains that the pain in her wrists is worse and 800 mg/day of ibuprofen does not give relief. You elect to try etanercept for her RA and send her off for a chest X-Ray. You caution your patient that a serious adverse effect of the drug is

(A) GI bleeding
(B) Hallucinations
(C) Infections
(D) Anemia
(E) Excessive tear production

Answers and Explanations

1. **The answer is C.** Fexofenadine is a potent histamine H_1-receptor antagonist; its poor central nervous system (CNS) penetration reduces sedative effects. Cetirizine is a second-generation antihistamine, but it still has some sedating effects. Ranitidine is a histamine H_2-receptor antagonist.

2. **The answer is C.** Methylergonovine produces powerful contraction of uterine smooth muscle that can reduce postpartum bleeding. The other agents also interact with serotonin receptors but would not be effective in this case.

3. **The answer is C.** The "triptans" as a class are effective against acute migraine attacks and all act as agonists at serotonin $5\text{-}HT_{1B}$ and HT_{1D} receptors. Agonists at α-adrenergic receptors like epinephrine cause vasoconstriction but are not effective for migraine; antihistamines and agents that interfere with the prostaglandin FP receptor would not be effective either.

4. **The answer is A.** NSAIDs as a class are associated with renal toxicity. Prednisone is effective in alleviating the inflammation in rheumatoid arthritis but is not associated with adverse renal effects. Colchicine and probenecid are used to treat gout, not rheumatoid arthritis.

5. **The answer is B.** E-series prostaglandins are responsible for maintenance of the ductus. Inhibitors of prostaglandin biosynthesis, indomethacin and celecoxib, cause closure of the ductus.

6. **The answer is A.** Diphenhydramine blocks H_1-receptors in the brain, thereby producing sedation. The release of dopamine and serotonin is modulated via H_3-receptors. Diphenhydramine readily crosses the blood–brain barrier. This agent has muscarinic-cholinergic agonist properties. It is not known to contain tryptophan.

7. **The answer is D.** Famotidine is an H_2-blocker that is used for symptoms of gastritis. Doxylamine is an H_1-blocker that is used as a sleep aid. Desloratadine is an H_1-blocker that is used for allergy symptoms. Cetrizine is used for allergy symptoms as well. Buspirone is a serotonin agonist that is prescribed for anxiety.

8. **The answer is B.** Sumatriptan is a $5\text{-}HT_{1D}$ agonist. An example of an agent known as a $5\text{-}HT_{1A}$ agonist would be buspirone, an antianxiety agent. Fluoxetine is an example of a serotonin-reuptake inhibitor. Ondansetron, an antinausea medication, is a $5\text{-}HT_3$ antagonist. The antipsychotic medication Risperdal is an example of a $5\text{-}HT_{2A}$ antagonist.

9. **The answer is B.** Bromocriptine is a dopaminergic agonist used to treat hyperprolactinemia, as with pituitary adenomas, or for suppression of normal lactation. It is also used for the management of Parkinson disease. Methysergide is used for the prophylaxis of migraine headaches. Ergotamine is used to treat acute migraine attacks. Aprotinin is used in cardiac surgery to reduce the amount of blood transfusions. Allopurinol is used to treat gout.

10. **The answer is C.** Carboprost tromethamine is used for induction of labor; it is a PGF_{2a} analog. PGG and PGH are prostaglandins that are inhibited by nonsteroidal anti-inflammatory drugs (NSAIDs). TXA_2 is a potent inducer of platelet aggregation. PGE_1 is used for the maintenance of patency of ductus arteriosus.

11. **The answer is E.** Aspirin has a much greater antithrombotic activity than other nonsteroidal anti-inflammatory drugs (NSAIDs), which is why this agent is used for the prevention of myocardial infarction (MI) in patients with a history of MI, angina, or cardiac surgery. Aspirin inhibits both COX-1 and COX-2; however, so do most other NSAIDs. Aspirin does not bind to COX but causes it to be covalently modified. Aspirin is a weak acid and is excreted by the kidneys; however, they are not the reason why aspirin is preferred over other NSAIDs in the setting of prevention of MI.

12. **The answer is A.** Mycophenolate mofetil is rapidly converted to mycophonolic acid which inhibits purine biosynthesis. It is a useful immunosuppressive in cases where cyclosporine or tacrolimus are not tolerated. Etanercept is a TNF-α antagonist used in RA and Crohn's disease. Tocilizumab is an anti-IL-6 antibody that would be of little benefit following an organ transplant. Colchicine inhibits leukocyte migration and is useful in acute gouty attacks. Basiliximab is an alternate immunosuppressive that can cause shortness of breath.

13. **The answer is C.** Infections are a common and potentially serious adverse effect of the DMARDs. NSAIDs cause GI bleeding. The DMARDs do not cause anemia. Cyclosporine can be used beneficially to increase tear production.

chapter 7

Drugs Used in Anemia and Disorders of Hemostasis

I. DRUGS USED IN THE TREATMENT OF ANEMIAS

A. **Iron deficiency anemias**
1. *Iron*
   a. **Structure and storage of iron (Fig. 7.1)**
      (1) Iron is an integral component of heme. Approximately 70% of total body iron is found in hemoglobin. Heme iron is also an essential component of muscle myoglobin and of several enzymes, such as catalase, peroxidase, cytochromes, and others.
      (2) Iron is stored in reticuloendothelial cells, hepatocytes, and intestinal cells as ferritin (a particle with a ferric hydroxide core and a surface layer of the protein apoferritin) and hemosiderin (aggregates of ferritin–apoferritin).
   b. **Absorption and transport**
      (1) Heme iron is much more readily absorbed across the intestine than inorganic iron.
      (2) Inorganic iron in the ferrous state (Fe^{2+}) is much more readily absorbed than that in the ferric state (Fe^{3+}); gastric acid and ascorbic acid promote the absorption of ferrous iron.
      (3) Iron is actively transported across the intestinal cell; it is then oxidized to ferric iron and stored as ferritin or transported to other tissues.
      (4) Iron is transported in the plasma bound to the glycoprotein transferrin; specific cell-surface receptors bind the transferrin–iron complex, and the iron is delivered to the recipient cell by endocytosis.
   c. **Regulation**
      (1) Except for menstruation and bleeding disorders, very little iron is lost from the body, and no mechanism exists for increasing excretion. Therefore, iron storage is regulated at the level of absorption.
      (2) When plasma iron concentrations are low, the number of transferrin receptors is increased, facilitating cellular absorption, and ferritin synthesis is decreased, reducing tissue iron storage.
      (3) When iron stores are high, intestinal absorption decreases; synthesis of transferrin receptors also decreases, inhibiting additional cellular uptake, and ferritin synthesis is increased.
2. *Causes of iron deficiency anemia*
   a. **Bleeding** (approximately 30 mg of iron is lost in a normal menstrual cycle).
   b. Dietary deficiencies.
   c. Malabsorption syndromes.
   d. Increased iron demands such as pregnancy or lactation.

FIGURE 7.1. Absorption and circulation of iron within the body.

3. *Iron salt supplements*
   a. **Oral agents**
      (1) Several ferrous iron salts are available for oral use. All are essentially equivalent therapeutically if doses are adjusted according to iron content (gluconate, sulfate, and fumarate forms are 12%, 20%, and 33% iron by weight, respectively; a polysaccharide–iron complex is also available).
      (2) Approximately 25% of orally administered iron is absorbed; a typical daily dose is 100–200 mg iron/day.
      (3) Oral iron treatment may require 3–6 months to replenish body stores.
   b. **Parenteral agents**
      (1) A colloidal suspension of ferrous hydroxide and dextran can be administered by intravenous (IV) infusion or intramuscular injection.
      (2) Parenteral agents may be useful in patients with iron absorption disorders caused by inflammatory bowel disease, small-bowel resection, gastrectomy, or hereditary absorption defects.
      (3) Parenteral agents are indicated for patients with hypersensitivity reactions to oral iron salts.
      (4) These agents are useful in severe anemic conditions in which rapid correction of iron deficiency is desired.
      (5) Parenteral agents may be used to reduce toxic reactions on initiation of erythropoietin (EPO; epoetin alfa) therapy in patients with renal disease.
   c. **Adverse and toxic effects**
      (1) Iron salt supplements produce gastrointestinal (GI) upset (nausea, cramps, constipation, and diarrhea).
      (2) These supplements may cause hypersensitivity reactions (most common with parenteral administration), including bronchospasm, urticaria, and anaphylaxis.
      (3) Fatal iron overdose (1–10 g) is possible; children are especially susceptible. **Deferoxamine** (Desferal), an iron-chelating agent, is used to treat iron toxicity. Administered systematically or by gastric lavage, deferoxamine binds iron and promotes excretion.

B. Red cell deficiency anemias

1. Red cell deficiency anemias are most commonly treated with erythropoiesis-stimulating agents (ESAs).

2. **EPO (Epogen, many others)**
   a. **Properties**
      (1) EPO is a glycoprotein produced mostly (90%) by the peritubular cells in the kidney; EPO is essential for normal reticulocyte production.
      (2) Synthesis of EPO is stimulated by hypoxia.
      (3) EPO is available as recombinant human EPO, **epoetin alfa, and darbepoetin. Darbepoetin** is a second-generation ESA with a half-life about twice that of epoetin alfa. Administered parenterally (IV or subcutaneously).
   b. **Mechanism of action**
      (1) EPO increases the rate of proliferation and differentiation of erythroid precursor cells in the bone marrow.
      (2) EPO induces the transformation of the most mature erythroid progenitor cell, erythroid colony-forming unit, to a proerythroblast.
      (3) EPO increases the release of reticulocytes from marrow.
      (4) EPO increases hemoglobin synthesis.
      (5) The action of EPO requires adequate stores of iron.
   c. **Therapeutic uses.** EPO is used to treat anemia in the following patients: acquired immune deficiency syndrome **patients** treated with zidovudine **(AZT),** cancer patients undergoing **chemotherapy,** and patients in **renal failure;** all of these conditions and treatments produce anemia. EPO is also used in surgical patients to reduce the need for transfusions. In a situation requiring a rapid increase in hematocrit, RBC transfusion is effective in 1–3 hours while EPO takes 2–6 weeks.
   d. **Adverse and toxic effects** of EPO include hypertension, seizures, and headache probably caused by rapid expansion of blood volume. ESAs have been shown to increase the risk of death and serious cardiovascular events, both arterial and venous thromboembolic events including myocardial infarction (MI), stroke, congestive heart failure, and hemodialysis graft occlusion, when administered to target a hemoglobin concentration >12 g/dL.

C. Sideroblastic anemias

1. Sideroblastic anemias are characterized by decreased hemoglobin synthesis and intracellular accumulation of iron in erythroid precursor cells. Iron is available but is not incorporated into hemoglobin in a normal manner.

2. Sideroblastic anemias are often caused by agents that antagonize or deplete pyridoxal phosphate.

3. Sideroblastic anemias are sometimes seen in alcoholics, in patients undergoing anti-tuberculin therapy with isoniazid and pyrazinamide, and in certain inflammatory and malignant disorders.

4. **Hereditary sideroblastic anemia** is an X-linked trait.

5. Sideroblastic anemia is treated with **pyridoxine** (vitamin B_6) administered orally (preferred route) or parenterally. Pyridoxine has variable efficacy with inherited forms of the disease.

D. Vitamin deficiency (megaloblastic) anemia

1. **Vitamin B_{12}**
   a. **Structure**
      (1) Vitamin B_{12} is a complex, cobalt-containing molecule. Various groups are covalently linked to the cobalt atom, forming the cobalamins. The endogenous cobalamins in humans are methylcobalamin and 5-deoxyadenosylcobalamin.
         (a) **Methylcobalamin** is a coenzyme essential for the production of methionine and S-adenosylmethionine from homocysteine and for the production of tetrahydrofolate from methyltetrahydrofolate.

    (b) Deoxyadenosylcobalamin participates in the mitochondrial reaction that produces succinyl-CoA from methylmalonyl-CoA; vitamin B_{12} deficiency leads to the production of abnormal fatty acids.

    (2) For pharmacologic use, vitamin B_{12} is supplied as the stable derivative cyanocobalamin or hydroxocobalamin (AlphaRedisol).

b. Transport and absorption

    (1) In the stomach, dietary vitamin B_{12} complexes with **intrinsic factor,** a peptide secreted by the parietal cells. The intrinsic factor–vitamin B_{12} complex is absorbed by active transport in the distal ileum.

    (2) Vitamin B_{12} is transported in the plasma bound to the protein transcobalamin II and is taken up by and stored in hepatocytes.

c. Actions and pharmacologic properties

    (1) Vitamin B_{12} is essential for normal DNA synthesis and fatty acid metabolism. A deficiency results in impaired DNA replication, which is most apparent in tissues that are actively dividing, such as the GI tract and erythroid precursors. The appearance of large macrocytic (megaloblastic) red cells in the blood is characteristic of this deficiency. Vitamin B_{12} deficiency can also result in irreversible neurologic disorders.

    (2) Vitamin B_{12}, along with vitamin B_6 and folic acid, participates in the metabolism of homocysteine to cysteine. Elevations in homocysteine are associated with accelerated atherosclerosis.

    (3) Loss of vitamin B_{12} from the body is very slow (2 µg/day), and hepatic stores are sufficient for up to 5 years. Vitamin B_{12} is not synthesized by eukaryotic cells and is normally obtained from microbial synthesis.

    (4) Parenteral administration of vitamin B_{12} is standard because the vast majority of situations requiring vitamin B_{12} replacement are due to malabsorption. Uncorrectable malabsorption requires life-long treatment.

    (5) Improvement in hemoglobin concentration is apparent in 7 days and normalizes in 1–2 months.

d. Therapeutic uses

    (1) Vitamin B_{12} is used to treat pernicious anemia (inadequate secretion of intrinsic factor with subsequent reduction in vitamin B_{12} absorption).

    (2) Vitamin B_{12} is used after partial or total gastrectomy to mitigate the loss or reduction of intrinsic factor synthesis.

    (3) Administration of vitamin B_{12} is used to replace vitamin B_{12} deficiency caused by dysfunction of the distal ileum with defective or absent absorption of the intrinsic factor–vitamin B_{12} complex.

    (4) Administration of vitamin B_{12} is necessary in patients with insufficient dietary intake of vitamin B_{12} (occasionally seen in strict vegetarians).

e. Adverse effects of vitamin B_{12} are uncommon, even at large doses. Hypokalemia and thrombocytosis can occur upon conversion of severe megaloblastic anemia to normal erythropoiesis with cyanocobalamin therapy.

2. *Folic acid (vitamin B₉) (Folacin, leucovorin)*

    a. Folic acid is composed of three subunits: pteridine, *para*-aminobenzoic acid (PABA), and one to five glutamic acid residues.

    (1) Folic acid typically occurs in the diet in a polyglutamate form that must be converted to the monoglutamyl form for absorption. Most folate is absorbed in the proximal portions of the small intestine and is transported to tissues bound to a plasma-binding protein. Folic acid requires reduction by dihydrofolate reductase to the active metabolite methyltetrahydrofolate.

    (2) Leucovorin is a racemic mixture of the *d/l* stereoisomers of 5-formyltetrahydrofolic acid. It does not require metabolism by dihydrofolate reductase.

    b. The cofactors of folic acid provide single carbon groups for transfer to various acceptors and are essential for the biosynthesis of purines and the pyrimidine **deoxythymidylate.** A deficiency in folic acid results in **impaired DNA synthesis;** mitotically active tissues such as erythroid tissues are markedly affected.

    c. Catabolism and excretion of vitamin B_9 are more rapid than that of vitamin B_{12}; hepatic reserves are sufficient for only 1–3 months.

    d. Folic acid and leucovorin are usually administered orally.

    e. Folic acid is used to correct dietary insufficiency (commonly observed in the elderly), as a supplement during pregnancy to decrease the risk of neural tube defects, during lactation, and in cases of rapid cell turnover, such as hemolytic anemia. Leucovorin may be used to reverse the effects of the folate antagonists (see Chapter 12) methotrexate, pyrimethamine, and trimethoprim.

E. Sickle cell anemias

    1. Hydroxyurea has been shown effective in reducing painful episodes by about 50%; the necessity of blood transfusions was also shown to be reduced. Hydroxyurea increases the production of **fetal hemoglobin,** which makes red cells resistant to sickling and reduces the expression of adhesion molecules such as L-selectin.

    2. Pentoxifylline (Trental) is a synthetic **dimethyxanthine** structurally similar to caffeine. The actions of pentoxifylline include increased erythrocyte flexibility and decreased blood viscosity. It is commonly used to treat intermittent claudication. Pentoxifylline appears to inhibit erythrocyte phosphodiesterase, which causes an increase in erythrocyte cyclic adenosine 5′-monophosphate activity and an increase in membrane flexibility.

II. DRUGS ACTING ON MYELOID CELLS

A. Myeloid growth factors are glycoproteins produced by many cells including fibroblasts, endothelial cells, macrophages, and immune cells that act to stimulate proliferation and differentiation of one or more myeloid lineage.

    1. *Sargramostim (granulocyte–macrophage colony-stimulating factor, GM-CSF, leukine)*

        a. Sargramostim is a recombinant protein expressed in yeast. Its principal action is to stimulate myelopoiesis in granulocyte–macrophage pathways as well as megakaryocytic and erythroid progenitor cells.

        b. Clinical uses

            (1) Reduce the duration of neutropenia and incidence of infection in patients receiving myelosuppressive chemotherapy or bone marrow transplantation.

            (2) Mobilize peripheral blood progenitor cells prior to collection.

            (3) For bone marrow graft failure.

        c. Sargramostim is **administered IV,** and the most common adverse effects are **granulocytosis,** bone pain, fever, nausea, and rash.

    2. *Filgrastim and pegfilgrastim (granulocyte colony-stimulating factor, G-CSF)*

        a. Filgrastim is a recombinant protein that stimulates bone marrow production of neutrophils without increasing the number of basophils, eosinophils, or monocytes.

        b. Pegfilgrastim is a filgrastim with a polypropylene glycol molecule added to the N-terminus.

        c. Its clinical uses are similar to those of sargramostim: reduction in the duration of neutropenia in patients on anticancer regimens and for patients with chronic severe neutropenia.

        d. Both GM-CSF and G-CSF play an important role in autologous stem-cell transplantation which is increasingly used instead of bone marrow transplantation.

    3. *Oprelvekin (interleukin-11)*

        a. Oprelvekin is a genetically engineered form of **human interleukin-11.** IL-11 has a number of biologic activities in hematopoietic, lymphopoietic, hepatic, adipose, neuronal, and osteoclast cells.

        b. It is used clinically to prevent **severe chemotherapy-induced thrombocytopenia** and to reduce the need for platelet transfusions following myelosuppressive chemotherapy for nonmyeloid malignancies.

4. Romiplostim is an engineered peptide that binds to the thrombopoietin receptor. It produces a dose-dependent increase in platelets after 4–6 following subcutaneous injection.

III. DRUGS USED IN HEMOSTATIC DISORDERS

A. Anticoagulants (Fig. 7.2)

1. *Heparin*

a. Structure

(1) Heparin is a polymeric mixture of sulfated mucopolysaccharides. Commercial heparin contains 8–15 repeats of *d*-glycosamine-*l*-iduronic acid and *d*-glucosamine-*d*-glucuronic acid. It is highly negatively charged at physiologic pH.

(2) Low-molecular-weight heparins are also available (dalteparin [Fragmin], enoxaparin [Lovenox]).

(3) Heparin is synthesized as a normal product of many tissues, including the lung, intestine, and liver. Commercial preparations are derived from bovine lung or porcine intestinal extracts.

b. Actions

(1) Increases the activity of antithrombin by 1,000-fold.

(a) Antithrombin inhibits activated serine proteases in the clotting cascade, including IIa (thrombin), IXa, and Xa.

(b) Heparin, antithrombin, and the clotting factors form a ternary complex. The clotting factor is inactivated, and intact heparin is released and recycled in a catalytic manner. Some evidence suggests that additional anti-clotting factors, such as heparin cofactor II, may also be activated by heparin.

(c) The lower-molecular-weight heparins act mainly via antithrombin to inhibit factor Xa; they have little effect on inhibition of thrombin.

(2) Heparin has a direct anticoagulant activity (can inhibit clotting in vitro).

(3) Heparin releases lipoprotein lipase from vascular beds, which accelerates postprandial clearing of lipoproteins from the plasma.

FIGURE 7.2. Sites of pharmacologic action of antithrombotic and fibrinolytic agents.

c. **Pharmacologic properties**
(1) Heparin must be given parenterally (by slow infusion or deep subcutaneous injection); it is not injected intramuscularly because of the potential for hematoma formation.
(2) The half-life ($t_{1/2}$) of heparin is dose-dependent. The principal advantage of the low-molecular-weight heparins is a greater pharmacokinetic predictability that allows once- or twice-a-day subcutaneous dosing without the need for monitoring.
(3) Heparin is metabolized in the liver by heparinase to smaller molecular weight compounds, which are excreted in the urine.

d. **Therapeutic uses**
(1) Heparin provides preoperative prophylaxis against deep vein thrombosis.
(2) Heparin is administered following acute MI (AMI) or pulmonary embolism.
(3) This agent reduces pulmonary embolism in patients with established thrombosis.
(4) Heparin prevents clotting in extracorporeal circulation devices.

e. **Adverse effects**
(1) Bleeding is a common adverse effect, especially in older women. An increased incidence of bleeding is also seen in patients with renal disease. Protamine sulfate, a highly positively charged mixture of peptides, can be administered IV if bleeding does not abate after the cessation of heparin therapy.
(2) Heparin causes thrombocytopenia in 25% of patients and severe platelet reductions in 5% of patients; heparin may induce antiplatelet antibodies and may also induce platelet aggregation and lysis.
(3) Heparin can cause hypersensitivity reactions, including chills, fever, urticaria, and anaphylaxis.
(4) Heparin may produce reversible alopecia.
(5) Osteoporosis and predisposition to fracture are seen with long-term use of heparin.

f. **Contraindications and drug interactions**
(1) Heparin is contraindicated in patients who are bleeding (internally or externally) and in patients with hemophilia, thrombocytopenia, hypertension, or purpura.
(2) Heparin is also contraindicated before and after brain, spinal cord, or eye surgery.
(3) Extreme caution is advised in the treatment of pregnant women; however, alternative agents (coumarin derivatives) are teratogenic.
(4) Heparin should not be administered with aspirin or other agents that interfere with platelet aggregation.
(5) Positively charged drugs, aminoglycosides, and some histamine-receptor antagonists can reduce the effectiveness of heparin therapy.

2. *Synthetic anticoagulants, fondaparinux*
a. Fondaparinux is a synthetic polysaccharide based on the antithrombin-binding region of heparin. Administered by subcutaneous injection, it behaves like the low-molecular-weight heparins in inactivating factor Xa.
b. Fondaparinux is approved for prophylaxis of thrombus formation in patients undergoing hip or knee surgery, treatment of pulmonary embolism, and deep vein thrombosis.

3. *Coumarin derivatives*
a. **Structure**
(1) Coumarin derivatives are derived from 4-hydroxycoumarin and include dicumarol, warfarin sodium, and phenprocoumon.
(2) Of these agents, warfarin has the best bioavailability and the least severe adverse effects.

b. **Actions and pharmacologic properties**
(1) Coumarin derivatives indirectly interfere with γ-carboxylation of glutamate residues in clotting factors II (prothrombin), VII, IX, and X, which is coupled to the oxidation of vitamin K. Continued production of functional clotting factors requires replenishment of reduced vitamin K from the oxidized form; this reduction is catalyzed by vitamin K epoxide reductase; which is directly inhibited by coumarin derivatives.

      (2) Clotting factors are still synthesized, but at reduced levels, and are undercarboxylated and have greatly reduced biologic activity; clotting factors produced before coumarin therapy decline in concentration as a function of factor half-life. This causes a latency period of 36–48 hours before effects are seen. It does not affect established thrombi.

        (a) Warfarin, administered orally, has 100% bioavailability. Highly teratogenic and fetotoxic, with a $t_{1/2}$ of 2.5 days, warfarin is extensively (99%) bound to plasma albumin and can displace many other drugs from this site.

        (b) Dicumarol is much less well absorbed; a $t_{1/2}$ of approximately 2–10 days increases the potential for bleeding episodes.

  c. Therapeutic uses

    (1) The therapeutic uses of coumarin derivatives are similar to those of heparin; they also include treatment and prophylaxis of venous thrombosis and of pulmonary embolism. Coumarin derivatives are also indicated to reduce thromboembolism in patients with mechanical heart valves.

    (2) Coumarin derivatives are also used to treat patients with atrial fibrillation, whose risk for a stroke is greatly increased.

  d. Adverse effects

    (1) Bleeding is a common adverse effect with oral anticoagulants; prothrombin times should be frequently monitored.

    (2) Warfarin causes hemorrhagic infarction in the breast, intestine, and fatty tissues; it also readily crosses the placenta and can cause hemorrhage in the fetus. Warfarin causes defects in normal fetal bone formation; its teratogenic potential is high.

  e. Drug interactions

    (1) Amiodarone and sulfinpyrazone inhibit the metabolism of the more active warfarin stereoisomer and increase drug activity.

    (2) Aspirin and salicylates increase warfarin action by inhibiting platelet function and displacement of warfarin from plasma-binding sites.

    (3) Antibiotics decrease microbial vitamin K production in the intestine.

    (4) Barbiturates and rifampin decrease warfarin effectiveness by inducing microsomal enzymes.

    (5) Oral contraceptives decrease warfarin effectiveness by increasing plasma clotting factors and decreasing antithrombin III.

 4. *Hirudin and analogs*

  a. Hirudin, a protein found in the saliva of the medicinal leech, directly binds to and **inhibits thrombin** in the circulation and within clots. It does not require antithrombin.

  b. Bivalirudin (Angiomax) is a synthetic 20-amino-acid peptide hirudin analog; desirudin and lepirudin are recombinant hirudin analogs made in yeast. All are administered parenterally.

  c. These drugs are used in patients with unstable angina pectoris undergoing percutaneous transluminal coronary angioplasty and when combined with additional antiplatelet drugs (see below) in patients undergoing percutaneous coronary interventions. Lepirudin is approved for anticoagulation in patients with heparin-induced thrombocytopenia.

 5. Argatroban is a small-molecule synthetic inhibitor of thrombin derived from arginine. They are useful in the management of patients at risk for heparin-induced thrombocytopenia and following coronary angioplasty.

 6. Dabigatran etexilate mesylate is the first oral direct thrombin inhibitor approved in the U.S. It is used to reduce the risk of stroke and peripheral embolism in patients with nonvalvular atrial fibrillation. Bleeding is the primary adverse effect.

B. Hemostatic agents

 1. *Vitamin K₁ (phytonadione)*

  a. Vitamin K₁ is found in foodstuffs and is available for oral or parenteral use. Adequate bile salts are required for oral absorption. **Vitamin K** is required for posttranslational modification of clotting factors II, VII, IX, and X.

    b. Administration of vitamin K to newborns reduces the incidence of **hypothrombinemia of the newborn,** which is especially common in premature infants.

    c. IV administration is typical for patients with **dietary deficiencies** and for replenishment of normal levels reduced by **antimicrobial therapy or surgery.**

    d. IV **vitamin K$_1$** is effective in reversing **bleeding episodes induced by oral hypoglycemic agents.**

2. *Plasma fractions*

    a. Plasma fractions must be administered IV.

    b. Plasma fractions are frequently prepared from blood or plasma pooled from multiple individuals; thus, they are associated with an increased risk of exposure to hepatitis and human immunodeficiency virus (HIV; approximately 80% of hemophiliacs over age 30 are infected with HIV). Recombinant DNA techniques that permit in vitro synthesis of these products eliminate this danger.

        (1) Plasma protein preparations include the following:

            (a) Lyophilized factor VIII concentrate and **recombinant factor VIII**.

            (b) Cryoprecipitate (plasma protein fraction obtained from whole blood).

            (c) Concentrates of plasma (contain variable amounts of factors II, IX, X, and VII).

            (d) Lyophilized factor IX concentrates, recombinant factor IX.

            (e) Recombinant factor VIIa.

            (f) Recombinant thrombin.

            (g) Antithrombin (Thrombate III).

            (h) Antiinhibitor coagulant complex—activated clotting factors.

        (2) Therapeutic uses. Therapeutic uses include the treatment of various congenital defects of hemostasis, including the following:

            (a) Hemophilia A (classic hemophilia, due to a deficiency in factor VIII).

            (b) Hemophilia B (Christmas disease, due to a deficiency in factor IX).

            (c) Hereditary antithrombin III deficiency.

3. *Other agents that increase clotting capacity*

    a. Desmopressin acetate (Stimate) increases factor VIII synthesis and can be used before minor surgery in patients with **mild hemophilia A.**

    b. Danazol is an impeded androgen that increases factor VIII synthesis. It is infrequently used in some anemias and refractory idiopathic thrombocytopenic purpura.

4. *Inhibitors of fibrinolysis*

    a. Aminocaproic acid

        (1) Aminocaproic acid is a synthetic agent similar in structure to lysine.

        (2) Aminocaproic acid competitively inhibits plasminogen activation.

        (3) This agent is used as an adjunct in the treatment of hemophilia, for postsurgical bleeding, and in patients with hyperfibrinolysis.

    b. Tranexamic acid (Cyklokapron). Tranexamic acid is a more potent analog of aminocaproic acid.

C. Antithrombotics

    1. *Aspirin (see Chapter 6)*

        a. Aspirin and aspirin-like agents **decrease thromboxane A$_2$ production** in platelets by **irreversibly** inhibiting cyclooxygenase, mostly COX-1.

        b. At higher doses (>325 mg/day), aspirin may **reduce antithrombotic action** by decreasing endothelial cell synthesis of prostaglandin I$_2$ (PGI$_2$), which requires cyclooxygenase (COX-2) activity. Low doses may impair PG synthesis in platelets to a greater extent than in endothelial cells and avoid this effect.

        c. Other NSAIDs (see Chapter 6) do not have comparable antithrombotic activity.

    2. *Dipyridamole (Persantine, Pyridamole)*

        a. Dipyridamole **inhibits the cellular uptake of adenosine,** which has vasodilating and antiaggregating activity.

        b. The use of dipyridamole as an antithrombotic agent is limited to prophylaxis (with warfarin) in patients with **prosthetic heart valves.**

3. *Ticlopidine (Ticlid), clopidogrel (Plavix), and prasugrel (Effient)*
   a. **Ticlopidine** irreversibly inhibits the platelet purinergic $P2Y_{12}$ receptor. This reduces the activation of glycoprotein IIb/IIIa and inhibits the binding of platelets to fibrinogen, thus **inhibiting platelet aggregation.** It is approved for the prevention of stroke and for the prevention of coronary stent thrombosis. Adverse effects include GI disturbances (frequent) and neutropenia (~1%).
   b. **Clopidogrel** is structurally similar and has the same mechanism of action but has fewer adverse effects and a very low frequency of neutropenia.
   c. **Prasugrel** is similar to clopidogrel but has a higher incidence of bleeding.
   d. These agents are used for arterial thromboembolism prophylaxis in high-risk patients, stroke prophylaxis in patients with noncardioembolic TIA or stroke, and **acute coronary syndrome.**
   e. Adverse effects also include bleeding, diarrhea, and rash. Maximal effects are seen after several days of therapy; effects persist several days after treatment.
4. **Anagrelide (Agrylin)** is an antithrombopenic agent that inhibits megakaryocytes for treatment of patients with thrombocythemia.
5. **Cilostazol** inhibits platelet aggregation and has antithrombotic and vasodilatory actions, mediated in part by inhibition of phosphodiesterase type III. It is approved for use in the treatment of claudication.
6. *GPIIb/IIIa inhibitors*
   a. The abundant platelet glycoprotein GPIIa/IIIb plays a critical role in platelet aggregation (Fig. 7.3). GPIIa/IIIb is an integrin that, when activated, binds to fibrinogen. There are two GPIIa/IIIb binding sites on a fibrinogen molecule, thus permitting fibrinogen-mediated platelet aggregation.
   b. **Abciximab** is the Fab fragment of a chimeric monoclonal antibody that contains human and mouse IgG components. It binds to GPIIa/IIIb and blocks fibrinogen binding. It also binds to the vitronectin receptor.
   c. **Eptifibatide** is a small **synthetic peptide** that competes for fibrinogen binding **to GPIIa/IIIb.**
   d. **Tirofiban** (Aggrastat) is a peptide mimetic of low molecular weight (mol. wt. = 495) that binds to the GPIIa/IIIb receptor (and the vitronectin receptor).
   e. These drugs have been approved for use in patients undergoing percutaneous coronary intervention, for unstable angina, and for post-MI.
   f. All are administered by infusion.

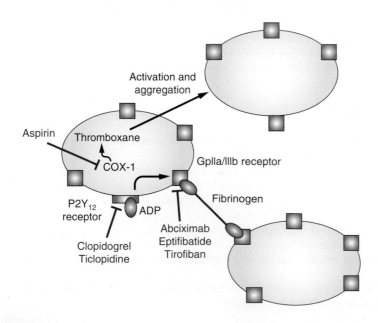

FIGURE 7.3. Sites of action of anti-platelet drugs.

    g. The most common adverse effect is bleeding, especially if used in combination with heparin.

  7. *Dextran 40 and dextran 70, 75*

    a. These agents are plasma volume expanders that reduce erythrocyte aggregation and **impair fibrin polymerization and platelet function** in vivo by an unclear mechanism.

    b. Adverse effects include **respiratory distress, urticaria,** and (rarely) anaphylaxis.

D. Thrombolytics (Table 7.1 and Fig. 7.4). Fibrin clots are dissolved by the serine protease plasmin. Inactive plasminogen is converted to plasmin by proteolysis in vivo by peptides called **tissue plasminogen activators.**

  1. *Tissue plasminogen activator (tPA), alteplase (Activase), reteplase (Retavase), and tenecteplase (TNKase)*

    a. tPA is an endogenous protease that preferentially activates plasminogen bound to fibrin. **Alteplase** is a recombinant human protein produced in cultured cells.

    b. tPA is most specific to **fibrin-bound plasminogen;** local activation of plasmin reduces the incidence of systemic bleeding.

    c. Reteplase and tenecteplase are genetically engineered forms of human tPA and have a longer half-life, higher specificity for fibrin, and greater resistance to plasminogen activator inhibitor-1 than native tPA. The increase in half-life permits administration as a bolus rather than by continuous infusion.

    d. Antithrombotics are used in patients with **acute arterial thrombosis** including AMI and **stroke**. The use of thrombolytics has reduced morbidity and mortality associated with AMI and acute ischemic stroke. Outcomes following AMI and stroke are improved if administration occurs promptly after the event; recommendations are usually within 3–6 hours. tPA has also been used in the treatment of pulmonary embolism and for deep vein thrombosis.

    e. The most common adverse effect of all thrombolytics is bleeding. Bleeding sites include both internal (intracranial, retroperitoneal, GI, genitourinary, respiratory) and superficial sites (venous cutdowns, arterial punctures, sites of recent surgical intervention).

  2. *Streptokinase*

    a. Streptokinase is a nonenzyme protein that is isolated from streptococci; it binds to plasminogen and activates it to plasmin nonenzymatically.

    b. Streptokinase acts on both circulating plasminogen and fibrin-bound plasminogen.

    c. Therapeutic uses of streptokinase include treatment of **AMI and stroke, acute pulmonary embolism, deep vein thrombosis,** and **reperfusion of occluded peripheral arteries.** It is also used, as are other thrombolytics, to **clear occluded venous catheters.**

table 7.1 Properties and Uses of Thrombolytics

Drug	Composition	Properties	Uses
Alteplase	Recombinant natural human tPA	Activity more localized to fibrin clot	AMI; stroke
Reteplase	Recombinant fragment of human tPA	Smaller than native tPA; in theory, diffuses into fibrin clot more readily	AMI
Duteplase	Recombinant human tPA with a single amino acid change	Activity more localized to fibrin clot	AMI
Streptokinase	Bacterial glycoprotein; activates plasminogen	Not targeted specifically to fibrin in clots	AMI; deep vein thrombosis
Urokinase	Produced in the kidney; activates plasminogen	Not targeted specifically to fibrin in clots	Acute massive pulmonary emboli; AMI
Anistreplase	Complex of streptokinase and plasminogen	Does not require endogenous plasminogen	AMI

AMI, acute myocardial infection; tPA, tissue plasminogen activator.

FIGURE 7.4. Actions of drugs acting on plasminogen.

    d. The major adverse effect associated with streptokinase is **systemic bleeding**. Many individuals have antistreptococcal antibodies because of prior exposure to the bacteria; this can reduce effectiveness and complicate treatment.

    e. Although streptokinase is commonly used in Europe, it is no longer marketed in the U.S.

  3. *Urokinase*

    a. Urokinase is a protease originally isolated from urine; the drug is now prepared in recombinant form from cultured kidney cells.

    b. Urokinase activates circulating and fibrin-bound plasminogen.

    c. Urokinase is approved for the treatment of pulmonary embolism. It is less antigenic than streptokinase and is indicated in patients sensitive to streptokinase.

  4. **Anistreplase** is a complex of streptokinase and plasminogen. It does not require circulating plasminogen and has a longer half-life than streptokinase.

▮ DRUG SUMMARY TABLE

Drugs Used for Anemias
Iron salts (Fe-Max, Femiron, Feostat, many others)
Epoetin alfa (Epogen, Procrit)
Darbepoetin Alfa (Aranesp)
Pyridoxine (vitamin B_6) (Neuro-K)
Cyanocobalamin (vitamin B_{12}) (Betalin, Redisol)
Hydroxocobalamin (vitamin B_{12}) (AlphaRedisol)
Folic acid (vitamin B_9) (Folacin, Folicet)
Leucovorin (generic)
Hydroxyurea (Mylocel, Droxia)
Pentoxifylline (Pentopak)

Myeloid Growth Stimulators
Sargramostim (Leukine)
Filgrastim (Neupogen)
Pegfilgrastim (Neulasta)
Oprelvekin (Neumega)

Anticoagulants
Heparin (Calciparine, others)
Fondaparinex (Arixtra)

Warfarin (Coumadin)
Phenprocoumon (Liquamar)
Dicumarol (generic)
Bivalirudin (Angiomax)
Desirudin (Iprivask)
Lepirudin (Refludan)
Antithrombin (Thrombate III)
Argatroban (generic)

Hemostatic Agents
Phytonadione (vitamin K_1) (AquaME- PHYTON, Mephyton)
Factor VIII (Kogenate, Helixate)
Factor IX (AlphaNine, Profilnine)
Factor VIIa (NovoSeven)
Thrombin (Recothrom)
AICC (Feiba)
Desmopressin acetate (DDAVP, Stimate)
Danazol (Danacrine)

Antifibrinolytics
Aminocaproic acid (Amicar)
Tranexamic acid (Cyklokapron)

Antithrombotics
Aspirin
Dipyridamole (Persantine, Pyridamole)
Ticlopidine (Ticlid)
Clopidogrel (Plavix)
Prasugrel (Effient)
Anagrelide (Agrylin)
Cilostazol (generic)
Dextran (Dextran 40, others)

GPIIb/IIIa Inhibitors
Abciximab (ReoPro)
Eptifibatide (Integrilin)
Tirofiban (Aggrastat)

Thrombolytics
Alteplase (Activase)
Reteplase (Retavase)
Tenecteplase (TNKase)
Streptokinase (Kabikinase, Streptase)
Urokinase (Abbokinase)
Anistreplase (Eminase)

Review Test

Directions: Each of the numbered items or incomplete statements in this section is followed by answers or by completions of the statement. Select the ONE lettered answer or completion that is BEST in each case.

1. A patient is admitted to the hospital for gallbladder surgery, and although the surgery is successful, a case of ileus develops. This necessitates feeding the patient parenterally for 8 days. A nurse observes that the surgical wound and IV sites have begun to ooze small but constant amounts of blood. Which of the following would be the most appropriate treatment of this patient?

(A) Ticlopidine
(B) Factor VIII concentrate
(C) Urokinase
(D) Vitamin K
(E) Folic acid

2. A man undergoing chemotherapy for lung cancer complains of shortness of breath when climbing stairs and generalized fatigue. An electrocardiogram (ECG) appears normal, but his hematocrit level is 8.1. Which of the following would be most appropriate for this patient?

(A) Erythropoietin
(B) Digoxin
(C) Ticlopidine
(D) Vitamin B_6
(E) Enalapril

3. A 56-year old woman has a temporary loss of peripheral vision and dizziness that lasts for approximately 10 minutes. Her family history reveals that her mother had thromboembolic disease, but her father was normal. Which of the following would be the best outpatient prophylactic regimen for this patient 2 days after these symptoms appeared?

(A) Anistreplase
(B) Clopidogrel
(C) Heparin
(D) Abciximab
(E) Streptokinase

4. A 53-year-old obese woman is brought into the emergency room by her concerned husband approximately 1 hour after complaining of constant abdominal pain, nausea, and shortness of breath. An electrocardiogram (ECG) and cardiac enzyme tests indicate a moderate myocardial infarction (MI) due to occlusion of the left descending coronary artery. Which of the following would be the best course of treatment for this patient?

(A) Reteplase
(B) Heparin
(C) Eptifibatide
(D) Lovastatin

5. A young couple present to their primary care physician stating that they are trying to conceive. They would like to know if the future mom-to-be needs to be on any supplements. Along with recommending a multivitamin with folic acid, the doctor also suggests an iron supplement. Pregnant women develop iron deficiency anemia because of

(A) Increased bleeding tendency
(B) Increased dietary deficiency
(C) Malabsorption
(D) Increased iron demands
(E) Increased excretion

6. A 65-year-old diabetic man develops end-stage renal disease. His glomerular filtration capacity is now low enough to require dialysis. His nephrologist also explains that the patient will require weekly injections of synthetic erythropoietin (EPO), since this protein is normally produced by the kidney. What is the mechanism of action of EPO?

(A) It increases proliferation of erythroid precursor cells in the bone marrow
(B) It decreases the release of reticulocytes from the bone marrow
(C) It decreases hemoglobin synthesis
(D) It is independent on the amount of iron stored in the body
(E) It participates in the mitochondrial reaction that produces succinyl-CoA

7. A 47-year-old man with a history of alcohol abuse presents to the urgent care clinic complaining of lightheadedness and dyspnea on exertion. His laboratory studies indicate a low hemoglobin level. Peripheral smear shows increased number of spherocytes. What agent could be used to treat this patient's anemia?

(A) Iron supplements
(B) Erythropoietin
(C) Vitamin B_6
(D) Vitamin B_{12}
(E) Folic acid

8. A 40-year-old morbidly obese woman undergoes gastric bypass surgery to help her lose weight. Her surgeon reminds her that now she will have to get a monthly injection of vitamin B_{12}, since the part of her stomach responsible for production of intrinsic factor has been removed. Which of the following is true about vitamin B_{12}?

(A) Loss of vitamin B_{12} from the body is a rapid process
(B) The molecule of vitamin B_{12} contains copper
(C) Vitamin B_{12} is not required for fatty acid metabolism
(D) A deficiency results in impaired DNA replication
(E) Neurologic deficits are not seen with this kind of anemia

9. A 31-year-old pregnant woman presents to her obstetrician for a routine visit. She has several questions for her doctor, one of which has to do with the supplements that she was advised to take at her first prenatal visit. She stated she leads a very busy lifestyle and sometimes forgets to take all the pills she is supposed to take. She wants to know the purpose of folic acid supplementation in pregnancy.

(A) It increases oxygen-carrying capacity of the blood
(B) It decreases the risk of neural tube defects
(C) It aids in bone growth of the maturing fetus
(D) It stimulates myelopoiesis of erythroid progenitor cells
(E) It reduces blood viscosity during pregnancy

10. A 29-year-old African-American man presents to the emergency department with a chief complaint of severe pain in his arms

and legs. Since this has happened to him before, he knows that what he is experiencing is a sickle crisis. He states that since he does not have medical insurance, he only comes to see a doctor when he experiences these "crises." Which pain medication is the emergency physician likely to prescribe?

(A) Indomethacin
(B) Hydrocodone
(C) Acetaminophen
(D) Celecoxib
(E) Hydroxyurea

11. A 74-year-old woman who is undergoing chemotherapy for advanced lung cancer presents to the infusion center for her next treatment. Before each treatment her white count, hemoglobin, and platelet counts are checked to make sure she is not experiencing chemotherapy-related cytotoxicity. Her blood sample is run in the analyzer, and her platelet count is reported to be at a dangerously low level. Which medication is her oncologist likely to prescribe in this situation, along with a platelet transfusion?

(A) Erythropoietin
(B) Oprelvekin
(C) Filgrastim
(D) Sargramostim
(E) Leucovorin

12. A 55-year-old woman undergoes an open cholecystectomy. She is admitted for postoperative observation and started on subcutaneous heparin treatment to prevent formation of deep venous thrombosis, a major risk factor for pulmonary embolism. Which of the following is true regarding the mechanism of action of heparin?

(A) Heparin increases activity of antithrombin
(B) Serine proteases of the clotting cascade are deactivated
(C) Heparin catalyzes clotting in vitro
(D) Heparin aids sequestration of lipoproteins
(E) Clotting factor is activated

13. A 63-year-old man has a history of atrial fibrillation. To reduce his risk of a stroke, his physician had given him an anticoagulant medication. This agent, while being of tremendous benefit to this patient, comes with its associated risks, such as spontaneous hemorrhage. To monitor the appropriateness of the current dosage of the medication, the patient comes in frequently to have the laboratory check his prothrombin level. Which medication must this patient be taking?

(A) Heparin
(B) Fragmin
(C) Lovenox
(D) Coumarin
(E) Protamine

14. A 75-year-old man is brought to the emergency department after being found on the floor of his room. His wife tells you that his medical history includes two prior strokes, for which he is now taking a "small pill that works on platelets." Your attending tells you that there are newer agents now that work by preventing platelet aggregation. He asks you if you know the names of any such agents. You are very excited, because you, in fact, had just reviewed your pharmacology. Which answer do you give?

(A) Heparin
(B) Coumarin
(C) Clopidogrel
(D) Alteplase
(E) Dextran

Answers and Explanations

1. **The answer is D.** After 6–7 days of parenteral feeding, vitamin K stores are depleted and clotting factor biosynthesis is impaired. Ticlopidine is an anticoagulant, and urokinase is a thrombolytic; both would be contraindicated in this circumstance. Folic acid would not improve the condition of the patient.

2. **The answer is A.** Erythropoietin (EPO) stimulates the production of erythrocytes, which are frequently diminished as a consequence of anticancer therapy, to correct the patient's hematocrit level. Digoxin is a cardiac glycoside that can improve contractility in impaired myocardium but would not be used in this circumstance. Enalapril is an angiotensin-converting enzyme (ACE) inhibitor that would have little effect on the patient's condition.

3. **The answer is B.** The patient has symptoms consistent with a transient ischemic attack (TIA). Prophylactic antiplatelet therapy should be instituted while the diagnosis is confirmed. Heparin is not suitable for outpatient use. Anistreplase and streptokinase are thrombolytics that may be used within hours of a thrombotic stroke but not after 2 days after a possible TIA.

4. **The answer is A.** Thrombolytics such as the recombinant tissue plasminogen activator (tPA) reteplase reduce morbidity and mortality if used shortly after an acute myocardial infarction (AMI). Heparin might be used after resolution of the AMI. If the patient is above recommended levels of low-density lipoprotein (LDL) cholesterol, she should be treated with a cholesterol-lowering drug such as lovastatin.

5. **The answer is D.** Pregnancy and lactation are the states of increased iron demands. While increased bleeding tendency, dietary deficiency, and malabsorption are all true causes of iron deficiency anemia, they are not the culprits during pregnancy. Iron storage is regulated at the level of absorption, and very little of it is lost from the body.

6. **The answer is A.** Erythropoietin (EPO) increases the rate of proliferation and differentiation of erythroid precursor cells in the bone marrow. It increases the release of reticulocytes. It also increases hemoglobin synthesis. Erythropoietin requires adequate iron stores. Participation in the mitochondrial reaction that produces succinyl-CoA refers to the mechanism of action of one of the natural cobalamins, deoxyadenosylcobalamin.

7. **The answer is C.** Sideroblastic anemia may develop in alcoholics and patients undergoing anti-tuberculin therapy. This condition is treated with vitamin B_6 supplements (pyridoxine). Iron supplements are used in iron deficiency anemia. Erythropoietin is used in anemia caused by acquired immune deficiency syndrome (AIDS), chemotherapy, and renal failure. Vitamin B_{12} and folic acid are used for megaloblastic anemias caused by depletion of the vitamin.

8. **The answer is D.** Deficiency of vitamin B_{12} results in impaired DNA replication. Loss of vitamin B_{12} is a very slow process, with hepatic stores being sufficient for up to 5 years. The molecule of vitamin B_{12} contains cobalt. Vitamin B_{12} is essential for normal fatty acid metabolism. Vitamin B_{12} deficiency causes irreversible neurologic disorders.

9. **The answer is B.** Folic acid supplementation has been shown to decrease the incidence of neural tube defects. Increasing the oxygen-carrying capacity of the blood refers to a possible role of iron supplements. Calcium is helpful in adding bone growth. Stimulating myelopoiesis of erythroid progenitor cells refers to the mechanism of action of erythropoietin. Finally, reduction of blood viscosity during pregnancy refers to pentoxifylline; however, this medication is not recommended during pregnancy.

10. **The answer is E.** Hydroxyurea increases the production of fetal hemoglobin and has been shown to be effective in reducing painful episodes of sickle crisis. Indomethacin is a nonsteroidal anti-inflammatory drug (NSAID) commonly used for pain associated with rheumatoid arthritis. Hydrocodone is a narcotic pain reliever that is only recommended in cases of severe pain, such as that caused by surgery. Acetaminophen is unlikely to be helpful in this patient's situation, as this agent is useful for mild-to-moderate pain. Celecoxib is a COX-2 inhibitor used in a variety of inflammatory conditions.

11. **The answer is B.** Oprelvekin has been shown to reduce the need for platelet transfusions following myelosuppressive chemotherapy. Erythropoietin is used for anemia. Filgrastim and sargramostim are used for neutropenia. Leucovorin is used in patients undergoing treatment with methotrexate, to prevent some of its side effects.

12. **The answer is A.** Heparin increases the activity of antithrombin by 1000-fold. Antithrombin, in turn, activates serine proteases of the clotting cascade. Heparin has a direct anticoagulant activity and can inhibit clotting in vitro. Heparin releases lipoprotein lipase from vascular beds, which accelerates clearing of lipoproteins from plasma. The clotting factor is inactivated, which releases heparin and allows it to be recycled.

13. **The answer is D.** Coumarin is commonly used in patients with atrial fibrillation for prevention of thromboembolic events, such as stroke. Prothrombin times should be frequently monitored in patients taking coumarin, as bleeding is a common adverse effect. Heparin is monitored with partial thromboplastin time. Fragmin and Lovenox are low-molecular-weight derivatives of heparin that do not require laboratory monitoring. Protamine is an agent used for heparin reversal.

14. **The answer is C.** Clopidogrel works by inhibiting platelet aggregation. Heparin works by increasing the activity of antithrombin. Coumarin interferes with γ-carboxylation of several clotting factors. Alteplase is a thrombolytic. Dextran impairs fibrin polymerization and platelet function.

8 Drugs Acting on the Gastrointestinal Tract

I. ANTIEMETICS

A. Vomiting reflex
1. The vomiting reflex is a coordinated reflex controlled by a bilateral **vomiting center** in the dorsal portion of the lateral reticular formation in the medulla.
2. Pharmacologic intervention relies on inhibition of inputs or depression of the vomiting center. The vomiting center receives inputs from several sources:
   a. **Area postrema** (chemoreceptor trigger zone, CTZ)
   b. **Vestibular apparatus**
   c. **Peripheral afferents** from the pharynx, gastrointestinal (GI) tract, and genitals
   d. **Higher cortical centers**

B. Antiemetics are useful in the treatment of vomiting associated with motion sickness, chemotherapy-induced emesis (CIE), radiation-induced emesis (RIE), postoperative nausea and vomiting (PONV), and other causes.
1. *Cholinoceptor antagonists*
   a. Cholinergic antagonists **reduce the excitability of labyrinthine receptors** and depress conduction from the vestibular apparatus to the vomiting center.
   b. Cholinergic antagonists like scopolamine are used to treat **motion sickness** and in **preoperative situations**. They are not useful in treating nausea caused by chemotherapy.
   c. Cholinergic antagonists produce adverse effects that include drowsiness, dry mouth, and blurred vision.
   d. **Scopolamine** (Trans-Scop) is a preferred agent because it has a relatively long duration of action and a more pronounced central nervous system (CNS) action. **Transdermal delivery** of scopolamine via a skin patch decreases the incidence of adverse effects and produces relief for 72 hours.
2. *Histamine H_1-receptor antagonists*
   a. Histamine H_1-receptor antagonists include **meclizine** (Antivert, Bonine), **cyclizine** (Marezine), **dimenhydrinate** (Dramamine), and **promethazine** (Phenergan).
   b. These agents act by inhibiting histamine pathways, and cholinergic pathways of the vestibular apparatus.
   c. Histamine H_1-receptor antagonists are used to treat **motion sickness** and **vertigo**.
   d. **Cyclizine** and **meclizine** are used for nausea and vomiting associated with **pregnancy**.
   e. These agents to varying degrees produce sedation and dry mouth and other anticholinergic side effects.
3. *Dopamine receptor antagonists*
   a. **Metoclopramide** (Reglan; see IV B)
   b. **Phenothiazines and butyrophenones**
      (1) These agents include the phenothiazine **prochlorperazine** (Compazine) and **promethazine** (Phenergan), and the butyrophone **droperidol** (Inapsine) that is only available in an intravenous (IV) formulation.

(2) These agents **block dopaminergic receptors in the CTZ** and appear to inhibit peripheral transmission to the vomiting center. They also **block α_1-adrenoceptors. Prochlorperazine** also **blocks muscarinic cholinoceptors.**

(3) These agents are used to treat **CIE, RIE, and PONY.**

(4) Adverse actions include anticholinergic effects such as drowsiness, dry mouth, and blurred vision (less pronounced with **droperidol**), **extrapyramidal effects**, and orthostatic hypotension. These agents are **contraindicated in Parkinson's disease** because of their extrapyramidal effects.

(5) Droperidol use is associated with **Q–T prolongation and torsade de pointes** and has a **black box warning.**

4. *Serotonin 5-hydroxy tryptamine 3 antagonists*

a. **Ondansetron** (Zofran), **dolasetron** (Anzemet), **granisetron** (Kytril), and **palonosetron** (Aloxi)

(1) These agents are **antagonists at serotonin 5-HT$_3$-receptors,** key components in the CNS and GI tract in triggering vomiting.

(2) These agents are very effective against acute **CIE** and **RIE,** and for PONY. They are **not effective for motion-sickness–induced** nausea and vomiting.

(3) These agents can be administered orally and parenterally, except **palonosetron** which is only administered intravenously.

(4) Palonosetron has a long duration of action with a half-life of 40 hours.

(5) Dose reduction of **ondansetron** may be necessary for patients with hepatic insufficiency.

(6) The most common adverse effects of these drugs are headache and mild constipation.

(7) Dolasetron prolongs the Q–T interval.

b. These agents are often combined with **corticosteroids, such as dexamethasone** (Decadron), to produce an enhanced antiemetic effect.

5. *Cannabinoids*

a. **Dronabinol** (Marinol) and **Nabilone** (Cesamet) are preparations of Δ-9-tetrahydrocannabinol, the active cannabinoid in marijuana.

b. These drugs act by **inhibiting the vomiting center through stimulation of a CB$_1$ subtype of cannabinoid receptors.**

c. They are alternative agents **used to control CIE.**

d. Adverse effects include sedation, tachycardia, hypotension, and behavioral alterations similar to those associated with the use of marijuana (see V X F).

6. *Benzodiazepines*

a. Benzodiazepines include **lorazepam** (Ativan) and **diazepam** (Valium).

b. Benzodiazepines act as anxiolytic agents to reduce **anticipatory emesis. Diazepam** is useful as a treatment of **vertigo,** and it controls symptoms in **Ménière disease** in 60%–70% of patients.

7. *Neurokinin 1 receptor antagonists*

a. **Aprepitant** (Emend; fosaprepitant is an IV prodrug formulation) is used to manage the **delayed phase of emesis caused by chemotherapy.**

b. Aprepitant is used in a combination with 5-HT$_3$ antagonists and corticosteroids.

c. It is metabolized by CYP3A4 and, therefore, may inhibit the metabolism of other drugs that use the same pathway. Drugs that inhibit CYP3A4 may increase its plasma levels.

d. Adverse effects include diarrhea and fatigue.

II. ANOREXIGENICS AND APPETITE ENHANCERS

A. General characteristics of anorexigenics

1. Anorexigenics are drugs that **decrease appetite** or **promote satiety**. They are used for the **adjunct treatment of obesity**.

2. Prolonged use of some anorexigenics may lead to physical or psychologic **dependence**.

B. **Amphetamines and amphetamine derivatives** (selected)
   1. *Amphetamine, methamphetamine, and phentermine* (Adipex) **act centrally** and elevate the synaptic concentration of catecholamines and dopamine, producing a **reduction in food-seeking behavior.** They have limited efficacy as anorexigenic agents, primarily during the first few weeks following initiation of therapy.
   2. These agents have a high risk of dependence.

C. **Orlistat (Xenical)**
   1. Orlistat is a reversible lipase inhibitor used for the **management of obesity** and is also available over the counter. It **inactivates the enzymes,** thus making them unavailable to digest dietary fats. Orlistat **inhibits absorption of fats by approximately 30%.**
   2. This agent is contraindicated in patients with **cholestasis** and **malabsorption syndromes**.
   3. **Fat-soluble vitamins** should be supplemented when taking Orlistat.
   4. Major side effects in GI are: fecal spotting, flatulence, and diarrhea.

D. *Dronabinol* (Δ-9-tetrahydrocannabinol) (Marinol) **stimulates appetite,** among its other activities. For this reason it may be used in patients with acquired immune deficiency syndrome (**AIDS**) **and cancer** who are malnourished due to lack of appetite.

E. *Megestrol* (Megace) is a progestational agent that has a side effect of **increased appetite.** It can be used in liquid form or, more commonly, in a pill form. Its use leads to **increased caloric intake and weight gain.** This agent is also used as a second- or third-line therapy for **breast cancer** patients who have progressed on tamoxifen (see Chapter 12).

III. AGENTS USED FOR UPPER GI TRACT DISORDERS

A. **Goal of therapy** for upper GI tract disorders **(peptic ulcers and gastroesophageal reflux disease [GERD])** is to **reduce gastric acid production,** to **neutralize gastric H$^+$,** or **to protect the walls of the stomach** from the acid and pepsin released by the stomach.

B. **Antacids**
   1. *General characteristics*
      a. Antacids are **weak bases** that are taken orally and that **partially neutralize gastric acid, reduce pepsin activity, and stimulate prostaglandin production.**
      b. Antacids **reduce the pain** associated with ulcers and may promote healing.
      c. Antacids have been largely **replaced for GI disorders by other drugs** but are still used commonly by patients as nonprescription remedies for dyspepsia.
   2. *Prototype agents*
      a. **Sodium bicarbonate** (Atka Seltzer)
         (1) Sodium bicarbonate reacts with gastric hydrochloric acid to form sodium chloride and carbon dioxide. It may cause nausea and belching.
         (2) Some unreacted sodium bicarbonate is absorbed systemically and can cause a metabolic alkalosis. **It should not be used for long-term treatment.**
         (3) Sodium bicarbonate is **contraindicated in hypertension, heart failure, and renal failure** because its high sodium content can increase fluid retention.
      b. **Calcium carbonate** (TUMS, Os-Cal)
         (1) Calcium carbonate reacts with gastric hydrochloric acid to form calcium chloride and carbon dioxide. It may also cause nausea and belching.
         (2) Calcium carbonate is partially absorbed from the GI tract and thus may cause some systemic effects like metabolic alkalosis. **It should not be used for long-term treatment.**
         (3) Calcium carbonate may stimulate gastrin release and thereby cause rebound acid production.

   c. Magnesium hydroxide
     (1) Magnesium hydroxide is not absorbed from the GI tract and therefore produces **no systemic effects.** This agent can be used for long-term therapy.
     (2) The most frequent adverse effect associated with magnesium hydroxide is **diarrhea.**
   d. Aluminum hydroxide
     (1) Aluminum hydroxide is **not absorbed** from the GI tract; it has no systemic effects.
     (2) Aluminum hydroxide causes **constipation.**
   e. Combination products (Maalox, Mylanta II, Gelusil) **combine magnesium hydroxide** and **aluminum hydroxide** to achieve a counteracting balance between each agents' adverse effects on the bowel.
   f. Sodium bicarbonate and calcium carbonate in the presence of dairy products containing calcium can cause hypercalcemia and metabolic alkalosis with renal insufficiency (**milk-alkali syndrome**).
  3. *Drug interactions.* Antacids alter the bioavailability of many drugs by the following mechanisms:
   a. The **increase in gastric pH** produced by antacids decreases the absorption of acidic drugs and increases the absorption of basic drugs.
   b. The **metal ion** in some preparations can **chelate other drugs** (e.g., **digoxin** and **tetracycline**) and **prevent** their **absorption.**

C. Inhibitors of gastric acid production (Fig. 8.1)
  1. *Histamine H₂-receptor antagonists*
   a. Mechanism of action. The H_2-receptor antagonists, **cimetidine** (Tagamet), **ranitidine** (Zantac), **famotidine** (Pepcid), and **nizatidine** (Axid), act as **competitive inhibitors of the histamine H_2-receptor on the parietal cell.** This results in a marked **decrease in histamine-stimulated gastric acid secretion.** Although other agents such as gastrin and acetylcholine may induce acid secretion, **histamine** is the predominant final mediator that **stimulates parietal acid secretion.** These drugs are rapidly absorbed, and effects are observed within **a few minutes to hours.**

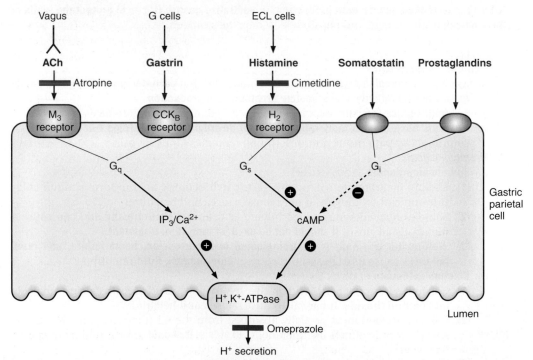

FIGURE 8.1. Site of action on parietal cells of three classes of antisecretory drugs. cAMP, cyclic adenosine monophosphate; H_2, histamine-2 receptor; M_1, muscarinic receptor.

   b. Therapeutic uses: Histamine H_2-receptor antagonists are used as sole agents to treat **peptic ulcer disease** (on discontinuation, recurrence is observed in 90% of patients), **GERD, stress-related gastritis** (administered IV in intensive care settings), and **non-ulcer-related dyspepsia.** Except for the latter condition, their use has been mostly supplanted by proton-pump inhibitors (PPIs) (see below).

   c. Adverse effects

      (1) Histamine H_2-receptor antagonists are associated with a low incidence of mild GI upset and headache. Confusion is seen with IV administration, especially in the elderly, and especially with **cimetidine.**

      (2) Cimetidine is also an **androgen-receptor antagonist** and can induce gynecomastia and impotence.

      (3) Cimetidine competes with other drugs for metabolism by the **cytochrome P-450** mixed-function oxidase system; it can **increase the half-life** of drugs that are metabolized by this system (e.g., **warfarin, theophylline, phenytoin,** and **benzodiazepines**).

      (4) Ranitidine, famotidine, and nizatidine do not bind to the androgen receptor; their effect on drug metabolism is negligible.

  2. *Proton-pump inhibitors*

   a. Omeprazole (Prilosec), **lansoprazole** (Prevacid), **dexlansoprazole** (Dexilant), **esomeprazole** (Nexium), **pantoprazole** (Protonix), and **rabeprazole** (Aciphex) are covalent, **irreversible inhibitors of the H^+/K^+-ATPase proton pump in parietal cells.** As lipophilic weak bases, these orally administered, delayed-release, **prodrugs** (to protect against their destruction by gastric acid) concentrate in the acidic compartments of parietal cells. There they are rapidly **converted to an active cation** which forms a covalent disulfide linkage to the H^+/K^+-ATPase proton pump that results in its inactivation, thereby blocking the transport of acid from the cell into the lumen.

   b. These agents **reduce both meal-stimulated and basal acid secretion.** Desired effects **may take 3–4 days** since not all proton pumps are inhibited with the first dose of these medications.

   c. Their bioavailability is decreased significantly by food and, ideally, should be administered 1 hour before a meal.

   d. These agents are the most effective drugs for treatment of all forms of **GERD.**

   e. PPIs, administered with the antibiotics (e.g., **clarithromycin** and **amoxicillin** or **metronidazole; "triple therapy"**), and perhaps bismuth subsalicylate, are preferred for the treatment of ***Helicobacter pylori*–associated ulcers**. (See Table 8.1 for information on their use in ulcer treatment regimens.)

   f. These agents are used to heal ulcers caused by **nonsteroidal anti-inflammatory drug therapy.**

   g. Omeprazole, by oral or IV administration, is FDA approved to reduce **stress-related mucosal bleeding.**

   h. These agents are useful in patients with untreatable hyper-acid secreting **gastrinomas.**

   i. Adverse effects include headaches and GI disturbances; the reduction in acid production may permit bacterial overgrowth with increased incidence of respiratory and enteric infections.

D. Protective agents

  1. *Sucralfate (Carafate)*

   a. Sucralfate, a polysaccharide complexed with aluminum hydroxide, has a particular affinity for exposed proteins in the crater of **duodenal ulcers;** it protects ulcerated areas from further damage and promotes healing. Sucralfate stimulates mucosal production of prostaglandins and inhibits pepsin. It is used in critical care settings to prevent **stress-related bleeding.**

   b. Sucralfate produces constipation and nausea.

  2. *Misoprostol (Cytotec)*, an analog of prostaglandin E_1 that acts in the GI tract to **stimulate bicarbonate and mucus production,** is used, rarely, to reduce the incidence of stress-related bleeding due to its adverse effect profile and its dosing schedule of four times daily.

  3. Bismuth subsalicylate (Pepto Bismol)—see VI B 2.

table 8.1 Combinations Approved by FDA or Recommended by the American College of Gastroenterology for Treatment of Peptic Ulcer Disease

Bismuth Compounds	Antibacterial 1	Antibacterial 2	Acid Inhibitor	Rx	Comments	Adverse Effects
Bismuth subsalicylate (Pepto Bismol), 4× daily	Metronidazole (Flagyl), 3× daily	Amoxicillin or tetracycline, 4× daily		14 days	"Triple therapy"; if not effective, resistance to metronidazole is assumed	Nausea, diarrhea, vomiting
Bismuth subsalicylate (Pepto Bismol), 4× daily	Clarithromycin (use when resistance to metronidazole occurs), 3× daily	Amoxicillin or tetracycline, 4× daily		14 days	Alternative "triple therapy"	Nausea, diarrhea, vomiting
Bismuth subsalicylate (Pepto Bismol), 4× daily	Metronidazole (Flagyl), 3× daily	Tetracycline, 4× daily	Omeprazole (Prilosec), 2× daily	7 days	15% greater cure rate than "triple therapy"	Significantly reduced incidence of GI side effects
Bismuth citrate, 2× daily	Clarithromycin (Biaxin), 3× daily		Ranitidine (Tritec), 2× daily	14 days	Bismuth combined with ranitidine (Tritec)	Nausea, diarrhea
Bismuth subsalicylate	Tetracycline plus metronidazole		Ranitidine or cimetidine	14 days	Bismuth combined with these antibiotics (Helidac)	Nausea, diarrhea, melena
	Clarithromycin, 3× daily	Metronidazole	Omeprazole	14 days	About as effective as "triple therapy"	Nausea, taste loss
	Clarithromycin, 3× daily	Amoxicillin	Omeprazole	14 days	About as effective as "triple therapy"	Nausea

IV. PROKINETIC AGENTS

A. Prokinetic drugs enhance the contractile force of the GI tract and increase transit of its contents.

B. Metoclopramide
1. Metoclopramide is a **dopamine-receptor antagonist.** Blockade of inhibitory dopamine receptors in the GI tract may allow stimulatory actions of ACh at muscarinic synapses to predominate. Metoclopramide also **blocks dopamine D_2-receptors within the CTZ.**
2. This agent **increases lower esophageal tone, stimulates gastric emptying, and increases the rate of transit through the small bowel.**
3. Metoclopramide is used to **treat reflux esophagitis, gastric motor failure,** and **diabetic gastroparesis;** it is also used to **promote placement of nasoenteric feeding tubes** in critically ill patients.
4. Metoclopramide is also used as an **antiemetic for nausea associated with chemotherapy** (e.g., cisplatin and doxorubicin) and **narcotic-induced vomiting.**
5. Metoclopramide produces sedation, **extrapyramidal effects,** and increased prolactin secretion.

V. DRUGS USED TO DISSOLVE GALLSTONES

A. Ursodiol (Actigall)
1. Ursodiol, an oral **naturally occurring bile acid,** requires administration for **months to reach** full effect.
2. This drug's conjugated form **reduces hepatic synthesis and secretion of cholesterol into bile, and its reabsorption by the intestine.** It effectively dissolves **cholesterol gallstones.**
3. This agent may be used for the prevention of gallstones in patients who are undergoing **rapid weight loss.**
4. Ursodiol has a low incidence of diarrhea.

VI. DIGESTIVE ENZYME REPLACEMENTS

A. Pancrelipase (Cotazym-S, Entolase, etc.)
1. Pancrelipase is a **digestive enzyme replacement** preparation of semipurified enzymes that contain various mixtures of lipase and proteolytic enzymes such as trypsin, and amylase.
2. It is used to treat **exocrine pancreatic insufficiency** associated with **cystic fibrosis** and **pancreatitis.**
3. Adverse effects are minimal with occasional GI upset and hyperuricosuria.

VII. AGENTS THAT ACT ON THE LOWER GI TRACT

A. Laxatives (stool softeners and antidiarrheals) act primarily on the large intestine to **promote an increase in the fluid** accumulated in the bowel, **decrease net absorption of fluid** from the bowel, or **alter bowel motility.** These actions facilitate the evacuation of fecal material. Laxatives should not be used chronically as they may induce "laxative dependence."
1. *Bulk-forming laxatives*
a. Bulk-forming laxatives include **psyllium** (Metamucil, etc.), **methylcellulose** (Citrucel), and **polycarbophil** (Fibercon and Fiber Lax).

     b. Bulk-forming laxatives are poorly absorbed from the bowel lumen and **retain water in the bowel.** The increased luminal mass **stimulates peristalsis** and produce laxation after 2–4 days; adequate hydration is required.

     c. These agents are the treatment of choice for **chronic constipation.**

     d. These agents may cause bloating and flatulence.

  2. *Osmotic agents.* These agents are used for both acute and chronic constipation.

     a. Salt-containing osmotic laxatives (saline laxatives)

       (1) Salt-containing osmotic laxatives include **magnesium citrate, magnesium hydroxide, and sodium phosphates.**

       (2) These agents are poorly absorbed ions that **retain water in the lumen by osmosis** and cause a **reflex increase in peristalsis.**

       (3) Salt-containing osmotic laxatives are taken orally. Sodium phosphates are also effective rectally. Onset of action typically occurs 3–6 hours after oral administration and 5–15 minutes after rectal administration. They require adequate hydration for effect.

       (4) Sodium phosphate may cause systemic adverse effects, especially in cases of renal dysfunction; these effects include phosphatemia and hypernatremia.

     b. Salt-free osmotic laxatives

       (1) Salt-free osmotic laxatives include **lactulose** (Chronulac) and **polyethylene glycol–electrolyte solutions** (Colyte, Go-Lytely).

       (2) These agents may be administered rectally (glycerin) or orally (lactulose). Go-Lytely is used for **preoperative colon preparation.**

  3. *Irritant (stimulant) laxatives*

     a. Irritant laxatives include **bisacodyl** (Modane, Dulcolax), **senna** (Senokot), and **cascara sagrada.**

     b. Irritant laxatives **stimulate smooth muscle contractions resulting from their irritant action on the bowel mucosa.** Local bowel **inflammation also promotes accumulation of water and electrolytes.** The increased luminal contents stimulate reflex peristalsis, and the irritant action stimulates peristalsis directly.

     c. The onset of action occurs in 6–12 hours; these agents require adequate hydration.

     d. Chronic use of irritant laxatives may result in **cathartic colon,** a condition of **colonic distention,** and development of **laxative dependence.**

  4. *Stool softeners*

     a. Stool softeners include **docusate sodium** (Colace, etc.), **glycerin,** and **mineral oil.**

     b. **Docusate** has a **detergent action** that facilitates the mixing of water and fatty substances to **increase luminal mass.**

     c. **Mineral oil coats fecal contents** and thereby inhibits absorption of water.

     d. **Mineral oil decreases the absorption of fat-soluble vitamins. Lipoid pneumonia** can develop if mineral oil is aspirated.

B. **Antidiarrheal agents** aim to decrease fecal water content by **increasing solute absorption and decreasing intestinal secretion and motility.** Increased transit time facilitates water reabsorption. Therapy with these drugs should be reserved for patients with significant and persistent symptoms of diarrhea.

  1. *Opioids* **act directly on opioid μ-receptors** to decrease transit rate, stimulate segmental (nonpropulsive) contraction, and inhibit longitudinal contraction.

     a. Diphenoxylate (Lomotil)

       (1) Diphenoxylate and its active metabolite, **difenoxin** (Motofen), are used for the treatment of diarrhea and not analgesia.

       (2) Diphenoxylate is used as a combination product with **atropine** to reduce the potential for abuse.

       (3) At high doses, this agent may produce CNS effects including nausea and vomiting, sedation, and constipation.

     b. Loperamide (Imodium)

       (1) Loperamide is an **opioid agonist** with **no CNS activity,** except at very high doses, but with marked effects on the intestine. It binds to opioid receptors in the GI tract.

(2) Loperamide has a faster onset and longer duration of action than diphenoxylate.

(3) Loperamide overdose can result in severe constipation, paralytic ileus, and CNS depression.

2. ***Bismuth subsalicylate (Pepto Bismol)***

   a. The salicylate in this agent **inhibits prostaglandin and chloride secretion in the intestine to reduce the liquid content of the stools.** It is effective for both treatment and prophylaxis of **traveler's diarrhea** and other forms of diarrhea.

   b. Bismuth subsalicylate forms a protective coating in the GI tract and has **direct antimicrobial activity.** It is used to treat *H. pylori* **infection.**

   c. Bismuth subsalicylate is also used effectively to **bind toxins produced by *Vibrio cholerae* and *Escherichia coli.*** The salicylate can be absorbed across the intestine.

   d. Bismuth subsalicylate produces adverse effects that include **tinnitus.** It may also produce **black stools** and staining of the tongue.

3. ***Octreotide (Sandostatin)***

   a. Octreotide is an **analog of somatostatin.** It is effective for the treatment of diarrhea caused by **short-gut syndrome and dumping syndrome.**

   b. Octreotide is used in cases of **severe diarrhea caused by excessive release of GI tract hormones,** including gastrin and vasoactive intestinal polypeptide. It is used in the treatment of **neuroendocrine tumors of the GI tract**.

   c. This agent must be administered parenterally.

   d. Octreotide causes mild GI dysfunction and formation of gallstones due to alteration of fat absorption.

C. **Agents used in inflammatory bowel disease (IBD): ulcerative colitis and Crohn's disease.**

   1. ***Mesalamine*** (Asacol, Pentasa), ***sulfasalazine*** (Azulfidine), ***olsalazine*** (Dipentum), and ***balsalazide*** (Colazal)

      a. **Mesalamine (5-aminosalicylic acid or 5-ASA),** the active agent for the treatment of IBD, is formulated as delayed-release microgranules (Penstasa), pH-sensitive resins (Asacol, Apriso, Lialda), a suspension enema (Rowasa), or wax suppository (Canasa) that present 5-ASA to different segments of the GI tract. **Sulfasalazine, olsalazine, and balsalazide** are dimers that **contain active 5-ASA bound by agents that prevent its absorption.** The bond is cleaved in the terminal ileum by bacterial enzyme. The released **5-ASA acts topically within the colon.** Although the exact mechanism of action of these agents is uncertain, these agents interfere with the production of inflammatory cytokines.

      b. These agents are most effective for the treatment of **mild-to-moderate ulcerative colitis.**

      c. **Sulfasalazine** is bound to **sulfapyridine** that when released and absorbed is responsible for a **high incidence of adverse effects** that include nausea, headaches, bone marrow suppression, general malaise, and **hypersensitivity. Slow acetylators** of sulfapyridine are most likely to experience adverse effects. The other agents are generally well tolerated. **Olsalazine** may cause a **secretory diarrhea.**

   2. ***Glucocorticoids*** and other **drugs reacting on the immune system**

      a. **Prednisone** and **prednisolone are** used most commonly in **acute exacerbation of the IBD,** as well as in **maintenance therapy.**

      b. **Budesonide** (Entocort) is an analog of prednisolone. It has low oral bioavailability, so enteric-coated, delayed-release formulations are more commonly used, particularly to treat Crohn's disease.

      c. The mechanism of action for these agents involves **inhibition of proinflammatory cytokines.** Glucocorticoids carry a high incidence of **systemic side effects,** so their use in maintenance therapy is limited.

      d. Up to **60% of patients with IBD are steroid unresponsive** or have only a partial response.

      e. Glucocorticoids **stimulate sodium absorption in the jejunum, ileum, and colon;** glucocorticoids such as budesonide and prednisone are also used to treat **refractory diarrhea** unresponsive to other agents (see VII B).

   3. ***Azathioprine*** (Imuran) and ***6-mercaptopurine*** (Purinethol)

      a. These agents are immune suppressants.

    b. Their onset of therapeutic action is **delayed by several weeks;** therefore, they are **not used in an acute setting.**

    c. These agents are used for **maintenance and remission of IBD in patients who do not respond well to steroids.**

    d. These drugs are **metabolized by thiopurine-*S*-methyltransferase,** of which levels are low in up to 12% of the population in whom dose reductions should be made. The enzyme is **absent in up to 0.3% of the population** to whom these drugs should not be administered.

    e. Their major side effect is **bone marrow depression.**

4. ***Methotrexate*** (Rheumatrex, Trexall) is another immune suppressant that acts via **inhibition of dihydrofolate reductase.** It is used to **induce and maintain remission in patients with Crohn's disease who do not respond well to steroids** (it is also used to treat rheumatoid arthritis and cancer). **Bone marrow suppression** is a major side effect when this drug is used at higher doses.

5. ***Infliximab*** (Remicade; administered intravenously), ***Adalimumab*** (Humira), ***Certolizumab*** (Cimzia), and **Natalizumab** (Tysabri).

    a. Infliximab, Adalimumab, and Certolizumab are monoclonal antibodies administered subcutaneously that bind to and **neutralize tumor necrosis factor,** a major cytokine that mediates the T_H1 immune response present during inflammation. Natalizumab is a monoclonal antibody that binds to **integrins** associated with circulating inflammatory cells.

    b. Infliximab is an approved alternative treatment for ulcerative colitis. All three are approved as alternative therapies for the acute and chronic treatment of Crohn's disease.

    c. Remission or improvement of symptoms is observed in two-thirds of patients. However, there is a significant loss of response over time in many of these patients.

    d. Serious adverse effects include numerous forms of **infections** (bacterial, fungal, etc.), including reactivation of **tuberculosis**, symptoms resembling serum sickness, hepatic dysfunction, exacerbation of congestive heart failure, additional risk of lymphoma and, with infliximab infusion, a myriad of reactions related to cardiovascular, respiratory, and skeletal muscle systems.

D. **Agents used in the treatment of irritable bowel syndrome (IBS):** ***Alosetron*** (Lotronex) is a **5-HT$_3$ antagonist** that blocks receptors on enteric neurons, thereby **reducing distention and inhibiting colonic motility,** thereby **reducing IBS-associated pain.** Its main approved use is in "diarrhea-predominant" IBS, specifically in women. Alosetron may cause **severe constipation with ischemic colitis that requires its discontinuation.** Therefore, its use is restricted to patients as an alternative treatment in women who have not responded to other therapies.

▮ DRUG SUMMARY TABLE

Antiemetics
Cholinoceptor, histamine receptor, and dopamine receptor antagonists
Scopolamine (Transderm Scop, Hyoscine)
Dimenhydrinate (Dramamine)
Cyclizine (Marezine)
Meclizine (Antivert, generic)
Promethazine (Phenergan, generic)
Diphenhydramine (Benadryl, etc.)
Trimethobenzamide (Tigan, generic)
Prochlorperazine (Compazine)
Droperidol (Inapsine)
Metoclopramide (Raglan, generic)
Serotonin receptor antagonists
Ondansetron (Zofran, generic)
Granisetron (Kytril, generic)
Dolasetron (Anzemet)

Magnesium and aluminum hydroxide (Maalox, Gelusil, etc.)
Histamine H$_2$-receptor antagonists
Cimetidine (Tagamet, generic)
Ranitidine (Zantac, generic)
Famotidine (Pepcid, generic)
Nizatidine (Axid, generic)
Proton pump inhibitors (PPIs)
Omeprazole (Prilosec)
Lansoprazole (Prevacid)
Pantoprazole (Protonix)
Rabeprazole (AcipHex)
Esomeprazole (Nexium)
Dexlansoprazole (Dexilant)
Mucosal protective agents
Sucralfate (Carafate, generic)
Misoprostol (Cytotec)

Alvimopan (Entereg)
Stool softeners
Docusate (Colace, etc.)
Mineral oil
Antidiarrheal agents: opioids
Loperamide (Imodium, generic)
Diphenoxylate (Lomotil, generic)
Difenoxin (Motofen)
Antidiarrheal agents
Bismuth subsalicylate (Pepto Bismol, Kaopectate, etc.)
Octreotide (Sandostatin, generic)
Agents for inflammatory bowel disease (IBD)
Sulfasalazine (Azulfidine, generic)
Mesalamine (Asacol, Pentasa)
Olsalazine (Dipentum)
Balsalazide (Colazal)
Budesonide (Entocort, generic)

Palonosetron (Aloxi)
Cannabinoids
Dronabinol (Marinol)
Nabilone (Cesamet)
Benzodiazepines
Lorazepam (Ativan, generic)
Diazepam (Valium, generic)
Neurokinin receptor antagonists
Aprepitant (Emend)

**Anorexigenics and Appetite
Enhancers**
Orlistat (Xenical, generic)
Dronabinol (Marinol)
Megestrol (Megace)

Agents Used for Upper GI
Antacids
Sodium bicarbonate (Alka Seltzer)
Calcium carbonate (TUMS,
    Rolaids, etc.)

Drugs Acting on Lower GI
Laxatives: bulk-forming agents
Psyllium (Metamucil, Serutan, etc.)
Methylcellulose (Citrucel, etc.)
Polycarbophil (Fibercon, etc.)
Laxatives: osmotic agents
Magnesium hydroxide (Milk of
    magnesia, etc.)
Magnesium citrate (Citroma, etc.)
Sodium phosphate (Visicol, etc.)
Lactulose (Chronulac, etc.)
PGE solutions (Go-Lytely, etc.)
Glycerin
Laxatives: irritant agents
Bisacodyl (Dulcolax, Correctol)
Senna (Senokot, etc.)
Cascara Sagrada
Lubiprostone (Amitiza)
Laxatives: Opioid-receptor
    antagonists
Methylnaltrexone (Relistor)

Prednisolone (Millipred, generic)
Methylprednisolone (Medrol, generic)
Azathioprine (Imuran, generic)
6-Mercaptopurine (Purinethol, generic)
Methotrexate (Rheumatrex, Trexall)
Infliximab (Remicade)
Adalimumab (Humira)
Certolizumab (Cimzia)
Natalizumab (Tysabri)
Agents for irritable bowel syndrome
(IBS)
Alosetron (Lotronex)

Prokinetic Agents
Metoclopramide (Reglan, generic)

Drugs Used to Dissolve Gallstones
Ursodiol (Actigal, generic)

Digestive Enzyme Replacements
Pancrelipase (Creon, generic)

Review Test

Directions: Each of the numbered items or incomplete statements in this section is followed by answers or by completions of the statement. Select the ONE lettered answer or completion that is BEST in each case.

1. A 54-year-old man with a 75-pack/year history of tobacco abuse and alcohol abuse has developed carcinoma of the larynx. His treatment includes concurrent high-dose cisplatin and radiation therapy. He has developed significant nausea and vomiting. Which would be the best agent to treat these side effects?

(A) Metoclopramide
(B) Ondansetron
(C) Meclizine
(D) Promethazine
(E) Loperamide

2. Aprepitant is which of the following?

(A) Cholinergic antagonist
(B) Dopaminergic agonist
(C) Histamine H_1-receptor antagonist
(D) Serotonin 5-HT_3 antagonist
(E) Substance P antagonist

3. A 74-year-old man went on a cruise to celebrate his 50th wedding anniversary. Concerned about a history of motion sickness, the patient saw his primary care physician about a medication to take. He is now seen by the onboard physician with complaints of blurred vision, confusion, constipation, and urinary retention. Which of the following did the primary care physician likely prescribe?

(A) Scopolamine
(B) Metoclopramide
(C) Haloperidol
(D) Dronabinol
(E) Ondansetron

4. Which of the following drugs would be best to use to treat irritable bowel syndrome (IBS) in a 53-year-old woman?

(A) Infliximab
(B) Diphenoxylate
(C) Cimetidine

(D) Alosetron
(E) Orlistat

5. A 35-year-old cancer patient is cachectic and has a poor appetite. You decide to start therapy with what agent?

(A) Granisetron
(B) Megestrol
(C) Dronabinol
(D) Phentermine
(E) Dextroamphetamine

6. As a gastroenterologist, you recommend the use of a histamine H_2-blocker for a patient who has a history of atrial fibrillation, for which he takes warfarin. Your office receives a call from his primary physician, who has admitted the patient for warfarin toxicity. Which of the following H_2-blockers has the patient likely been taking?

(A) Cimetidine
(B) Ranitidine
(C) Scopolamine
(D) Famotidine
(E) Nizatidine

7. A 34-year-old man is seen over multiple visits for complaints of "ulcers," despite the use of ranitidine. Further studies, finding elevated levels of gastrin and evidence of ulcers involving the jejunum, suggest a diagnosis of Zollinger-Ellison syndrome. Which of the following agents would be most useful in the management of this patient?

(A) Famotidine
(B) Lansoprazole
(C) Misoprostol
(D) Propantheline
(E) Pepto Bismol

8. A 63-year-old man with long-standing, poorly controlled diabetes is admitted for yet another episode of ketoacidosis. Now that he is out of the intensive care unit and beginning to eat, he complains of regurgitation of food following even small meals. You suspect the development of diabetic gastropathy, a consequence of his autonomic neuropathy. Which of the following might help his condition?

(A) Sucralfate
(B) Metoclopramide
(C) Scopolamine
(D) Misoprostol
(E) Pepto Bismol

9. A 78-year-old woman sees her primary care physician with complaints of "heartburn." Her history includes only hypertension. She lives on a fixed income and has no prescription coverage. Her doctor recommends over-the-counter antacids to be used regularly. Which of the following would be a good choice and why?

(A) Sodium bicarbonate because it is good for long-term use
(B) Calcium carbonate because it is good for long-term use and she could use the calcium
(C) Magnesium hydroxide for short-term use only because of her hypertension
(D) A combined agent to balance the constipation associated with magnesium hydroxide and the diarrhea associated with aluminum hydroxide
(E) A combined agent to balance the diarrhea associated with magnesium hydroxide and the constipation associated with aluminum hydroxide

10. An otherwise healthy 33-year-old man sees his physician for a routine physical examination. The patient has no complaints and is planning on vacationing in Mexico next month. However, he is afraid of developing traveler's diarrhea. You recommend that he take which of the following drugs for prophylaxis?

(A) Glucocorticoids
(B) Loperamide
(C) Bismuth subsalicylate
(D) Kaolin
(E) Diphenoxylate

11. A 72-year-old man with a 150-pack/year history of cigarette smoking presents for further workup of a large mass seen on a recent chest X-ray. The patient reports a 50-lb unintentional weight loss over the last 3 months and a poor appetite. In addition to beginning chemotherapy, the oncologist decides to add which agent to promote his appetite?

(A) Aprepitant
(B) Lorazepam
(C) Ondansetron
(D) Megestrol

12. A 65-year-old man presents to his family physician with a 3-month history of watery diarrhea. He is referred to a gastroenterologist, who finds that the patient is also hypokalemic and achlorhydric and has an elevated serum level of vasoactive intestinal peptide due to a pancreatic islet cell tumor (VIPoma). Which agent would be best to treat the patient's symptoms?

(A) Gastrin
(B) Octreotide
(C) Glucagon
(D) Bismuth subsalicylate
(E) Sulfasalazine

Answers and Explanations

1. **The answer is B.** Ondansetron is a 5-HT$_3$ antagonist that is highly effective in the treatment of cisplatin-induced chemotherapy, better so than metoclopramide. Both meclizine and promethazine are antagonists of H$_1$-receptors used in the treatment of motion sickness, true vertigo, and pregnancy-associated nausea. Loperamide is an antidiarrheal agent.

2. **The answer is E.** Aprepitant is the first available substance P antagonist used for the prevention of both sudden and delayed chemotherapy-induced nausea and vomiting. It can be used synergistically with serotonin 5-HT$_3$ antagonists such as ondansetron. The other antagonists, cholinergic (i.e., scopolamine), histaminic (i.e., promethazine), and dopaminergic (i.e., metoclopramide), are used to treat nausea and vomiting, although not in this setting.

3. **The answer is A.** Scopolamine is a cholinergic antagonist that is likely associated with all the patient's new symptoms. Metoclopramide can cause extrapyramidal effects, as can haloperidol. Dronabinol can cause sedation, dry mouth, psychotic effects, and orthostatic hypotension. Ondansetron can cause mild headache.

4. **The answer is D.** Alosetron has been shown to provide some relief of irritable bowel syndrome (IBS). Infliximab is a biologic agent used in the management of inflammatory bowel disease (IBD). Diphenoxylate is a morphine analog used to treat diarrhea. Cimetidine is used to treat esophageal reflux. Orlistat is an agent used to manage obesity.

5. **The answer is B.** Megestrol is used to stimulate appetite in patients with cancer-related cachexia. Dronabinol is used in the treatment of AIDS wasting, specifically to increase appetite. Granisetron is effective for nausea and vomiting in chemotherapy. The other agents, phentermine and dextroamphetamine, are used to aid in weight loss.

6. **The answer is A.** Cimetidine is a competitive inhibitor of the P-450 system, which thereby increases the half-life of warfarin. This can lead to supratherapeutic levels of the drug and bleeding problems. The other H$_2$-blockers, including ranitidine, famotidine, and nizatidine, are not metabolized by the P-450 system.

7. **The answer is B.** Lansoprazole is an H$^+$/K$^+$-ATPase proton pump inhibitor useful in the treatment of patients who have failed histamine H$_2$-blocker therapy and patients with Zollinger-Ellison syndrome. Famotidine is a histamine H$_2$-blocker. Misoprostol is used to prevent ulcers in patients taking nonsteroidal anti-inflammatory drugs (NSAIDs). Propantheline is a cholinergic agent used in conjunction with other agents, and rarely alone. Ulcers associated with *Helicobacter pylori* can be treated with Pepto Bismol.

8. **The answer is B.** Poor gastric emptying is a manifestation of the neuropathy that accompanies long-standing diabetes. Metoclopramide is a prokinetic agent used in the treatment of diabetic gastroparesis. Sucralfate, scopolamine, and misoprostol are used to treat gastric ulcers. Pepto Bismol is added in the case of peptic ulcers due to *Helicobacter pylori*.

9. **The answer is E.** Both sodium bicarbonate and calcium carbonate are not for long-term use. In addition, sodium bicarbonate is contraindicated in patients with hypertension. A combined agent like Maalox or Mylanta II provides a balance between the diarrhea associated with magnesium hydroxide and the constipation associated with aluminum hydroxide.

10. **The answer is C.** Bismuth subsalicylate is effective for both the treatment and prophylaxis of traveler's diarrhea, most often due to *Escherichia coli (E. coli)*-contaminated water. Loperamide and diphenoxylate are good to treat diarrhea, but generally are not used for prophylaxis. Glucocorticoids are for diarrhea refractory to normal treatment.

11. **The answer is D.** Megestrol acetate is used as an appetite stimulant and results in weight gain in some patients with cancer. Aprepitant, lorazepam, and ondansetron, while having different mechanisms, are all used for nausea and vomiting, which he may experience eventually with his chemotherapy.

12. **The answer is B.** Octreotide is used in the treatment of endocrine tumors such as gastrinomas, glucagonomas, and VIPomas to help alleviate the diarrhea. Bismuth subsalicylate is used to treat traveler's diarrhea, and sulfasalazine is used treat such inflammatory bowel disease, such as Crohn's disease. Gastrin is a GI hormone.

chapter 9

Drugs Acting on the Pulmonary System

I. INTRODUCTION TO PULMONARY DISORDERS

In **asthma, chronic bronchitis**, and **rhinitis**, the effective diameter of the airways is decreased. The goal of therapy is to decrease airway resistance by increasing the diameter of the bronchi and decreasing mucus secretion or stagnation in the airways.

A. Asthma

1. ***Asthma is characterized by acute episodes of bronchoconstriction caused by underlying airway inflammation***. A hallmark of asthma is bronchial hyperreactivity to numerous kinds of endogenous or exogenous stimuli. In asthmatic patients, the response to various stimuli is amplified by persistent inflammation.

2. ***Antigenic stimuli trigger the release of mediators*** (leukotrienes, histamine, PGD_2, and many others) that cause a bronchospastic response, with smooth muscle contraction, mucus secretion, and recruitment of inflammatory cells such as eosinophils, neutrophils, and macrophages (early-phase response).

3. Late-phase response (which may occur in hours or days) is an inflammatory response; the levels of histamine and other mediators released from inflammatory cells rise again and may induce bronchospasm. Eventually, fibrin and collagen deposition and tissue destruction occur. Smooth muscle hypertrophy occurs in chronic asthma.

4. Nonantigenic stimuli (cool air, exercise, and nonoxidizing pollutants) can trigger nonspecific bronchoconstriction after early-phase sensitization.

5. **Methacholine** (a muscarinic cholinergic agonist) **challenge test** is frequently used in the diagnosis of asthma.

B. Chronic obstructive pulmonary disease (COPD)

1. **Chronic bronchitis**

   a. Chronic bronchitis is characterized by pulmonary obstruction caused by excessive production of mucus due to hyperplasia and hyperfunctioning of mucus-secreting goblet cells; this causes a chronic (>2 months) cough.

   b. Chronic bronchitis is often induced by smoking or an environmental irritant.

2. **Emphysema**

   a. Emphysema is a type of COPD characterized by irreversible loss of alveoli due to destruction of cell walls. This decreases the surface area available for gas exchange.

C. Rhinitis

1. Rhinitis is a decrease in nasal airways due to thickening of the mucosa and increased mucus secretion.

2. Rhinitis may be caused by allergy, viruses, vasomotor abnormalities, or rhinitis medicamentosa.

II. AGENTS USED TO TREAT ASTHMA AND OTHER BRONCHIAL DISORDERS (TABLE 9.1)

Treatment of persistent asthma is a two-pronged approach: controller therapy typically using inhaled corticosteroids and long-acting β_2-agonists, and relief therapy with short-acting β_2-agonists for acute exacerbations

A. Adrenergic agonists
   1. *General characteristics*
      a. Adrenergic agonists stimulate β_2-adrenoceptors, causing an increase in cyclic adenosine monophosphate (cAMP) levels, which leads to relaxation of bronchial smooth muscle. These agents also inhibit the release of mediators and stimulate mucociliary clearance.
      b. Adrenergic agonists arc useful for the treatment of the acute bronchoconstriction (exacerbations) of asthma.
      c. Depending on biologic half-life of the drug, these agents are used both for quick relief and for controller therapy.
      d. The use of short-acting, inhaled β_2-adrenoceptor agonists on a daily basis, with increasing necessity of use, indicates the need for additional long-term pharmacotherapy.
   2. *Short-acting β_2-adrenoceptor agonists*
      a. **Albuterol, terbutaline, pirbuterol, and metaproterenol**
         (1) These agents have enhanced β_2-receptor selectivity.
         (2) These agents are generally administered by inhalation and their onset of action is 1–5 minutes. Some preparations are available for oral administration.
         (3) Long-term use of these agents for the treatment of chronic asthma is associated with diminished control, perhaps due to β-receptor down-regulation.
      b. **Nonselective agents**
         (1) **Isoproterenol** is a relatively nonselective β-receptor agonist and a potent bronchodilator. Isoproterenol is most effective in asthmatic patients when administered as an inhalant. During an acute attack, dosing every 1–2 hours is typically required; oral preparations are administered 4 times daily (qid).
         (2) **Epinephrine** is available over-the-counter (OTC) and acts as a β_1-, β_2-, and α_1-adrenoceptor agonist. Epinephrine can be administered as an inhalant or subcutaneously (in emergency circumstances); onset of action occurs within 5–10 minutes and duration is 60–90 minutes.
   3. *Long-acting β_2-adrenoceptor agonists*
      a. **Salmeterol (Serevent) and formoterol (Foradil)**
         (1) These agents are administered as inhalants but have a slower onset of action and a longer duration of action than the short-acting preparations. Both have very lipophilic side chains that slow diffusion out of the airway.

t a b l e **9.1** Drugs for the Management of Asthma	
Bronchodilators	**Anti-inflammatory Agents**
Short-acting	Inhaled corticosteroids: beclomethasone, fluticasone, budesonide, mometasone
Inhaled β_2-agonists: terbutaline, pirbuterol, albuterol	Oral antileukotrienes: montekulast and zafirkulast
Long-acting	Anti-IgE: parenteral omalizumab
Inhaled β_2-agonist: salmeterol, formoterol	
Inhaled anticholinergics: tiotropium, ipratropium	

(2) These agents are very effective for prophylaxis of asthma but should not be used to treat an acute attack.

(3) Salmeterol can cause arrhythmias.

b. Albuterol and terbutaline can be administered orally for controller therapy. As with the other mixed β-adrenoceptor agonists, systemic use is cardiostimulatory.

4. *Adverse effects of adrenergic agonists*

   a. The adverse effects of adrenergic agonists are based on receptor occupancy.

   b. These adverse effects are minimized by inhalant delivery of the adrenergic agonists directly to the airways.

   (1) Epinephrine and isoproterenol have significant β_1-receptor activity and can cause cardiac effects, including tachycardia and arrhythmias, and the exacerbation of angina.

   (2) The most common adverse effect of β_2-adrenoreceptor agonists is skeletal muscle tremor.

   (3) The adverse effects of α-adrenoceptor agonists include vasoconstriction and hypertension.

   (4) Tachyphylaxis, a blunting in the response to adrenergic agonists on repeated use, can be countered by switching to a different agonist or by adding a methylxanthine or corticosteroid to the regimen.

B. Methylxanthines

1. *General characteristics*

   a. For asthma, the most frequently administered methylxanthine is theophylline (1,3-dimethylxanthine). Additional members of this family include theobromine and caffeine.

   b. Because of the limited solubility of theophylline in water, it is complexed as a salt, as in aminophylline and oxtriphylline.

2. *Mechanism of action* (Fig. 9.1)

   a. Methylxanthines cause bronchodilation by action on the smooth muscles in the airways. The exact mechanism remains controversial; some data suggest that it is an **adenosine-receptor antagonist** (adenosine causes bronchoconstriction and promotes the release of histamine from mast cells). In addition, these drugs may decrease the intracellular Ca^{2+}. Theophylline analogs that lack adenosine-antagonist activity maintain bronchodilator activity.

   b. Theophylline inhibits phosphodiesterases, mostly PDE3 and PDE4 (leading to increased cAMP), but this effect requires rather high doses. Inhibition of PDE4 seems to be the most important for airway effects.

   c. Theophylline also has some anti-inflammatory properties and reduces airway responsiveness to agents such as histamine and to allergens.

   d. Theophylline is effective in reducing the synergistic effect of adenosine and antigen stimulation on histamine release.

3. *Pharmacologic effects*

   a. Respiratory system. Methylxanthines affect a number of physiologic systems, but they are most useful in the treatment of asthma because of the following:

   (1) These agents produce rapid relaxation of bronchial smooth muscle.

   (2) Methylxanthines decrease histamine release in response to reaginic (IgE) stimulation.

   (3) These agents stimulate ciliary transport of mucus.

   (4) Methylxanthines improve respiratory performance by improving the contractility of the diaphragm and by stimulating the medullary respiratory center.

   b. Other systems

   (1) Methylxanthines have positive chronotropic and inotropic actions on the heart.

   (2) These agents cause pulmonary and peripheral vasodilation but cerebral vasoconstriction.

   (3) Methylxanthines cause an increase in alertness and cortical arousal at low doses; at high doses, this can proceed to severe nervousness and seizures due to medullary stimulation.

FIGURE 9.1. An overview of the mechanism of action of antiasthma drugs.

(4) These agents stimulate gastric acid and pepsinogen release.
(5) Methylxanthines cause diuresis.

4. **Pharmacologic properties**
   a. **Methylxanthines have a narrow therapeutic index**; blood levels should be monitored on initiation of therapy.
   b. Methylxanthines can readily permeate into all tissue compartments; these agents cross the placenta and can enter breast milk.
   c. Methylxanthines are metabolized extensively in the liver and are excreted by the kidney.

5. **Prototype drug: theophylline**
   a. Theophylline is available in a microcrystalline form for inhalation and as a sustained-release preparation; it can be administered intravenously (IV).

    b. Theophylline has a variable half-life ($t_{1/2}$), approximately 8–9 hours in adults, but shorter in children. Clearance of theophylline is affected by diet, drugs, and hepatic disease.

6. *Therapeutic uses*

    a. Methylxanthines are considered adjuncts to inhaled corticosteroids and are used to treat acute or chronic asthma that is unresponsive to inhaled corticosteroids or β-adrenoceptor agonists; they can be administered prophylactically.

    b. These agents are used to treat chronic bronchitis and emphysema.

    c. These agents are used to treat apnea in preterm infants (based on stimulation of the central respiratory center); usually, caffeine is the agent of choice for this therapy.

7. *Adverse effects*

    a. The adverse effects of methylxanthines include **nausea and vomiting** (central emetic effect), arrhythmias, nervousness, and gastrointestinal bleeding.

    b. Methylxanthines may cause behavioral problems in children.

    c. The combined use of these agents with β_2-adrenoceptor agonists is now suspected to be responsible for recent rises in asthma mortality.

C. Muscarinic antagonists

1. Muscarinic antagonists include **ipratropium bromide** (Atrovent) and atropine.

2. Muscarinic antagonists are competitive antagonists of acetylcholine (ACh) at the muscarinic receptor. They inhibit ACh-mediated constriction of bronchial airways. Anticholinergics also decrease vagal-stimulated mucus secretion.

3. These agents are somewhat variable in their effectiveness as bronchodilators in asthma, but they are useful in patients who are refractory to, or intolerant of, sympathomimetics or methylxanthines.

4. **Ipratropium**, a quaternary amine that is poorly absorbed and does not cross the blood–brain barrier, is administered as an aerosol; its low systemic absorption limits adverse effects. It isused in asthma and COPD.

5. **Tiotropium (Spiriva)** is a long-acting muscarinic antagonist approved for maintenance in COPD.

6. **Atropine** is readily absorbed into the systemic circulation. The adverse effects of atropine include drowsiness, sedation, dry mouth, and blurred vision; these effects limit its use as an antiasthmatic.

D. Glucocorticoids (Fig. 9.2)

1. Glucocorticoids include beclomethasone (Beclovent, Vanceril), triamcinolone acetate (Azmacort), budesonide (Rhinocort), flunisolide (AeroBid), and fluticasone propionate (Flovent). These are **first-line agents for the treatment of persistent asthma**.

2. Glucocorticoids produce a significant increase in airway diameter, probably by attenuating prostaglandin and leukotriene syntheses via annexin 1a and by generally inhibiting the immune response including production of cytokines and chemoattractants. They increase responsiveness to sympathomimetics and decrease mucus production.

3. Glucocorticoids are available as oral, topical, and inhaled agents.

    a. The use of inhaled glucocorticoids is recommended for the initial treatment of asthma, with additional agents added as needed. They are used prophylactically rather than to reverse an acute attack. The most common adverse effects of inhaled glucocorticoids are hoarseness and **oral candidiasis**; the most serious adverse effects are adrenal suppression and osteoporosis.

    b. Inhaled glucocorticoids are partially absorbed.

    c. Because of their systemic adverse effects, **oral glucocorticoids** (see Chapter 10) are usually reserved for patients with severe persistent asthma.

    d. Inhaled glucocorticoids are poorly effective in COPD.

E. Leukotriene inhibitors

1. *Zafirlukast (Accolate) and montelukast (Singulair)*

    a. Zafirlukast and montelukast are antagonists of the leukotriene receptor LT_1. This blocks the action of the cys-leukotrienes C_4, D_4, and E_4 (LTC_4, LTD_4, LTE_4, respectively).

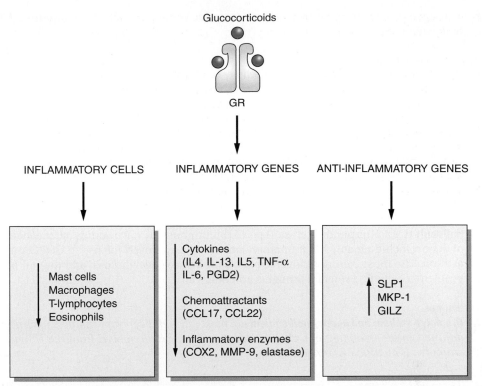

FIGURE 9.2. Effects of glucocorticoids in asthma. SLP-1, secretory leukoprotease inhibitor 1; MAKP1, MAP kinase phosphatase; GILZ, glucocorticoid-induced leucine zipper.

    b. The drugs reduce bronchoconstriction and inflammatory cell infiltration.

    c. Most studies with this class of drugs have been done with mild persistent asthma, and they appear to be moderately effective.

    d. These drugs are recommended as an alternative to medium-dose inhaled glucocorticoids in moderate and severe persistent asthma.

    e. Adverse effects of zafirlukast include headache and elevation in liver enzymes.

    f. Zafirlukast and montelukast are administered orally, 1–2 times per day.

    g. Zafirlukast inhibits the metabolism of warfarin.

2. ***Zileuton (Zyflo)***

    a. Zileuton inhibits 5-lipoxygenase, the rate-limiting enzyme in leukotriene biosynthesis.

    b. Zileuton causes an immediate and sustained 15% improvement in forced expiratory volume in patients with mild persistent asthma.

    c. This agent relieves bronchoconstriction from exercise.

    d. Zileuton is administered orally, usually 4 times per day.

    e. Zileuton may cause liver toxicity; hepatic enzymes should be monitored; elderly women appear to be at highest risk. Zileuton may cause flu-like symptoms: chills, fatigue, and fever.

    f. Zileuton inhibits microsomal P-450s and thereby decreases the metabolism of terfenadine, warfarin, and theophylline.

F. α_1-**Proteinase inhibitor (Prolastin, Aralast)**

    1. α_1-Proteinase inhibitor is used to treat emphysema caused by a deficiency in α_1-proteinase, a peptide that inhibits elastase. In patients with the deficiency, elastase destroys lung parenchyma.

2. This agent is administered by weekly IV injection to treat patients homozygous for this deficiency.

G. **Anti-IgE antibody (Fig. 9.3)**
   1. **Omalizumab binds to human IgE's high-affinity Fc receptor (Fcε8RI),** blocking the binding of IgE to mast cells, basophils, and other cells associated with the allergic response. It also lowers free serum IgE concentrations by as much as 90% and, since it does not block the allergen–antibody reaction, leads to a reduction in allergen concentrations.
   2. These activities reduce both the early-phase degranulation reaction of mast cells and the late-phase release of mediators.
   3. Omalizumab is approved for the treatment of asthma in patients over 12 years old who are refractory to inhaled glucocorticoids and those asthmatic patients with allergies.
   4. The drug is administered by subcutaneous injection every 2–4 weeks.

H. **Roflumilast (Daliresp)**
   1. **Roflumilast** is a phosphodiesterase Type 4 inhibitor but may have additional mechanisms of action including anti-inflammatory activity. It is approved for use in COPD but not asthma. The most common adverse effects are nausea, weight loss, and mental health problems, including suicidal thoughts and behavior.

I. **Chromones**
   1. *Cromolyn sodium and nedocromil sodium are mast cell stabilizers and inhalers were used as adjuncts in the treatment of asthma. Nedocromil has been removed from the US market; cromolyn is available as a nasal spray.*

FIGURE 9.3. The mechanism of action of anti-IgE antibodies.

III. DRUGS USED TO TREAT RHINITIS AND COUGH

A. Rhinitis
   1. *Characteristics of rhinitis*
      a. Congestion is caused by increased mucus production, vasodilation, and fluid accumulation in mucosal spaces.
      b. Mucus production, vasodilation, and parasympathetic stimulation and airway widening are produced by inflammatory mediators (histamine, leukotrienes, prostaglandins, and kinins).
   2. *Selected drugs*
      a. **Antihistamines** (see Chapter 6 for a detail discussion)
         (1) Antihistamines are histamine (H_1)-receptor antagonists; they include first-generation diphenhydramine, brompheniramine, chlorpheniramine, and second-generation loratadine, which are useful in allergic rhinitis but have little effect on rhinitis associated with colds.
         (2) Antihistamines reduce the parasympathetic tone of arterioles and decrease secretion through their anticholinergic activity. Anticholinergics might be more effective in rhinitis, but the doses required produce systemic adverse effects. **Ipratropium bromide** (Atrovent), a poorly absorbed ACh antagonist administered by nasal spray, is approved for rhinorrhea associated with the common cold or with allergic or nonallergic seasonal rhinitis.
      b. **α-Adrenoceptor agonists**
         (1) α-Adrenoceptor agonists act as nasal decongestants.
         (2) These agents include epinephrine and oxymetazoline, which are administered as nasal aerosols; pseudoephedrine, which is administered orally; and phenylephrine, which may be administered orally or as a nasal aerosol.
         (3) Administration as an aerosol is characterized by rapid onset, few systemic effects, and an increased tendency to produce rebound nasal congestion. Oral administration results in longer duration of action, increased systemic effects, and less potential for rebound congestion and dependence.
         (4) These agents reduce airway resistance by **constricting dilated arterioles in the nasal mucosa**.
         (5) α-Adrenoceptor agonists produce adverse effects that include nervousness, tremor, insomnia, dizziness, and rhinitis medicamentosa (chronic mucosal inflammation due to prolonged use of topical vasoconstrictors, characterized by rebound congestion, tachyphylaxis, dependence, and eventual mucosal necrosis).
      c. **Inhaled corticosteroids**
         (1) Topical corticosteroids include beclomethasone (Beconase, Vancenase) and flunisolide (Nasalide).
         (2) Topical corticosteroids are administered as nasal sprays to reduce systemic absorption and adverse effects.
         (3) These agents require 1–2 weeks for full effect.

B. Cough
   1. *Characteristics of cough.* **Cough is produced by the cough reflex, which is integrated in the cough center in the medulla.** The initial stimulus for cough probably arises in the bronchial mucosa, where irritation results in bronchoconstriction. "Cough" receptors, specialized stretch receptors in the trachea and bronchial tree, send vagal afferents to the cough center and trigger the cough reflex.
   2. *Selected drugs*
      a. Antitussive agents
         (1) **Opioids: Codeine, hydrocodone, and hydromorphone**
            (a) Codeine, hydrocodone, and hydromorphone decrease sensitivity of the central cough center to peripheral stimuli and decrease mucosal secretions. Antitussive actions occur at doses lower than those required for analgesia.

      (b) These agents produce constipation, nausea, and respiratory depression.

  (2) Dextromethorphan

      (a) Dextromethorphan is the l-isomer of an opioid; it is active as an antitussive but has less analgesic activity or addictive liability than codeine.

      (b) Dextromethorphan is less constipating than **codeine**.

  (3) Benzonatate (Tessalon)

      (a) Benzonatate is a glycerol derivative chemically similar to **procaine** and other ester-type anesthetics.

      (b) Benzonatate reduces the activity of peripheral cough receptors and also appears to reduce the threshold of the central cough center.

  (4) Diphenhydramine

      (a) Diphenhydramine is an H_1-receptor antagonist; however, antitussive activity is probably not mediated at this receptor.

      (b) Diphenhydramine acts centrally to decrease the sensitivity of the cough center to afferents.

  b. Expectorants stimulate the production of watery, less-viscous mucus; they include **guaifenesin**.

    (1) Guaifenesin acts directly via the gastrointestinal tract to stimulate the vagal reflex.

    (2) Near-emetic doses of guaifenesin are required for beneficial effect; these doses are not attained in typical OTC preparations.

  c. Mucolytics: ***N*-Acetylcysteine**

    (1) *N*-Acetylcysteine reduces the viscosity of mucus and sputum by **cleaving disulfide bonds**.

    (2) *N*-Acetylcysteine is delivered as an **inhalant** and modestly reduces COPD exacerbation rates by roughly 30%.

    (3) Intravenous *N*-acetylcysteine is used as an antidote for acetaminophen toxicity (quite apart from its mucolytic activity).

DRUG SUMMARY TABLE

Short-Acting β_2-Adrenoceptor Agonists
Albuterol (Proventil, Ventolin)
Levalbuterol (Xopenex)
Pirbuterol (Maxair)
Metaproterenol (Alupent)
Epinephrine (Primatene Mist, Bronkaid Mist)
Isoproterenol (Isuprel)

Long-Acting β_2-Adrenoceptor Agonists
Salmeterol (Serevent)
Formoterol (Foradil)
Terbutaline (generic)

Other Adrenoceptor Agonists for Asthma
Epinephrine (Asthmahaler, Epifrin, others)
Isoproterenol (Isuprel)
Ephedrine (Broncholate, Primatene)

Methylxanthines
Theophylline (Elixophyllin, others)

Muscarinic Antagonists
Ipratropium bromide (Atrovent)
Tiotropium (Spirva)
Atropine (generic)

PDE4 Inhibitors
Roflumilast (Daliresp)

Inhaled Glucocorticoids
Beclomethasone (Beclovent, Vanceril)
Triamcinolone acetate (Azmacort)
Budesonide (Rhinocort)
Flunisolide (AeroBid)
Fluticasone propionate (Flovent)
Ciclesonide (Alvesco)
Mometasone (Flovent)

Leukotriene Inhibitors
Zafirlukast (Accolate)
Montelukast (Singulair)
Zileuton (Zyflo)

Enzyme Inhibitors
α_1-Proteinase inhibitor (Prolastin, Aralast)

Anti-IgE Antibody
Omalizumab (Xolair)

Antihistamines (selected H_1-receptor antagonists, see Chapter 6)
Diphenhydramine (Benadryl, Compose, generic)
Loratadine (Claritin)
Fexofenadine (Allegra)

Chlorpheniramine (generic)
Brompheniramine (generic)

α-Adrenoceptor Agonists (selected, see Chapter 2)
Oxymetazoline (Afrin, others)
Phenylephrine (Neo-Synephrine, others)
Pseudoephedrine (Sudafed, Afrinol, others)

Antitussives
Codeine (generic)
Hydrocodone (Tussigon, Hycodan, others)
Hydromorphone (Dilaudid)
Dextromethorphan (generic)
Benzonatate (Tessalon)

Expectorants
Guaifenesin (Extussive, Fenesin, others)

Mucolytics
N-Acetylcysteine (Acetadote, Mucomyst)

Chromone
Chromolyn Sodium (Nasalcrom)

Review Test

Directions: Each of the numbered items or incomplete statements in this section is followed by answers or by completions of the statement. Select the ONE lettered answer or completion that is BEST in each case.

1. A 17-year-old patient is brought to your allergy practice complaining of chronic cough that gets quite severe at times. The condition occurs about twice a week and is beginning to interfere with his studies. Which of the following would be the most appropriate treatment for this patient?

(A) Oral prednisone
(B) Omalizumab
(C) Diphenhydramine
(D) Inhaled budesonide
(E) Theophylline

2. A woman who has asthma and is recovering from a myocardial infarction is on several medications including a baby aspirin a day. She complains of large bruises on her arms and legs and some fatigue. A standard blood panel reveals markedly elevated alanine aminotransferase (ALT). Which of the following is most likely responsible for the increase in liver enzymes?

(A) Heparin
(B) Zileuton
(C) Zafirlukast
(D) Albuterol
(E) Aspirin

3. A 20-year-old college student participates in several intramural athletic programs but is complaining that his asthma, which you have been treating with inhaled glucocorticoids for 5 years, is getting worse. In the last month, he has used his albuterol inhaler at least 20 times following baseball practice, but he has not been waking much at night. You elect to change his treatment regimen. Which of the following would be the best change in treatment for this patient?

(A) Oral triamcinolone
(B) Zileuton
(C) Salmeterol
(D) Etanercept

4. Which of the following statements regarding the pharmacokinetics of theophylline is correct?

(A) It is primarily metabolized by the kidney
(B) Its metabolism depends on age
(C) It is poorly absorbed after oral administration
(D) It has a wide therapeutic index

5. Which of the following statements correctly describes the action of theophylline?

(A) It stimulates cyclic adenosine monophosphate (AMP) phosphodiesterase
(B) It is an adenosine-receptor antagonist
(C) It does not cross the blood–brain barrier
(D) It blocks the release of acetylcholine (ACh) in the bronchial tree

6. Which of the following statements regarding opiate action is correct?

(A) It triggers a vagal reflex to suppress cough
(B) It can cause diarrhea
(C) Its expectorant action is caused by stimulation of mucus production
(D) It acts centrally to suppress the medullary cough center

7. Which of the following statements about the mechanism of action of ipratropium is correct?

(A) It acts centrally to decrease vagal acetylcholine (ACh) release
(B) It inhibits pulmonary ACh receptors
(C) It decreases mast cell release of histamine
(D) It blocks the action of histamine at H_1 receptors

8. Zileuton is useful in the treatment of asthma because it

(A) Inhibits prostaglandin biosynthesis
(B) Inhibits leukotriene synthesis
(C) Inhibits leukotriene receptors
(D) Inhibits 12-lipoxygenase

9. A 49-year-old man with a 15-year history of 2-pack a day smoking come to your office complaining of difficulty in breathing. You immediately notice a wheezing when he breathes. Following pulmonary function tests and lung diffusion studies, you and a pulmonologist colleague diagnose his condition as chronic obstructive pulmonary disease (COPD) and prescribe inhaled tiopropium twice a day. He returns 6 months later, pleased that he has quit smoking, but complaining he is having about 1 episode of serious shortness of breath per day. Which of the following might you add to his treatment?

(A) Oral dexamethasone
(B) Roflumilast
(C) Inhaled beclomethasone
(D) Zileuton

Answers and Explanations

1. **The answer is D.** This is a fairly classical presentation of asthma, which should be confirmed with further pulmonary testing. Mild persistent asthma can be treated in several ways (Table 9.1), but inhaled glucocorticoids are very effective. Oral prednisone has many side effects, especially in a young person. Omalizumab is for patients who are refractory to other treatments and those with allergies. Antihistamines such as diphenhydramine are poorly effective in asthma, and theophylline is only moderately effective.

2. **The answer is B.** Zileuton is a leukotriene synthesis inhibitor that can cause increases in hepatic enzymes and altered liver function. It decreases the rate of heparin metabolism, leaving patients prone to easy bruising. Zafirlukast and albuterol are antiasthmatic agents but do not alter liver enzymes. Aspirin might cause bleeding disorders, but the low dose this patient is taking is unlikely to be responsible for the liver enzyme abnormalities.

3. **The answer is C.** The patient's asthma is worsening, especially in response to exercise or increased allergen exposure, and the excess of short-acting β_2-agonists requires a change in medication. The best choice would be a long-acting β_2-agonist like salmeterol. Oral glucocorticoids have many adverse effects, and zileuton is unlikely to be sufficiently efficacious in the worsening asthma. Etanercept is an anti-inflammatory used in rheumatoid arthritis.

4. **The answer is B.** The metabolism of theophylline depends on age; the half-life of the drug in children is much shorter than in adults. The methylxanthines are all well absorbed and are metabolized in the liver.

5. **The answer is B.** Theophylline may have several mechanisms of action, but its adenosine-receptor antagonist activity and the inhibition of phosphodiesterase are the best understood.

6. **The answer is D.** Opioids such as codeine act centrally to decrease the sensitivity of the cough center; they also decrease propulsion in the bowel.

7. **The answer is B.** Ipratropium is an acetylcholine (ACh) muscarinic receptor antagonist; it is poorly absorbed, so most of its effect is in the lung. It does not cross the blood–brain barrier and does not block mediator release or H_1-receptors.

8. **The answer is B.** By inhibiting 5-lipoxygenase, zileuton reduces leukotriene biosynthesis; it does not inhibit (and in fact it might increase) prostaglandin synthesis.

9. **The answer is B.** Roflumilast is a fairly specific PDE4 inhibitor, useful to decrease exacerbations in patients with chronic obstructive pulmonary disease (COPD). Oral glucocorticoids such as dexamethasone pose serious risks when used chronically and inhaled glucocorticoids are not recommended in early-stage COPD although they might be of benefit in patients with severe disease. Zileuton is ineffective in COPD.

chapter 10

Drugs Acting on the Endocrine System

I. HORMONE RECEPTORS

All known hormones, and drugs that mimic hormones, act via one of **two basic receptor systems:** membrane-associated receptors and intracellular receptors (see Chapter 1).

A. Membrane-associated Receptors

1. Membrane-associated receptors bind hydrophilic hormones (which penetrate the plasma membrane poorly), such as insulin, adrenocorticotropic hormone (ACTH), and epinephrine, outside the cell.
2. Membrane-associated receptors transmit signals into the cell by a variety of "second messenger" mechanisms, including the following:
   a. Changes in cyclic adenosine monophosphate (cAMP) or cyclic guanosine monophosphate (cGMP) caused by changes in the activity of cyclases.
   b. Increased phosphoinositide turnover via increased phosphoinositide kinase activity.
   c. Changes in intracellular Ca^{2+} by acting on intracellular stores or membrane Ca^{2+} channels.
   d. Changes in intracellular ions by action on specific channels. These include Na^+, Ca^{2+}, K^+, and Cl^-.
   e. Increased tyrosine phosphorylation on specific proteins by the action of tyrosine kinases.

B. Intracellular Receptors

1. Intracellular receptors bind hydrophobic hormones (which penetrate the plasma membrane easily) such as cortisol, retinol, and estrogen inside the cell—either in the cytoplasm or the nucleus.
2. Intracellular receptors modulate the transcription rate of specific target genes to change the levels of cellular proteins.

II. THE HYPOTHALAMUS

A. Agents Affecting Growth Hormone

1. Growth hormone-releasing hormone (GHRH)
   a. GHRH is an active peptide of 44 amino acids produced by the hypothalamus within the arcuate nucleus.
   b. GHRH binds to specific membrane GHRH receptors on pituitary somatotrophs.
   c. GHRH rapidly elevates serum growth hormone (somatotropin) levels with high specificity.

d. A GHRH analog composed of the amino-terminal 24 residues, sermorelin, was available for use to diagnose pituitary responsiveness and growth hormone secretory capacity but has been removed from the U.S. market.

e. GHRH release from the arcuate nucleus is also modulated by "GH secretagogues" via a unique GH secretagogue receptor which is actually the ghrelin receptor. Ghrelin is a peptide secreted by the stomach in response to fasting. Ghrelin also stimulates appetite.

2. *Somatotropin release-inhibiting hormone (SST, somatostatin)*

   a. SST has two forms, a 14-amino acid peptide and a 28-amino acid peptide that are produced by differential proteolysis from the same precursor. These peptides are produced in the hypothalamus and other areas of the brain and by pancreatic D cells, as well as by other cells in the gastrointestinal (GI) tract.

   b. SST binds to specific somatostatin receptors in the plasma membrane of target tissues.

   c. At least five different isoforms of somatostatin receptors (SSTR1–SSTR5) are expressed, with marked differences in their tissue distribution.

   d. Somatostatin **inhibits** the release of **growth hormone** and **thyroid-stimulating hormone** (TSH) from the pituitary and the release of **glucagon** and **insulin** from the pancreas. Somatostatin also inhibits secretion of a number of gut peptides such as **vasoactive intestinal polypeptide** (VIP), and **gastrin**, and it inhibits the growth and proliferation of many cell types. It also inhibits the secretion of vasodilator hormones, especially within the gut.

   e. **Octreotide** is an octapeptide SST analog available for use in the United States It is administered by subcutaneous (SC), intramuscular (IM), or intravenous (IV) injection.

   f. Octreotide is used to treat **acromegaly**; severe diarrhea associated with hypersecretory states such as VIP-secreting tumors **(VIPomas)**; **gastrinoma**; **glucagonoma**; variceal and upper GI bleeding; and TSH-secreting adenomas.

   g. Lanreotide (Somatuline) is a long-acting somatostatin analog approved for the treatment of acromegaly.

   h. Adverse effects of octreotide include nausea, cramps, and increased gallstone formation. Both hypo- and hyperglycemia have been reported following its use.

B. Gonadotropin-releasing Hormone (GnRH) and Analogs

   1. Endogenous GnRH is a 10-amino acid peptide secreted from the pre-optic area of hypothalamus. It binds to specific receptors on pituitary gonadotrophs.

   2. Short-term or **pulsatile administration of GnRH agonists (every 1–4 h) increases the synthesis and release of both luteinizing hormone (LH) and follicle-stimulating hormone (FSH).** This occurs by modulating the function of the hypophyseal-pituitary gonadal axis (Fig. 10.1, left-hand side).

   3. Chronic administration (2–4 weeks of daily administration) of GnRH inhibits the release of both LH and FSH by causing a reduction in the number of GnRH receptors.

   4. GnRH analogs have two main uses

   a. Chemical castration, requiring chronic administration, is useful in the treatment of hormone-dependent cancers and hyperplasias such as prostate cancer, breast cancer, endometriosis, and fibroids

   b. Treatment of infertility requires pulsatile administration to stimulate FSH and LH.

   5. Adverse effects include a transient worsening of symptoms, hot flashes, and induction of ovarian cysts in the first months of long-term treatment.

   6. GnRH analogs are listed in Table 10.1

   a. Gonadorelin hydrochloride or acetate

      (1) Decapeptide identical in sequence to endogenous GnRH

      (2) Hydrochloride is used in the diagnosis of hypogonadism; acetate is used for the treatment of infertility.

   b. Nafarelin acetate

      (1) Nafarelin acetate is a synthetic decapeptide of GnRH with one modified amino acid. It is about 200 times more potent than GnRH and is administered as a nasal spray.

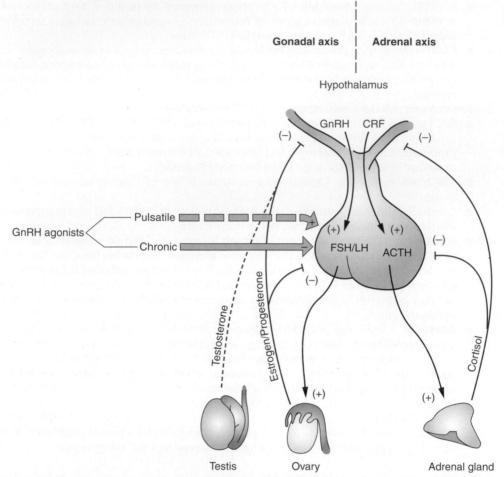

FIGURE 10.1. The hypothalamic-pituitary axis. The pituitary releases trophic hormones such as follicle-stimulating hormone *(FSH)* and luteinizing hormone *(LH)* or adrenocorticotropic hormone *(ACTH)* in response to releasing hormones produced in the hypothalamus. The trophic hormones act on peripheral organs such as the ovary or testis to increase the production of gonadal steroids. Gonadal steroids in turn exert negative feedback on the hypothalamus and pituitary. *CHF,* corticotropin-releasing factor; *GnRH,* gonadotropin-releasing hormone.

t a b l e **10.1** Gonadotropin Analogs		
Drug	**Administration**	**Uses**
GnRH Receptor Agonists		
Leuprolide (Lupron, Eligard)	SC, IM, implant	PC, BC, Endo, Fibro, PP
Gonadorelin (Factrel, Lutrepulse)	IV, SC	DA, Fert
Triptorelin (Trelstar)	IM	Fert, Endo, PC, H
Nafarelin (Synarel)	Intranasal	PP, Endo, Fibr, H
Goserelin (Zoladex)	SC implant	PC, BC, Endo, Fib
Histrelin (Vantas)	SC implant	PC
GnRH Receptor Antagonists		
Ganirelix (Antagon)	SC	Fert
Abarelix (Plenaxis)	IM	PC
Cetrorelix (Cetrotide)	SC	Fert

PC, prostate cancer; BC, breast cancer; Endo, endometriosis; Fibr, fibroids; Fert, fertility; PP, precocious puberty; DA, diagnostic agent; H, hirsutism.

(2) Nafarelin is used for the management of endometriosis and central precocious puberty.

c. Triptorelin (Trelstar Depot), a decapeptide that is more potent than GnRH.

d. Goserelin

(1) Goserelin acetate contains two amino acid substitutions that increase its half-life compared with that of endogenous GnRH.

(2) This peptide is injected either SC, as a long-acting implant, or by IV infusion. The half-life of the peptide is approximately 10–20 minutes following IV administration. Peak response is achieved 15 minutes after IV administration and 30–60 minutes after SC injection. The therapeutic effectiveness of the implant is 28 days.

e. Leuprolide acetate

(1) Leuprolide acetate is a synthetic 9-amino acid GnRH analog with increased potency.

(2) Leuprolide is administered parenterally, and a long-acting (up to 6 months) controlled release preparation is available.

(3) Leuprolide acetate may be used to treat prostate cancer, prostatic hypertrophy, breast cancer, endometriosis, and fibroids.

f. Histrelin is a nonpeptide GnRH analog; implant delivers drug continuously for 1 year.

g. GnRH antagonists

(1) Cetrorelix, ganirelix, and degarelix are a class of GnRH analogs that act as **pure antagonists**; they do not cause a surge of testosterone or estradiol on initiation of therapy.

(2) All are decapeptides and administered SC or IM.

(3) An advantage of the GnRH antagonists over the GnRH agonists (e.g., leuprolide) is a reduction in the required fertility therapy cycle from several weeks (i.e., 3 weeks with leuprolide) to only several days. Secondarily, the effects of GnRH antagonists start and reverse rapidly, allowing pituitary function to return to baseline within 1–4 days after drug discontinuation.

(4) These drugs are used as part of an assisted reproductive technology procedure, for endometriosis, and prostatic hyperplasia. Degarelix is approved for advanced prostate cancer.

C. Prolactin-releasing factor (PRF) and prolactin-inhibiting factor (PIF). Secretion of **prolactin** from the pituitary is controlled by both **inhibition** (mediated by PIF, which is dopamine) and **stimulation** (mediated by PRF).

1. *PRF*

a. Several peptides, including thyrotropin-releasing hormone (TRH), that increase the synthesis and release of prolactin have been identified in the hypothalamus and placenta; however, their physiologic role is unclear.

b. Drugs that reduce central nervous system (CNS) dopaminergic activity cause an increase in prolactin secretion, as will dopamine antagonists. These include

(1) Antipsychotics, including chlorpromazine and haloperidol

(2) Antidepressants, including imipramine

(3) Antianxiety agents, including diazepam

c. Various hormones also stimulate prolactin secretion; these include testosterone, estrogen, TRH, and VIP.

d. Drugs that promote prolactin secretion are used to treat lactation failure.

2. *PIF*

a. Inhibition of prolactin secretion can be produced by a number of dopamine agonists.

(1) Bromocriptine acts as an agonist of dopamine D_2-receptors and an antagonist of D_1-receptors.

(2) Cabergoline is a potent D_2 agonist with greater D_2 selectivity. It is more effective in reducing hyperprolactinemia than bromocriptine and has a long half-life that permits twice-weekly dosing.

b. Therapeutic uses of these agents include the inhibition of prolactin secretion in amenorrhea, galactorrhea, and prolactin-secreting tumors; the correction of female infertility secondary to hyperprolactinemia; and the treatment of Parkinson disease.

D. Corticotropin-releasing Hormone (CRH), Corticorelin
1. CRH is a 41-amino acid peptide found in the hypothalamus and the gut; a recombinant peptide, corticorelin, is available for diagnostic use.
2. CRH stimulates ACTH synthesis and release in pituitary corticotrophs by binding to specific membrane receptors.
3. CRH is subject to rapid proteolysis; it must be given IV.
4. Corticorelin is used diagnostically to discriminate between pituitary or ectopic sources of ACTH production and to differentiate between hypothalamic-hypophyseal or primary adrenal disease.

E. Thyrotropin-releasing Hormone
1. TRH is a tripeptide (Glu-His-Pro) found in the hypothalamus and other locations in the brain.
2. TRH binds to specific membrane receptors and stimulates the secretion of TSH from the pituitary and induces prolactin secretion.
3. TRH is no longer available in the United States.

III. THE ANTERIOR PITUITARY

A. Growth hormone agonists (GH, somatotropin), methionyl-growth hormone **(somatrem), and antagonists (Pegvisomant)**
1. *Structure*
    a. Growth hormone is a 191-amino acid protein produced in the anterior pituitary.
    b. Secretion of GH is controlled by hypothalamic factors: GHRH and SST (see above).
2. *Actions and pharmacologic properties*
    a. The effects of GH are mediated by specific membrane receptors. GH has two independent receptor interaction domains, and one molecule of GH tethers two GH receptors together and the homodimer activates a tyrosine kinase, Jak2.
    b. GH has both direct actions and indirect actions mediated by the induction of insulin-like growth factor-1 (IGF-1) synthesis in and release from the liver and the kidney.
        (1) Direct actions of GH include
            (a) Antagonism of the action of insulin
            (b) Stimulation of triglyceride hydrolysis in adipose tissue
            (c) Increased hepatic glucose output
            (d) Positive calcium balance
            (e) Renal reabsorption of sodium and potassium
            (f) Production of somatomedins or IGFs in the liver and other tissues
        (2) Indirect actions of GH mediated by IGF-1 include
            (a) Longitudinal growth of bones and growth of soft tissue
            (b) Increased amino acid transport, DNA and RNA synthesis, and proliferation of many tissues
            (c) Increased protein synthesis and positive nitrogen balance
    c. GH is administered by IM or SC injection. Peak blood levels are obtained in 2–4 hours; activity persists for 36 hours after administration, because of the relatively long half-life of somatomedins. A depot preparation (Nutropin Depot) composed of microspheres of somatropin embedded in biodegradable polyactide-coglycodide microspheres is designed to decrease the number of injections required.

3. ***Therapeutic uses***
   a. GH is used for replacement therapy in children with GH deficiency before epiphyseal closure.
   b. GH stimulates growth in patients with Turner syndrome.
   c. Other approved uses include long-term replacement of GH deficiency in adults, treatment of cachexia and acquired immune deficiency syndrome (AIDS) wasting, positive nitrogen balance in patients with severe burns, Prader-Willi syndrome in children, and short bowel syndrome.

4. ***Adverse effects and contraindications***
   a. In about 2% of the patients, anti-GH antibodies develop. Edema, metabolic disturbances, and injection site reactions have been reported with GH treatment.
   b. Administration of GH is contraindicated in obese patients, patients with closed epiphyses who do not have GH deficiency, and patients with neoplastic disease.

B. **GH Antagonists, Pegvisomant**
   1. Pegvisomant is a GH receptor antagonist. It is a recombinant GH that contains nine mutations that allow it to bind to one GH receptor, but it fails to bind a second GH receptor. This blocks the action of endogenous GH.
   2. Used specifically for the treatment of acromegaly.
   3. Pegvisomant is administered SC.

C. **Gonadotropins**
   1. ***Luteinizing hormone and follicle-stimulating hormone***
      a. Structure
         (1) LH and FSH are glycoproteins found in the anterior pituitary.
         (2) **LH, FSH, and TSH are all composed of an identical α subunit** and a β subunit unique to each hormone.
      b. Actions and pharmacologic properties
         (1) The activity of LH and FSH is mediated by specific membrane receptors that cause an increase in intracellular cAMP.
         (2) In women, LH increases estrogen production in the ovary and is required for progesterone production by the corpus luteum after ovulation. FSH is required for normal development and maturation of the ovarian follicles.
         (3) In men, LH induces testosterone production by the interstitial (Leydig) cells of the testis. FSH acts on the testis to stimulate spermatogenesis and the synthesis of androgen-binding protein.
      c. Therapeutic uses. FSH and LH of pituitary origin are not used pharmacologically. Rather, the menopausal and chorionic gonadotropins described below are used as the source of biologically active peptides.
   2. ***Human menopausal gonadotropins (menotropins) and human chorionic gonadotropin (hCG)***
      a. **Menotropins** are isolated from the urine of postmenopausal women and contain a mixture of LH and FSH. Urofollitropin (Bravelle) is immunologically purified FSH from the urine of pregnant women.
      b. **hCG** is produced by the placenta and can be isolated and purified from the urine of pregnant women. hCG is nearly identical in activity to LH, but differs in sequence and carbohydrate content.
      c. Recombinant human FSH (follitropin-α and follitropin-β are available). They have less batch-to-batch variability than preparations derived from urine. Recombinant LH is also available (Lutropin alpha).
      d. Menotropins and hCG must be administered parenterally.
      e. Therapeutic uses
         (1) Menotropins are used in concert with hCG to stimulate ovulation in women with functioning ovaries; approximately 75% of women treated with these peptides ovulate.
         (2) hCG can be used in both men and women to stimulate gonadal steroidogenesis in cases of LH insufficiency.

      (3) hCG can be used to induce external sexual maturation and spermatogenesis in men with secondary hypogonadism, but this may require months of treatment.

      (4) In the absence of an anatomic block, hCG can also promote the descent of the testes in cryptorchidism.

  f. Adverse effects and contraindications

      (1) Menotropins and hCG cause ovarian enlargement in about 20% of treated women.

      (2) Menotropins and hCG may cause **ovarian hyperstimulation syndrome** in up to 1% of patients, resulting in acute respiratory distress, ascites, hypovolemia, and shock.

D. Thyroid-stimulating Hormone (TSH, Thyrotropin α) (Thyrogen)

  1. TSH is a 211-amino acid glycoprotein with two subunits that is secreted from the anterior pituitary.

  2. TSH stimulates the production and release of triiodothyronine (T_3) and thyroxine (T_4) from the thyroid gland. The effect is mediated by stimulation of specific TSH receptors in the plasma membrane, thereby increasing intracellular cAMP.

  3. Thyrotropin-α is available for use in diagnosing the cause of thyroid deficiency.

E. Adrenocorticotropic Hormone (ACTH, Corticotropin) and Cosyntropin

  1. *Structure*

    a. ACTH is a 39-amino acid peptide secreted from the anterior pituitary. The N-terminal 24-amino acid portion of the peptide has full biologic activity.

    b. The N-terminal 13-amino acids of ACTH are identical to those in α-melanocyte-stimulating hormone (α-MSH).

  2. *Actions and pharmacologic properties*

    a. ACTH stimulates the adrenocortical secretion of glucocorticoids and, to a lesser extent, mineralocorticoids and androgens. Effects are mediated by specific membrane-bound ACTH receptors coupled to an increase in intracellular cAMP.

    b. Excess ACTH levels may produce hyperpigmentation because of activity of the intrinsic α-MSH portion of the peptide.

    c. ACTH is available in both human and bovine purified preparations, as well as synthetic 1-24-ACTH (cosyntropin).

    d. All preparations of ACTH are administered parenterally.

  3. *Therapeutic uses*

    a. ACTH is used in the evaluation of primary or secondary hypoadrenalism.

    b. ACTH may be used in special circumstances when an increase in glucocorticoids is desired. However, the direct administration of steroids is usually preferred.

  4. *Adverse effects and contraindications*

    a. The adverse effects associated with ACTH are similar to those of glucocorticoids.

    b. Allergic reactions, acne, hirsutism, and amenorrhea have also been reported.

IV. THE POSTERIOR PITUITARY

A. Antidiuretic Hormone (ADH, Vasopressin)

  1. *Structure*

    a. ADH is a nine-amino acid peptide synthesized in the hypothalamus and stored in the posterior pituitary.

    b. ADH is released in response to increasing plasma osmolarity or a fall in blood pressure.

  2. *Actions*

    a. The actions of ADH are mediated by three types of specific receptors: V_{1a}, located in vascular smooth muscle, myometrium, and kidney; V_{1b}, located in the CNS and adrenal medulla; and V_2, located in renal tubules. V_1 receptors are coupled to increased inositide turnover and increased intracellular Ca^{2+}; V_2 receptors are coupled to an increase in cAMP.

b. In renal tubules, ADH causes the **permeability of water to increase** because of the insertion of water channels composed of the protein **aquaporin-2** into the apical and basolateral membranes. ADH also increases the transport of urea in the inner medullary collecting duct, which increases the urine-concentrating ability of the kidney.

c. ADH causes vasoconstriction (via V_{ia} receptors) at higher doses.

d. ADH stimulates the hepatic synthesis of **coagulation factor VIII and von Willebrand factor.**

3. *Pharmacologic properties of ADH preparations*

a. Aqueous vasopressin (Pitressin), a short-acting preparation that acts on both V_1 and V_2 receptors, is administered parenterally and lasts 2–6 hours.

b. Desmopressin acetate (DDAVP, Stimate) is a longer lasting (10–20 h) preparation administered intranasally, parenterally, or orally.

4. *Therapeutic uses*

a. Desmopressin is the most effective treatment for severe diabetes insipidus because its V_2 activity is 3,000 times greater than its V_1 activity; but it **is not effective in the nephrogenic** form of the disease.

b. Vasopressin is included in the advanced cardiac life support protocol as a substitute for epinephrine in cardiac arrest with asystole. It has been useful in treating some types of GI bleeding, especially esophageal variceal bleeding and bleeding caused by colonic diverticula, but this use is no longer approved.

c. Desmopressin is useful in **nocturnal enuresis** by reducing nighttime urine production

5. Adverse effects. ADH preparations produce headache, nausea, and cramps, and they may cause constriction of coronary arteries.

6. **ADH antagonists**

a. The vaptans are non-peptide antagonists of vasopressin receptors.

   1. **Conivaptan** (Vaprisol) blocks both V_{1a} and V_2 receptors. It is administered IV and is approved for the use for hypervolemic and euvolemic hyponatremia in SIADH (syndrome of inappropriate ADH) and as an adjunct for diuretic therapy in CHF.

   2. The oral **tolvaptan** (Samsca) is specific for V_2 receptors and is approved for the same indications.

7. *Drug interactions*

a. Clofibrate increases secretion of ADH from the pituitary and can be used to treat mild forms of diabetes insipidus.

b. Chlorpropamide and tricyclic antidepressants increase the sensitivity of the tubular cells to ADH.

c. Li^+ and **demeclocycline inhibit** the action of ADH. Demeclocycline is used more often than Li^+ because of fewer side effects, but use of either of these drugs in SIADH has been replaced with the specific vaptans.

B. **Oxytocin**

1. *Structure*

a. Oxytocin is a nine-amino acid peptide synthesized in the hypothalamus and secreted by the posterior pituitary.

b. Oxytocin differs from ADH by only two amino acids.

2. *Actions and pharmacologic properties*

a. Elicits milk ejection from the breast.

b. Stimulates contraction of uterine smooth muscle.

c. Oxytocin has been associated with parental, mating, and social behaviors.

d. Is infused IV, administered IM, or delivered intranasally. The plasma $t_{1/2}$ of oxytocin is 5–10 minutes.

3. *Therapeutic uses*

a. Is used for **induction and maintenance of labor.**

b. **Stimulates milk ejection** from the breast.

c. Is sometimes used to **control postpartum uterine bleeding** (more readily controlled with ergot alkaloids).

4. *Adverse effects and contraindications*
   a. Oxytocin can produce hypertension and water intoxication (ADH activity).
   b. Oxytocin can cause uterine rupture and should not be used after uterine surgery or if signs of fetal distress are present.

V. DRUGS ACTING ON THE GONADAL AND REPRODUCTIVE SYSTEM

A. Estrogens
   1. *Structure*
      a. Natural estrogens (Fig. 10.2)
         (1) Natural estrogens include 17β-estradiol, estrone, and estriol, each of which contains 18 carbon atoms. **The most potent natural estrogen is 17β-estradiol**.
         (2) Natural estrogens are produced by the metabolism of cholesterol; testosterone is the immediate precursor of estradiol. Conversion of testosterone to 17β-estradiol is catalyzed by the enzyme aromatase.
         (3) Estrone and estriol are produced in the liver and other peripheral tissues from 17β-estradiol and are frequently conjugated by esterification to sulfates.
         (4) Equilin, an estrone derivative, is a pharmacologically useful estrogen purified from horse urine.

Estradiol
   R_1: -H; R_2: -OH

Ethinyl estradiol
   R_1: -C≡CH; R_2: -OH

Mestranol
   R_1: -C≡CH; R_2: -OCH$_3$

Diethylstilbestrol

FIGURE 10.2. Structures of estrogens.

    b. Synthetic estrogens

        (1) A variety of synthetic estrogens have been produced.

        (2) Frequently used synthetic estrogens include the steroidal agents **ethinyl estradiol** and **mestranol** and the nonsteroidal compounds diethylstilbestrol (DES) and dienestrol.

2. *Mechanism of action.* Estrogens bind to specific intracellular receptors. The hormone–receptor complex interacts with specific DNA sequences and alters the transcription rates of target genes (Fig. 1.1F) by recruiting coactivators and corepressors. They may also affect the half-life of specific messenger RNAs. These events lead to a change in the synthesis of specific proteins within a target cell. There are two estrogen receptors, ER-α and ER-β, that differ in their tissue distribution; while both receptors have about the same affinity for 17β-estradiol, they have differential affinities for other ligands and affect target genes in a differential manner.

3. *Metabolism*

    a. 17β-Estradiol is extensively (98%) bound to sex steroid-binding globulin (SSBG) and serum albumin.

    b. Estrone sulfate is frequently combined with α-equilin or with other estrogenic sulfates, is effective orally, but natural estrogens are subject to a large first-pass effect. Synthetic estrogens may be administered orally, topically, transdermally, or by injection.

    c. All estrogens are extensively metabolized in the liver and are conjugated with either glucuronic acid or sulfate, hydroxylated or O-methylated. Most metabolites are excreted in the urine, with approximately 10% undergoing enterohepatic circulation and eventual elimination in the feces.

4. *Actions*

    a. Growth and development

        (1) Estrogens are required for the development and maturation of female internal and external genitalia, growth of the breasts, linear bone growth at puberty, and closure of the epiphyses. Typical female distribution of SC fat and pubic and axillary hair is also influenced by estrogens.

        (2) Estrogens are required in the uterus for growth of myometrium and for growth and development of the endometrial lining. Continuous exposure can lead to **endometrial hyperplasia** and bleeding.

    b. Menstrual cycle. Estrogens are required for ovarian follicular development and regulation of the menstrual cycle.

    c. Systemic metabolism

        (1) Estrogens promote a positive nitrogen balance, increase plasma triglycerides, and tend to decrease serum cholesterol by decreasing low-density lipoprotein (LDL) and increasing high-density lipoprotein (HDL) concentrations.

        (2) Estrogens decrease total serum proteins but increase levels of transferrin, steroid- and thyroid-binding globulins (TBG), plasminogen, fibrinogen, and **coagulation factors** II, VII, VIII, IX, and X. Antithrombin III, protein C, and protein S levels are decreased. **Overall, estrogens increase the coagulability of blood.**

        (3) Estrogens **decrease bone resorption**, with little effect on bone formation.

        (4) Estrogens increase leptin release from adipose tissue.

    d. Influence libido and mood

5. *Therapeutic uses*

    a. Hypogonadism. Estrogens are used for estrogen replacement therapy in ovarian failure or after castration.

    b. Menstrual abnormalities

    c. Menopausal therapy

        (1) Menopausal hormone therapy (MHT) can be achieved with oral, parenteral, topical (intravaginal), or transdermal estrogens, in various combinations with or without progestins.

        (2) Postmenopausal estrogen therapy improves hot flashes, sweating, and atrophic vaginitis.

(3) Postmenopausal estrogen therapy slows the rate of bone loss.

(4) Estrogens are usually administered in a cyclical manner to avoid long periods of continuous exposure.

(5) Concomitant use of estrogen therapy with a progestin reduces the incidence of endometrial carcinoma.

(6) Transdermal delivery of 17β-estradiol using a skin patch is effective and long-lasting in treating menopausal symptoms.

d. Oral contraception (see V E 1)

e. Androgen-dependent prostatic tumors are effectively treated by DES.

6. *Adverse effects and contraindications*

a. Estrogens are associated with nausea, headaches, cholestasis, hypertension, and gall-bladder disease.

b. Estrogens present an increased risk (5–15 times) of endometrial cancer that is dose and duration dependent. Risk is reduced by periodic withdrawal of estrogen therapy and replacement by progestin treatment, or concomitant treatment with both drugs.

c. Estrogen therapy is the major cause of postmenopausal bleeding and may mask bleeding due to endometrial cancer.

d. DES is associated with adenocarcinoma of the vagina; incidence in women exposed in utero to DES is 1:1,000; genital malformation is much more common.

e. Estrogens are contraindicated in the presence of estrogen-dependent or estrogen-responsive carcinoma, liver disease, or thromboembolic disease.

f. Recent large clinical trials indicate that some regimens of MHT are associated with increased risk of myocardial infarction, stroke, breast cancer, and dementia. Whether this risk is solely attributable to the estrogenic component and whether or not all estrogenic preparations at all doses share these liabilities are unresolved.

B. **Antiestrogens** interfere with the binding of estrogen with its specific receptor, and they may also alter the conformation of the estrogen receptor such that it fails to activate target genes. This class of compounds is distinguished from progestins and androgens, which also possess physiologic antiestrogenic activity.

1. *Clomiphene, fulvestrant*

a. Clomiphene and fulvestrant are nonsteroidal agents.

b. Clomiphene and fulvestrant bind competitively to the estrogen receptor and may also reduce the levels of some mitogens. Clomiphene has partial agonist activity in some tissues including the ovary and endometrium; fulvestrant appears to be an antagonist is all tissues.

c. These agents eventually reduce the number of functional receptors available for endogenous estrogens and **diminish estrogen action both along the hypothalamic-pituitary axis and in peripheral tissues.**

d. **Clomiphene is used to treat infertility** in cases of anovulation in women with an intact hypothalamic-pituitary axis and sufficient production of estrogen. **Fulvestrant is used to treat women with progressive breast cancer** after tamoxifen (see below).

e. These agents may cause ovarian enlargement, hot flashes, nausea, and vomiting.

2. *Danazol*

a. Danazol is a testosterone derivative with antiandrogen and antiestrogenic activities.

b. Danazol **inhibits** several of the enzymes involved in **steroidogenesis**, but **does not inhibit aromatase**; may also bind to estrogen and androgen receptors; and inhibits gonadotropin release in both men and women.

c. **Danazol is used to inhibit ovarian function, treat endometriosis and fibrocystic disease of the breast.**

d. This agent may cause edema, masculinization (deepening of the voice and decreased breast size) in some women, headache, and **hepatocellular disease.**

e. Danazol is contraindicated in pregnant women or in patients with hepatic disease.

C. **Selective Estrogen Receptor Modulators (SERMs)** (Fig. 10.3)

    1. SERMs are ligands for the estrogen receptor that have agonist activity in one tissue but may have antagonist activity or no activity in another tissue. The response of a tissue is determined by the conformation that the ligand confers upon the estrogen receptor, and the set of coactivators that are expressed in that tissue (Fig. 10.4). Currently, there are three SERMs approved for use in the United States: tamoxifen, raloxifene, and toremifene; many others are in clinical trial.

        a. **Tamoxifen is an estrogen antagonist in the breast** and in the brain but is an agonist in the uterus and in bone. It is used in the **treatment of advanced, hormone receptor-positive breast cancer and for primary prevention of breast cancer in women at high risk** of the disease. Tamoxifen increases the risk of endometrial cancer.

        b. **Raloxifene is an agonist in bone** but has no effect on the uterus or breast and is an estrogen antagonist in the brain. **It is used for the treatment and prevention of osteoporosis and for uterine fibroids.** Raloxifene has been shown to reduce the risk of estrogen receptor-positive invasive breast cancer by 66%–76%.

        c. **Toremifene is used to treat metastatic breast cancer.**

    2. Common adverse effects of SERMs are edema, hot flashes, nausea, vomiting, vaginal bleeding, and vaginal discharge. There is an increase in thromboembolic events with raloxifene but not with tamoxifen.

D. **Aromatase Inhibitors (see Fig. 10.4)**

    1. Aromatase is the enzyme that catalyzes the final step in the production of estrogens from androgenic precursors within the ovary or in peripheral tissues.

    2. Aromatase inhibitors are a new class of oral estrogen synthesis inhibitors.

        a. **Exemestane** is a steroidal, **irreversible aromatase inhibitor**. It is approved for use in the treatment of breast cancer. Testolactone is another irreversible aromatase inhibitor.

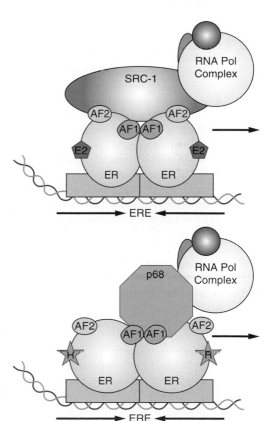

FIGURE 10.3. Mechanism of action of SERMs. Two cell types, uterine and breast epithelia, are illustrated. *Top:* 17β-Estradiol binds to the estrogen receptor (ER) and induces a conformational change. Some coactivators *(blue shapes)* can interact with this conformation and thus increase transcription of specific genes *(arrow)*. Both cell types express a coactivator that can respond to the 17β-estradiol-induced conformation. *Bottom:* Tamoxifen induces a different conformation of ER. Uterine epithelia expresses a coactivator that increases transcription; breast epithelia do not express such coactivators.

FIGURE 10.4. Enzymatic conversion of andro-gens to estrogens and dihydrotestosterone. 17β-HSD is hydroxysteroid dehydrogenase. There are multiple isoforms of this enzyme: types 1 and 3 catalyze reactions that make more-active steroids; types 2 and 4 make less active metabolites.

Major adverse effects include hot flashes, fatigue, and CNS effects such as insomnia, depression, and anxiety.

b. Anastrazole and **letrozole** are nonsteroidal **competitive inhibitors of aromatase**. These drugs are used as first- or second-line agents in the treatment of breast cancer. Adverse effects include hot flashes, vaginal bleeding, insomnia, bone pain, and GI disturbances.

E. Progestins

1. Structure

    a. The most important natural progestin is progesterone, which is synthesized by the ovaries, testes, and adrenals.

    b. Synthetic progestins include the **19-nor compounds**, such as norethindrone, norg-estrel, and levonorgestrel. All of these agents are potent oral progestins derived from testosterone; some have androgenic activity (Fig. 10.5).

    c. Several synthetic derivatives of progesterone have progestin activity, including **megestrol** (Megace), **medroxyprogesterone acetate** (Amen, Provera, others), and hydroxyprogesterone caproate. Gonanes include norgestimate and desogestrel; these agents have reduced androgenic activity. **Drospirenone is a spironolactone analog** with antimineralocorticoid, antiandrogenic, and progestational activity.

2. Actions and pharmacologic properties

    a. Progestins bind to intranuclear receptors that alter the transcription of target genes. There are two isoforms of the progesterone receptor: PR-A and PR-B. Both are derived from the same gene. **Progestins slow the mitotic activity of the estrogen-stimulated uterus, cause vascularization of the endometrium, and induce a more glandular appear-ance and function.**

    b. Progestins slightly decrease triglycerides and HDL, but they slightly increase LDL, depending on the preparation and dose. Progestins also increase lipoprotein lipase.

    c. Progestins increase basal and stimulated insulin secretion, and stimulate appetite.

    d. Progesterone is extensively bound to corticosteroid-binding globulin in the plasma and is not administered orally because of rapid hepatic metabolism.

    e. Progestins are eliminated by hydroxylation to pregnanediol and conjugation with glucuronic acid and subsequent urinary excretion.

Progesterone   **Medroxyprogesterone acetate**

Testosterone   **Norethindrone**

FIGURE 10.5. Structures of some progestins and androgens.

3. Therapeutic uses

a. Progestins are used for contraception, alone or in combination with estrogens.

b. Progestins may be administered orally, by depot injection, as a vaginal gel, and as a slow-release intrauterine device.

c. These agents are used in the **treatment of endometrial cancer and endometrial hyperplasia.**

d. Progestins control abnormal uterine bleeding.

e. Progestins are used to delay menstruation for surgical or postoperative reasons.

f. Megace is used to stimulate appetite in patients with cancer or AIDS.

g. These agents are used diagnostically to evaluate endometrial function in amenorrhea.

F. Antiprogestins, Mifepristone (RU-486)

1. Mifepristone is a norethindrone derivative with potent antiprogestin and antiglucocorticoid activities.

2. Mifepristone acts as a competitive antagonist of progesterone and glucocorticoid receptors.

3. Mifepristone has been approved for use to induce medical abortion in the first trimester.

a. Mifepristone is combined with a parenteral or intravaginal application of a prostaglandin 48 hours after the antiprogestin to induce abortion.

b. Mifepristone causes myometrial contractions and blastocyst detachment and expulsion.

c. This combination is approximately 99% effective.

4. Mifepristone is used as an emergency postcoital contraceptive and is very effective if used within 72 hours of intercourse.

5. Relatively infrequent side effects of mifepristone include bleeding, nausea, and abdominal pain.

G. Hormonal Contraceptives

1. ***Oral contraceptives* represent the primary use of estrogens and progestins.**

   a. Types of oral contraceptives

      (1) Combination pills

         (a) Combination pills contain mixtures of estrogens and a progestin. The estrogen component (20–50 µg/day) is either **ethinyl estradiol** or **mestranol** (mestranol is metabolized to ethinyl estradiol); it is combined with a progestin (0.05–2.5 mg/day), such as **norethindrone, norgestrel, levonorgestrel, norethindrone acetate, ethynodiol diacetate, drospirenone, or desogestrel.**

         (b) Combination pills reduce the level and cyclicity of both LH and FSH, **resulting in failure to ovulate.**

         (c) Combination pills are typically taken continuously for 21 days, followed by a 7-day withdrawal (or placebo) period to induce menses. Biphasic and triphasic formulations, which try to mimic the endogenous ratio of estrogen/progestin, are available.

         (d) "Continuous dosage products" are available that contain ethinyl estradiol and levonorgestrel and are taken every day for 84 days followed by 7 days of inert tablets (Seasonale) or 7 days of low-dose ethinyl estradiol (Seasonique), thus producing four menstrual periods per year. Lybrel contains the same hormones taken continuously for 365 days to suppress menstruation completely.

         (e) These pills also affect the genital tract in ways that are unfavorable for conception: thickening cervical mucus, speeding ovum transport through the fallopian tubes, and making the endometrium less favorable for implantation.

      (2) Progestin-only preparations ("mini pills")

         (a) Progestin-only oral preparations contain **norethindrone.**

         (b) These preparations are taken daily on a continuous schedule.

         (c) Progestin-only preparations do **not** completely suppress ovulation, resulting in irregular fertile periods. They are not as effective as the combination preparations.

         (d) The mechanism of contraception is unclear, but it is likely **due to the formation of a relatively atrophic endometrium** (which impairs implantation) and **viscous cervical mucus**.

         (e) **Breakthrough bleeding is as high as 25%.**

   b. Adverse effects

      (1) Cardiovascular

         (a) Oral contraceptives are associated with a twofold to fourfold increase in morbidity and mortality due to myocardial infarction; this may be age dependant.

         (b) The incidence of hypertension is three to six times higher among women taking oral contraceptives.

         (c) Oral contraceptives produce a marked increase (up to 50%) in triglyceride levels, depending on the relative doses of estrogens and progestins in the individual preparation.

         (d) The risk of cardiovascular complications increases markedly in women over age 35 and in women who smoke.

      (2) Thromboembolic disease

         (a) The risk of stroke is 2–10 times higher in individuals taking oral contraceptives.

         (b) Estrogens increase levels of fibrinogen and coagulation factors II, VII, VIII, IX, and X, while decreasing concentrations of antithrombin III.

      (3) Genitourinary tract. Oral contraceptives **reduce the incidence of ovarian and endometrial cancers. They also reduce the incidence of pelvic inflammatory disease.**

      (4) Hepatobiliary system. Oral contraceptives increase the incidence of **gallbladder disease and gallstones.**

      (5) Other adverse effects of oral contraceptives include weight gain, edema, breast tenderness, headache, mood alteration, breakthrough bleeding, and amenorrhea on discontinuation.

   c. Oral contraceptives are contraindicated in cardiovascular disease, thromboembolic disease, estrogen-dependent or estrogen-responsive cancer, impaired liver function, undiagnosed bleeding, and migraine.

2. *Progestin injections*
   a. Medroxyprogesterone acetate (Depo-Provera) is available as a suspension for SC or IM injections. This preparation provides contraception for 3 months.

3. *Subcutaneous progestin implants*
   a. Implanon is a synthetic progestin, **etonogestrel**, surrounded by a biomatrix coating. A single rod is placed under the skin and provides effective contraception for up to 3 years. Actual effectiveness is superior to that of combination oral contraceptives. Rods must be removed after 3 years.
   b. Adverse effects are dominated by menstrual and bleeding irregularities.

4. *Intrauterine devices (IUDs)*
   a. Levonorgestrel-containing IUDs are available as a means of contraception.
   b. Contraception is achieved mostly by local actions on the endometrium with hypotrophic glands and pseudodecidualization. Ovulation occurs in about 50% of menstrual cycles.
   c. These devices should be implanted by a trained physician.

5. *Postcoital (emergency) oral contraceptives*
   a. Plan A (Yuzpe regimen): 100–120 µg of ethinyl estradiol with 0.5–0.75 mg of levonorgestrel, taken twice, 12 hours apart, has been found very effective if taken within 72 hours of coitus. At least 18 oral contraceptive preparations contain these two drugs.
   b. Plan B: 0.750 mg of levonorgestrel, within 72 hours after unprotected intercourse, one dose taken as soon as possible; a second dose must be taken 12 hours after the initial dose. Plan B: One Step is one 1.5 mg dose of levonorgestrel and is equally effective.
   c. Nausea and vomiting are common with the use of postcoital oral contraceptives and can be severe. The risk of cancer in female offspring precludes this treatment if pregnancy is suspected.

H. **Androgens and Anabolic Steroids**
1. *Testosterone*
   a. Testosterone is synthesized primarily in the Leydig cells of the testis under the influence of LH. Testosterone is metabolized to the more potent 5α-dihydrotestosterone by **5α-reductase**. There are two isoforms of this enzyme: type I, which is expressed in skin and liver; and type II, which is expressed in prostate, seminal vesicles, and hair follicles.
   b. Testosterone is extensively bound (98%), mostly to SSBG and also to albumin.
   c. Natural testosterone can be administered transdermally or intramuscularly.

2. *Synthetic androgens*
   a. The 17-substituted testosterone esters (testosterone propionate, testosterone enanthate, and testosterone cypionate) are administered by injection, usually as a depot in oil.
   b. 17-Alkyl testosterone derivatives include methyltestosterone, fluoxymesterone, and oxymetholone. Absorption of these oral agents is greater if they are administered sublingually, thus avoiding the large hepatic first-pass effect.
   c. Nandrolone (Hybolin, Deca-Durabolin) and oxandrolone (Oxandrine, others) are testosterone derivatives with about a **5- to 10-fold higher anabolic-to-androgenic ratio** than testosterone itself. Nandrolone is administered parenterally; oxandrolone is an oral agent.

3. *Actions.* Androgens form a complex with a specific intracellular receptor (a member of the nuclear-receptor family) and interact with specific genes to modulate differentiation, development, and growth. (See Fig. 1.1F.)
   a. Androgenic actions
      (1) Androgens stimulate the **differentiation and development of Wolffian structures**, including the epididymis, seminal vesicles, prostate, and penis.
      (2) Androgens stimulate the development and maintenance of male secondary sexual characteristics.

b. Anabolic actions

   (1) Anabolic steroids cause acceleration of epiphyseal closure, and they result in linear growth at puberty.

   (2) Anabolic steroids cause an increase in muscle mass and lead to a positive nitrogen balance.

   (3) Behavioral effects of anabolic steroids include aggressiveness and increased libido.

4. *Uses*

   a. Prepubertal and postpubertal hypogonadism. Androgens promote linear growth and sexual maturation and maintain male secondary sexual characteristics, libido, and potency.

   b. Anemia

   (1) Androgens stimulate secretion of erythropoietin.

   (2) Androgens have largely been supplanted by recombinant erythropoietin (epoetin) for anemia, but they may be effective in some cases of bone marrow hypoplasia.

   c. Estrogen-dependent breast cancers

   d. Wasting disorders in AIDS or after severe burns

   e. Illicit use by athletes. Large doses of androgens increase the extent and rate of muscle formation and may increase the intensity of training.

   f. Hereditary angioedema. Androgens are used to treat hereditary angioedema based on androgen-dependent increases in C_1 complement inhibitor.

   g. The combination of testosterone or methyltestosterone with estrogens (either esterified estrogens or estradiol) may be used for MHT when estrogens alone have not provided adequate therapeutic responses.

5. *Adverse effects and contraindications*

   a. Androgens and anabolic steroids produce decreased testicular function, edema, and altered plasma lipids (increased LDL and decreased HDL levels).

   b. These agents cause masculinization in women.

   c. Androgens increase plasma fibrinolytic activity, causing severe bleeding with concomitant anticoagulant therapy.

   d. **17-Alkyl substituted androgens** (but not testosterone ester preparations) are **associated with increases in hepatic enzymes**, hyperbilirubinemia, and cholestatic hepatitis, which may result in jaundice. Long-term use is associated with liver tumors.

   e. Androgens and anabolic steroids are contraindicated in pregnant women and in patients with carcinoma of the prostate or hepatic, renal, or cardiovascular disease.

I. Antiandrogens are agents that impair the action or synthesis of endogenous androgens.

   1. *Flutamide, bicalutamide, nilutamide*

   a. **Flutamide is a steroidal oral antiandrogen** that acts as a competitive androgen-receptor antagonist. Nilutamide and bicalutamide are **nonsteroidal androgen-receptor antagonists** with better specificity for the androgen receptor and have a longer half-life that permits once-a-day dosing rather than three times a day for finasteride.

   b. These drugs are useful in the treatment of prostatic carcinoma and are highly efficacious when combined with long-term GnRH agonist therapy.

   c. Adverse effects include gynecomastia, elevation in liver enzymes, chest pain, and GI disturbances. These agents are highly teratogenic.

   2. *Finasteride (Proscar)*

   a. Finasteride inhibits type II 5α-reductase, thereby reducing the production of the potent androgen 5α-dihydrotestosterone.

   b. Finasteride is used to treat benign prostatic hypertrophy (BPH) and male pattern baldness.

   c. Finasteride decreases prostate volume and increases urine flow.

   3. *Dutasteride*

   a. Dutasteride inhibits both type I and II 5α-reductase and is more potent than finasteride. Serum dihydrotachysterol (DHT) levels can be reduced by more than 90% in 2 weeks.

   b. Dutasteride is used to treat BPH and baldness.

4. ***Ketoconazole***
   a. Ketoconazole is an antifungal agent that blocks multiple P-450-dependent steps in steroidogenesis, including desmolase.
   b. Ketoconazole can be used to treat precocious puberty and is used to treat hirsutism, in for example PCOS.
5. ***Spironolactone***
   a. Spironolactone antagonizes the binding of both androgen and aldosterone at their respective receptors; it also decreases the activity of the steroidogenic enzyme 17-hydroxylase.
   b. Spironolactone is used as a potassium-sparing diuretic (see Chapter 3) and to treat hirsutism in women (usually in combination with estrogen).

VI. THE ADRENAL CORTEX

A. Corticosteroids
1. *Natural adrenocortical steroids*
   a. Glucocorticoids are synthesized under the control of ACTH (Fig. 10.6). **Cortisol (hydrocortisone) is the predominant natural glucocorticoid in humans**. The 3-keto and 11-hydroxyl groups are important for biologic activity.
   b. **The major mineralocorticoid of the adrenal cortex is aldosterone**. 11-Deoxycorticosterone, an aldosterone precursor, has both mineralocorticoid and glucocorticoid activity.
   c. The adrenals also synthesize various androgens, predominantly dehydroepiandrosterone and androstenedione.

FIGURE 10.6. Biosynthesis of adrenal steroids.

2. *Synthetic adrenocortical steroids*

   a. A wide array of steroid compounds with various ratios of mineralocorticoid to glucocorticoid properties has been synthesized. The most important of these compounds are listed in Table 10.2.

   b. Cortisone acetate and prednisone are 11-keto steroids that are converted to 11-hydroxyl groups by the liver to give cortisol and prednisolone, respectively.

   c. A C_1-C_2 double bond, as in prednisolone and prednisone, increases glucocorticoid activity without increasing mineralocorticoid activity.

   d. The addition of a 9α-fluoro group (e.g., dexamethasone or fludrocortisone) increases activity.

   e. Methylation or hydroxylation at the 16α position abolishes mineralocorticoid activity with little effect on glucocorticoid potency.

3. *Mechanism of action.* The effects of mineralocorticoids and glucocorticoids are mediated by two separate and **specific intracellular receptors**, the **MR** (mineralocorticoid receptor) and **GR** (glucocorticoid receptor), respectively. Natural and synthetic steroids enter cells rapidly and interact with these intracellular receptors. The resulting complexes modulate the transcription rate of specific genes and lead to an increase or decrease in the levels of specific proteins.

4. *Pharmacologic properties*

   a. Plasma binding

      (1) Eighty percent of circulating cortisol is bound to corticosteroid-binding globulin (CBG); 10% is bound to plasma albumin.

      (2) Some of the potent synthetic glucocorticoids, such as dexamethasone, do not bind to CBG, leaving all of the absorbed drug in a free state.

   b. Both natural and synthetic steroids are excreted by the kidney following reduction and formation of glucuronides or sulfates.

   c. All of the steroids listed in Table 10.2 (except aldosterone) may be administered orally. A variety of glucocorticoids, including cortisol, prednisolone, and dexamethasone,

table **10.2**	Properties of Adrenocortical Steroids			
Agent	Equivalent Dose (mg)	Metabolic Potency	Anti-Inflammatory Potency	Sodium-retaining Potency
Oral Glucocorticoids				
Cortisol	20	20	1	1
Cortisone	25	20	1	1
Prednisone	5	5	4	0.5
Prednisolone	5	5	4	0.5
Dexamethasone	0.75	1	30	0.05
Betamethasone	0.6	1.0–1.5	25–40	0.05
Triamcinolone	4	4	5	0.1
Aldosterone		0.3		3,000
Fludrocortisone	0.01	0.1		125–250
Topical Glucocorticoids				
Betamethasone	Highest potency			
Clobetasol	Highest potency			
Halobetasol	Highest potency			
Amcinonide	High potency			
Fluocinonide	High potency			
Triamcinolone	High potency			
Beclomethasone	Medium potency			
Fluticasone	Medium potency			
Hydrocortisone	Medium potency			
Dexamethasone	Low potency			
Desonide	Low potency			

can be injected IM or SC. Various glucocorticoid preparations are available for otic, rectal, or topical administration. As discussed in Chapter 9, glucocorticoids administered as inhalants are used to treat asthma.

   d. Agents with the longest half-life tend to be the most potent.

   (1) Short-acting agents such as cortisol are active for 8–12 hours.

   (2) Intermediate-acting agents such as prednisolone are active for 12–36 hours.

   (3) Long-acting agents such as dexamethasone are active for 39–54 hours.

   e. Drug administration attempts to pattern the circadian rhythm: A double dose is given in the morning, and a single dose is given in the afternoon.

   f. Alternate-day therapy relieves clinical manifestations of the disease state while causing less severe suppression of the adrenal-hypothalamic-pituitary axis. In this therapy, large doses of short-acting or intermediate-acting glucocorticoids are administered every other day.

   g. Patients removed from long-term glucocorticoid therapy **must be weaned off the drug over several days**, using progressively lower doses to allow recovery of adrenal responsiveness.

5. *Glucocorticoids*

   a. Actions. Glucocorticoids affect virtually all tissues. Therapeutic actions and adverse effects are extensions of these physiologic effects.

   (1) Physiologic effects

   (a) The physiologic effects of glucocorticoids are mediated by increased protein breakdown, leading to a **negative nitrogen balance.**

   (b) Glucocorticoids **increase blood glucose levels** by **stimulation of gluconeogenesis.**

   (c) These agents **increase** the **synthesis** of several **key enzymes** involved in glucose and amino acid metabolism.

   (d) Glucocorticoids **increase plasma fatty acids** and **ketone body formation** via increased lipolysis and decreased glucose uptake into fat cells and redistribution of body fat.

   (e) These agents **increase kaliuresis** via increasing renal blood flow and glomerular filtration rate; increased protein metabolism results in release of intracellular potassium.

   (f) Glucocorticoids decrease intestinal absorption of Ca^{2+} and inhibit osteoblasts.

   (g) Glucocorticoids promote Na^+ and water retention.

   (2) Anti-inflammatory effects. The anti-inflammatory effects of glucocorticoids are produced by the inhibition of all of the classic signs of inflammation (erythema, swelling, soreness, and heat). Specific effects include:

   (a) Inhibition of the antigenic response of macrophages and leukocytes.

   (b) Inhibition of vascular permeability by reduction of histamine release and the action of kinins.

   (c) Inhibition of arachidonic acid and prostaglandin production by inhibition of phospholipase A_2 (mediated by annexin 1) and the cyclooxygenases.

   (d) Inhibition of cytokine production, including IL-1, IL-2, IL-3, IL-6, tumor necrosis factor-α, and granulocyte-macrophage colony-stimulating factor.

   (3) Immunologic effects

   (a) Glucocorticoids decrease circulating lymphocytes, monocytes, eosinophils, and basophils.

   (b) Glucocorticoids increase circulating neutrophils.

   (c) Long-term therapy results in involution and atrophy of all lymphoid tissues.

   (4) Other effects

   (a) Inhibition of plasma ACTH and possible adrenal atrophy

   (b) Inhibition of fibroblast growth and collagen synthesis

   (c) Stimulation of acid and pepsin secretion in the stomach

   (d) Altered CNS responses, influencing mood and sleep patterns

   (e) Enhanced neuromuscular transmission

   (f) Induction of surfactant production in the fetal lung at term

b. Therapeutic uses

(1) Glucocorticoids are used in **replacement therapy** for primary or secondary insufficiency (Addison disease); this therapy usually requires the use of both a mineralocorticoid and a glucocorticoid.

(2) Inflammation and immunosuppression

(a) Glucocorticoids are used to treat the following disorders: rheumatoid arthritis, bursitis, lupus erythematosus, and other autoimmune diseases; asthma; nephrotic syndrome; ulcerative colitis; and ocular inflammation.

(b) These agents are also used in hypersensitivity and allergic reactions.

(c) Glucocorticoids can reduce organ or graft rejection.

(3) Sarcoidosis

(4) Dermatologic disorders

(5) Idiopathic nephrosis of children

(6) Neuromuscular disorders, such as Bell's palsy

(7) Shock

(8) Adrenocortical hyperplasia

(9) Stimulation of surfactant production and acceleration of lung maturation in a preterm fetus

(10) Neoplastic diseases, including adult and childhood leukemias

(11) Diagnosis of Cushing syndrome **(dexamethasone suppression test)**

(a) This test measures the suppression of plasma cortisol following the administration of dexamethasone which normally binds to GR in the pituitary and inhibits ACTH production. Failure to suppress cortisol may indicate primary Cushing syndrome or ectopic ACTH production.

c. Adverse effects and contraindications

(1) Most of the adverse effects of glucocorticoids are exaggerated physiologic effects leading to a state of iatrogenic Cushing disease.

(2) Certain glucocorticoids have mineralocorticoid activity, potentially causing sodium retention, potassium loss, and eventual hypokalemic, hypochloremic alkalosis.

(3) Adverse effects of glucocorticoids include the following:

(a) Adrenal suppression

(b) Hyperglycemia and other metabolic disturbances including steroid-induced diabetes mellitus and weight gain

(c) Osteoporosis

(d) Peptic ulcer

(e) Cataracts and increased intraocular pressure leading to glaucoma

(f) Edema

(g) Hypertension

(h) Increased susceptibility to infection and poor wound healing

(i) Muscle weakness and tissue loss

6. *Mineralocorticoids*

a. Actions

(1) Mineralocorticoids primarily affect the kidney, regulating salt and water balance and increasing sodium retention and potassium loss.

(2) Fludrocortisone (Florinef) is the agent of choice for long-term mineralocorticoid replacement.

(3) Adverse effects include sodium retention and hypokalemia, edema, and hypertension.

b. Therapeutic uses. Mineralocorticoids are used in replacement therapy to maintain electrolyte and fluid balance in hypoadrenalism.

B. Adrenocortical Antagonists

1. *Mitotane (o,p′-DDD)*

a. Mitotane causes selective atrophy of the zona fasciculata and zona reticularis and can reduce plasma cortisol level in Cushing syndrome produced by adrenal carcinoma.

    b. Mitotane use is limited to adrenal carcinomas when other therapies are not feasible.

    c. Severe adverse effects of mitotane are not unusual and may include GI distress, mental confusion, lethargy, and dermal toxicity.

2. *Aminoglutethimide*

    a. Aminoglutethimide blocks the conversion of cholesterol to pregnenolone and reduces adrenal production of aldosterone, cortisol, and androgens. The reduction in plasma cortisol triggers a compensatory increase in ACTH that antagonizes the effect of aminoglutethimide. ACTH release may be prevented by coadministration of a glucocorticoid such as cortisol.

    b. Aminoglutethimide is useful in treating hyperadrenalism due to adrenal carcinoma or congenital adrenal hyperplasia.

    c. Adverse effects of aminoglutethimide include drowsiness, rashes, and nausea.

3. *Metyrapone*

    a. Metyrapone blocks the activity of 11-hydroxylase, thereby reducing cortisol production.

    b. Metyrapone is used diagnostically to assess adrenal and pituitary function.

4. *Ketoconazole*

    a. Ketoconazole is an antifungal agent that, at high doses, is a potent inhibitor of several of the P-450 enzymes involved in steroidogenesis in the adrenals and gonads.

    b. Ketoconazole is useful in treating hirsutism and Cushing syndrome.

VII. THE THYROID

A. Thyroid Hormone Receptor Agonists

    1. *Synthesis of natural thyroid hormones*

        a. Natural thyroid hormones are formed by the iodination of tyrosine residues on the glycoprotein thyroglobulin. A tyrosine residue may be iodinated at one (monoiodotyrosine, MIT) or two (diiodotyrosine, DIT) positions. Two iodinated tyrosines are then coupled to synthesize triiodothyronine (T_3; formed from one molecule each of MIT and DIT) or thyroxine (T_4; formed from two DIT molecules). T_4 synthesis exceeds T_3 synthesis fivefold. Eighty percent of circulating T_3 is derived from deiodination of T_4.

        b. Biosynthesis is stimulated by TSH, which acts by a membrane-associated G-protein coupled receptor that increases follicular cell cAMP.

        c. I^- is a potent inhibitor of thyroid hormone release.

    2. *Thyroid hormone preparations*

        a. Thyroid hormone preparations include the following:

            (1) Levothyroxine sodium, a synthetic sodium salt of T_4 that maintains normal T_4 and T_3 levels.

            (2) Liothyronine sodium, a synthetic sodium salt of T_3.

            (3) Liotrix, a 4:1 mixture of the above T_4 and T_3 preparations.

            (4) Thyroid USP, which is prepared from dried and defatted animal thyroid glands and contains a mixture of T_4, T_3, MIT, and DIT.

        b. The potency of animal-based thyroid hormone preparations can vary.

        c. Given the availability of synthetics, thyroid USP is not recommended for initial therapy.

    3. *Mechanism of action.* Thyroid hormones interact with specific nuclear receptor proteins located in the nucleus of target cells and alter the synthesis rate of specific mRNAs, leading to increased production of specific proteins, including Na^+/K^+-ATPase. Increased ATP hydrolysis and oxygen consumption contribute to the effects of thyroid hormones on basal metabolic rate and thermogenesis. T_3 is the most important ligand for the thyroid receptor; T_4 binds very weakly. Thyroid hormones affect virtually all tissues.

    4. *Pharmacologic properties*

        a. More than 99% of circulating T_4 is bound to plasma proteins; only 5%–10% of T_3 is protein bound. Most T_3 and T_4 are bound to TBG. T_4 also binds to prealbumin, and both T_4 and T_3 bind weakly to albumin.

b. T_3 has a $t_{1/2}$ of approximately 1 day; T_4 has a $t_{1/2}$ of approximately 5–7 days.

c. Levothyroxine sodium and liothyronine sodium can be administered orally or IV. Oral absorption rates range from 30% to 65%. Levothyroxine sodium is preferred to liothyronine because it has better oral absorption, has a longer $t_{1/2}$, and produces a favorable T_4:T_3 ratio.

d. Metabolism

    (1) T_3 and T_4 are inactivated by deiodination.

    (2) Conjugation of T_3 and T_4 with glucuronic acid or sulfate occurs in the liver, and these metabolites are secreted in the bile.

    (3) Some enterohepatic circulation of the metabolites occurs; 20%–40% of T_4 is eliminated in the feces.

5. *Actions*

  a. Thyroid hormones are essential for **normal physical and mental development** of the fetus. Linear growth of the long bones, growth of the brain, and normal myelination depend on thyroid hormone. **Hypothyroidism in infants leads to cretinism** (myxedema with physical and mental retardation).

  b. These agents increase the basal metabolic rate and blood sugar levels. They also increase the synthesis of fatty acids **and decrease plasma cholesterol** and triglyceride levels.

  c. Thyroid hormones **increase the heart rate** and peripheral resistance.

  d. These agents inhibit TRH and TSH release from the hypothalamus and pituitary, respectively.

  e. Thyroid hormones exert **maintenance effects** on the CNS, reproductive tract, GI tract, and musculature.

6. *Therapeutic uses*

  a. Primary, secondary, or tertiary hypothyroidism caused by

    (1) Hashimoto disease

    (2) Myxedema

    (3) Simple goiter (thyroid gland enlargement without hyperthyroidism)

    (4) Following surgical ablation of the thyroid gland

  b. TSH-dependent carcinomas of the thyroid may be treated with thyroid hormones if other therapies are not feasible.

7. *Adverse effects*

  a. Thyroid hormones produce iatrogenic hyperthyroidism, **nervousness, anxiety, and headache**.

  b. These agents induce **arrhythmias, angina, or infarction** in patients with underlying cardiovascular disease.

  c. Thyroid hormones should be used cautiously in the elderly.

B. Antithyroid Drugs

  1. *Thioamides*

    a. Thioamides include **propylthiouracil** (PTU) and **methimazole;** methimazole is approximately 10 times more potent than PTU.

    b. Thioamides interfere with the **organification and coupling of iodide by inhibiting the peroxidase** enzyme. PTU inhibits the conversion of T_4 to T_3.

    c. PTU can be used during pregnancy; **methimazole is teratogenic** and cannot.

    d. Thioamides remain active after oral administration; 50%–80% is absorbed.

    e. These agents have a $t_{1/2}$ of approximately 1–2 hours; they are concentrated in the thyroid gland and inhibit thyroid hormone biosynthesis for 6–24 hours. They do not affect T_3/T_4 already within the thyroid; attaining euthyroid status when initiating therapy may take 2–4 months.

    f. Thioamides are eliminated in the urine as glucuronides.

    g. Thioamides treat hyperthyroidism from a variety of causes, including Graves disease and toxic goiter. Thioamides are also used to control hyperthyroidism prior to thyroid surgery.

    h. These agents commonly cause rashes, headache, or nausea; they may also induce leukopenia or agranulocytosis.

2. **Anion inhibitors of thyroid function**
   a. Anion inhibitors of thyroid function include thiocyanate, perchlorate, and fluoborate.
   b. These agents are monovalent anions with a hydrated radius similar in size to that of iodide.
   c. Anion inhibitors competitively inhibit the transport of iodide by the thyroid gland.
   d. These agents are limited by severe toxicities (including fatal aplastic anemia) to occasional diagnostic use for thyroid function.

3. **Iodide**
   a. In high intracellular concentrations, iodide inhibits several steps in thyroid hormone biosynthesis, including iodide transport and organification (Wolff-Chaikoff effect).
   b. Iodide inhibits the release of thyroid hormone.
   c. Iodide is usually combined with a thioamide; it is rarely used as sole therapy.
   d. This agent is used before thyroid surgery, causing firming of thyroid tissues and decreased thyroid vascularity, and in the treatment of spirotrichosis.
   e. Iodide may cause angioedema, rash, a metallic taste on administration, and hypersensitivity reactions.

4. **Radioactive iodine ^{131}I**
   a. Radioactive iodine ^{131}I emits beta particles and x-rays and has a radioactive $t_{1/2}$ of approximately 8 days. ^{131}I is transported and concentrated in the thyroid like the nonradioactive isotope. High-energy radioiodine emissions are toxic to follicular cells.
   b. Radioactive iodine ^{131}I treats hyperthyroidism via nonsurgical ablation of the thyroid gland or reduction of hyperactive thyroid gland without damage to the surrounding tissue.
   c. This agent is helpful (in low doses) in the diagnosis of hyperthyroidism, hypothyroidism, and goiter; it may be used to assess thyroid responsiveness.
   d. Overdosage of this agent commonly induces hypothyroidism.

VIII. THE PANCREAS AND GLUCOSE HOMEOSTASIS

A. Insulin
   1. **Structure and synthesis**
      a. Insulin is a polypeptide hormone produced by the **pancreatic β cell**. Insulin consists of two chains, A and B, linked by two disulfide bridges.
      b. Human insulin contains 51 amino acids. Bovine insulin differs from human insulin at three amino acid sites; porcine insulin differs in only one amino acid.
      c. Insulin is stored as a complex with Zn^{2+}; two molecules of zinc complex six molecules of insulin.
      d. Insulin synthesis and release are modulated by the following:
         (1) The most important stimulus is glucose. Amino acids, fatty acids, and ketone bodies also stimulate release.
         (2) The islets of Langerhans contain several cell types besides β cells that synthesize and release peptide humoral agents (including glucagon and somatostatin) that can modulate insulin secretion.
         (3) **α-Adrenergic pathways inhibit secretion of insulin**; this is the predominant inhibitory mechanism.
      e. **β-Adrenergic stimulation increases insulin** release.
      f. Elevated intracellular Ca^{2+} acts as an insulin secretagogue.
   2. **Mechanism of action**
      a. Insulin binds to specific high affinity receptors with tyrosine kinase activity located in the plasma membrane. Specific tyrosine residues of the insulin receptor become phosphorylated (auto-phosphorylation); other substrates for phosphorylation include IRS-1-4 (insulin receptor substrates-1 to -4). The increase in glucose transport in muscle and adipose tissue is mediated by the recruitment of hexose transport molecules (GLUT-1 and GLUT-4) into the plasma membrane.

    b. Insulin alters the phosphorylation state of key metabolic enzymes, leading to enzymatic activation or inactivation.

    c. Insulin induces the transcription of several genes involved in increasing glucose catabolism and specifically inhibits transcription of other genes involved in gluconeogenesis.

3. *Actions.* **Insulin promotes systemic cellular K$^+$ uptake.**

    a. Liver

        (1) Inhibits glucose production and increases glycolysis

        (2) Inhibits glycogenolysis and stimulates glycogen synthesis

        (3) Increases the synthesis of triglycerides

        (4) Increases protein synthesis

    b. Muscle

        (1) Increases glucose transport and glycolysis

        (2) Increases glycogen deposition

        (3) Increases protein synthesis

    c. Adipose tissue

        (1) Increases glucose transport

        (2) Increases lipogenesis and lipoprotein lipase

        (3) Decreases intracellular lipolysis

4. *Pharmacologic properties*

    a. Insulin has a $t_{1/2}$ of 5–10 minutes.

    b. Insulin is degraded by hepatic glutathione-insulin transhydrogenase, which reduces the disulfide linkages between the A and B chains, producing two biologically inactive peptides.

5. *Insulin preparations* (Table 10.3)

    a. Historically, insulin preparations were derived from bovine and porcine glands. Bovine insulin was removed from the U.S. market due to concern about "mad cow" disease; preparation of porcine insulin was stopped in 2005. Human insulin is prepared by recombinant DNA techniques to produce the human peptide in bacteria.

    b. Insulin preparations are often mixed to control blood sugar levels: A single morning injection of a lente or ultralente form is typically supplemented with preprandial injections of a rapid-acting product. Dosage regimens must be individualized.

        (1) Rapid acting. **Insulin glulisine, insulin aspart,** and **insulin lispro** are human insulins that have been modified at 1–2 amino acids in the B chain to increase their solubility. These insulins dissociate into monomers almost instantly upon SC injection. They provide better postprandial control of glucose levels than regular insulin.

        (2) Short acting. **Regular insulin** is prepared as a recombinant human protein.

        (3) Intermediate acting. **Isophane insulin (or Neutral Protamine Hagedorn)** is prepared by precipitating insulin-zinc complexes with protamine, a mixture of basic peptides. This slows absorption and extends the duration of action.

        (4) Long acting

            (a) **Ultralente insulin** has a larger particle size than Lente products.

            (b) **Glargine insulin** has a single amino acid in the A chain and two additional amino acids in the B chain that differ from regular insulin. This causes it to form a stable, slowly dissolving precipitate upon injection.

            (c) **Detemir** insulin has a 14-carbon fatty acid (myristic acid) added to the A chain and an amino acid removed from the B chain; this also causes it to form a stable, slowly dissolving precipitate.

6. *Therapeutic uses.* Insulin is used to treat all of the manifestations of hyperglycemia in **both type I (insulin-dependent)** and **type II (non-insulin-dependent) diabetes mellitus.** Most type II diabetics are treated with dietary changes and oral hypoglycemic agents. In serious cases of type II diabetes in which these treatments are inadequate to control blood glucose levels, insulin may be required.

table 10.3	Pharmacologic Properties of Agents Used for Long-Term Management of Hyperglycemia		
Agent	**Route of Administration**	**Onset of Action**	**Duration of Action**
Insulins			
Rapid acting			
Insulin glulisine	SC	20 min	1–2 h
Insulin aspart	SC	15 min	3–5 h
Insulin lispro	SC	15 min	3–5 h
Short acting			
Regular	SC, IM, IV	15 min	2–5 h
Intermediate acting			
Isophane	SC	2 h	24 h
Slow acting			
Insulin glargine	SC	1.5	24 h
Insulin detemir	SC	1.5	12–20 h
Ultralente	SC	4 h	36 h
Sulfonylureas			
Tolbutamide	Oral	20 min	6–10 h
Acetohexamide	Oral	20 min	12–20 h
Tolazamide	Oral	20 min	10–14 h
Glipizide	Oral	30 min	16–24 h
Glyburide	Oral	1–2 h	24 h
Glimepiride	Oral	1–2 h	24 h
Chlorpropamide	Oral	1–2 h	>24 h
Biguanines			
Metformin	Oral	-2 h	6 h
Meglitinides			
Repaglinide	Oral	20 min	1 h
Nateglinide	Oral	30 min	1–2 h
α-Glucosidase inhibitors			
Acarbose	Oral	30 min	2 h
Miglitol	Oral		
Thiazolidinediones			
Pioglitazone	Oral	3 h	12 h
Rosaglitazone	Oral	3 h	12–18 h
Incretins			
Exenatide	SC	1 h	2–3 h
DPP-IV inhibitor			
Sitagliptin	Oral	2 h	12 h
Amylin analog			
Pramlintide	SC	30 min	3 h

7. **Adverse effects**
   a. Hypoglycemia may occur from insulin overdose, insufficient caloric intake, strenuous exercise, or when combined with ethanol. Sequelae include tachycardia, sweating, and sympathetic and parasympathetic actions that can progress to coma.
   b. Hypokalemia
   c. Anaphylactoid reaction
   d. Lipodystrophy or hypertrophy of SC fat at the injection site
   e. Weight gain

B. **Oral hypoglycemic Agents**
   1. *Sulfonylureas*
      a. Structure
         (1) **First-generation** compounds include **tolbutamide, acetohexamide, tolazamide,** and **chlorpropamide.**
         (2) Second-generation compounds include glyburide and glipizide; they are up to 200 times more potent than first-generation agents.
         (3) Third-generation **compounds, such as glimepiride,** may be used in conjunction with insulin. These compounds may interact with different cellular proteins than other sulfonylureas.
         (4) All of the sulfonylureas are well absorbed after oral administration and bind to plasma proteins, notably albumin.
      b. Mechanism of action
         (1) Sulfonylureas cause an increase in the amount of insulin secreted by the β cells in response to a glucose challenge. Sulfonylureas block K^+ channels in β cells, leading to depolarization, increased Ca^{2+} entry via voltage-dependent calcium channels, and increased insulin secretion.
         (2) These agents increase sensitivity to insulin, perhaps by increasing the number of insulin receptors. However, sulfonylureas do not decrease the insulin requirements of patients with type I diabetes.
         (3) Sulfonylureas decrease serum glucagon, which opposes the action of insulin.
      c. Pharmacologic properties (see Table 10.3). Pharmacologic failure with oral antidiabetic agents is common, initially affecting 15%–30% of patients and as many as 90% after 6–7 years of therapy.
         (1) Short-acting agents
            (a) Short-acting sulfonylureas include **tolbutamide.**
            (b) Short-acting sulfonylureas are rapidly absorbed; absorption is not affected if taken with food.
            (c) As with all sulfonylureas, **hypoglycemia** is a potentially dangerous adverse effect of these short-acting agents. Other adverse effects include dermatologic disorders and GI disturbances, including nausea and heartburn.
         (2) Intermediate-acting agents
            (a) **Acetohexamide**
               (i) Acetohexamide is rapidly absorbed.
               (ii) Acetohexamide is metabolized to hydrohexamide, which is biologically active and has a $t_{1/2}$ of 6 hours.
               (iii) Acetohexamide has uricosuric properties, making it useful in diabetic patients with gout.
            (b) **Tolazamide**
               (i) Tolazamide is slowly absorbed.
               (ii) Tolazamide is about five times more potent on a milligram basis than tolbutamide
               (iii) Tolazamide exerts a **mild diuretic effect.**
            (c) **Glipizide**
               (i) Glipizide is rapidly absorbed, but absorption can be delayed by food.
               (ii) Glipizide becomes highly protein-bound in the plasma.
            (d) **Glyburide**
               (i) Glyburide is rapidly absorbed.
               (ii) Glyburide inhibits hepatic glucose production.
               (iii) Glyburide exerts a **mild diuretic effect.**
         (3) Long-acting agents
            (a) Long-acting sulfonylureas include **chlorpropamide** and **glimepiride.**
            (b) Long-acting sulfonylureas are rapidly absorbed.
            (c) These agents are extensively reabsorbed in the kidney; reabsorption is slowed under basic pH conditions.

      (d) Long-acting sulfonylureas cause adverse effects more frequently than other sulfonylureas. Water retention is common, and alcohol consumption produces a **disulfiram-like reaction** in some patients.

      (e) These agents are contraindicated in elderly patients, in whom toxicities seem to be exacerbated.

  d. Therapeutic uses

    (1) Sulfonylureas are very useful in treating type II diabetes mellitus but are **not effective against type I diabetes.**

    (2) Sulfonylureas should not be used in patients with renal or liver disease.

2. *Biguanine hypoglycemics* include **metformin**.

  a. Metformin reduces hepatic glucose production and intestinal absorption of glucose; it does not alter insulin secretion. These effects are believed to be due to an increase in the activity of AMP kinase, a key intracellular regulator of energy homeostasis.

  b. Metformin increases peripheral insulin sensitivity.

  c. Metformin may be used alone or in combination with sulfonylureas and thiazolidinediones.

  d. Metformin has been found useful in the treatment of polycystic ovary syndrome; it lowers serum androgens and restores normal menstrual cycles and ovulation.

  e. **Metformin rarely causes hypoglycemia** or weight gain.

  f. Adverse effects of metformin include **lactic acidosis**.

3. *Meglitinides: repaglinide and nateglinide*

  a. These agents are oral insulin secretagogues that **act by blocking ATP-dependent K$^+$ channels**, leading to increased insulin secretion by pancreatic β-cells.

  b. Nateglinide has a more rapid onset of action and is more specific for pancreatic K$^+$ channels than repaglinide.

  c. These drugs are metabolized by the liver and should not be used in patients with hepatic insufficiency.

  d. The major adverse effect of these drugs is **hypoglycemia**.

4. α-*Glucosidase inhibitors* include **acarbose and miglitol**.

  a. Acarbose and miglitol are oligosaccharides or oligosaccharide derivatives.

  b. They act as competitive, **reversible inhibitors of pancreatic α-amylase and intestinal α-glucosidase enzymes**; they act in the lumen of the intestine.

  c. Inhibition of α-glucosidase prolongs digestion of carbohydrates and reduces peak plasma glucose levels.

  d. Miglitol is a more potent inhibitor of sucrase and maltase than is acarbose. Unlike acarbose, miglitol does not inhibit pancreatic α-amylase but does inhibit isomaltose.

  e. These drugs are usually combined with a sulfonylurea or another oral hypoglycemic agent.

  f. α-Glucosidase inhibitors rarely cause hypoglycemia.

5. *Thiazolidinediones* include **pioglitazone and rosiglitazone**.

  a. Thiazolidinediones are a new class of oral hypoglycemic agents that act by increasing **tissue sensitivity to insulin**.

  b. These drugs bind to a specific intracellular receptor (PPAR-γ), a member of the nuclear-receptor family. Rosiglitazone has about 10-fold higher affinity for PPAR-γ than does pioglitazone.

  c. Thiazolidinediones predominantly affect liver, skeletal muscle, and adipose tissue.

    (1) In the liver, thiazolidinediones **decrease glucose output** and insulin levels.

    (2) In muscle, thiazolidinediones **increase glucose uptake**.

    (3) In adipose tissue, these **drugs increase glucose uptake and decrease fatty acid release** and may increase the release of hormones such as adiponectin and resistin.

  d. The actions of these drugs require the presence of insulin.

  e. Thiazolidinediones reduce plasma glucose and triglycerides.

  f. Thiazolidinediones do not cause hypoglycemia.

  g. Thiazolidindiones are associated with exacerbating or causing congestive heart failure.

6. *Incretin mimetics*
   a. Endogenous human incretins, such as **glucagon-like peptide-1 (GLP-1),** are released from the gut and enhance insulin secretion.
   b. **Exenatide** is a synthetic 39-amino acid GLP-1 analog; **liraglutide** is longer acting and more resistant to metabolism . They also reduce appetite.
   c. Incretins decrease glucagon secretion, slow gastric emptying, reduce food intake, and promote β-cell proliferation.
   d. SC injection of incretins may improve glycemic control in patients with type II diabetes mellitus who have not achieved adequate glycemic control on metformin, a sulfonylurea, or a combination of metformin and a sulfonylurea.
   e. Pancreatitis has been observed as a serious adverse effect.

7. *Dipeptidyl peptidase 4 (DPP-IV) inhibitors*
   a. **Sitagliptin, saxagliptin, and linagliptin** are members of a class of antidiabetic agents that act by **inhibiting dipeptidyl peptidase 4**, a serine protease.
   b. Dipeptidyl peptidase 4 is responsible for the proteolysis of the incretins, including GLP-1 and glucose-dependent insulinotropic peptide.
   c. **DPP-IV inhibitors** may also improve β-cell function.
   d. In monotherapy or in combination with metformin, DPP-IV inhibitors decrease fasting and postprandial plasma glucose concentrations and plasma HbA1c concentration.
   e. Administered orally; most common side effects are headache and nausea.

8. *Amylin analogs.* **Pramlintide** is a synthetic amylin analog. Amylin is a polypeptide stored and secreted by β-cells of the pancreas, and it acts in concert with insulin to reduce blood sugar.
   a. Pramlintide acts to slow gastric emptying, decrease glucagon secretion, and decreases appetite.
   b. Administered SC, typically with insulin. Common side effects are hypoglycemia and nausea.

C. Agents that Increase Blood Glucose (Hyperglycemics)
   1. *Glucagon*
      a. Structure and synthesis
         (1) Glucagon is a single-chain polypeptide of 29 amino **acids produced by the α cells of the pancreas.**
         (2) Glucagon shares a structural homology with secretin, VIP, and gastric inhibitory peptide.
         (3) Secretion of glucagon is inhibited by elevated plasma glucose, insulin, and somatostatin.
         (4) Secretion of glucagon is stimulated by amino acids, sympathetic stimulation, and sympathetic secretion.
      b. Actions and pharmacologic properties
         (1) Membrane-bound receptors are most abundant in the liver; response is coupled to an increase in cAMP.
         (2) **Glucagon stimulates the use of glycogen stores and gluconeogenesis**; in general, its actions oppose those of insulin.
         (3) Large doses produce marked relaxation of the smooth muscle.
         (4) Glucagon is extensively degraded in the liver and kidney and is also subject to hydrolysis in plasma. Plasma $t_{1/2}$ of glucagon is approximately 3–5 minutes.
      c. Therapeutic uses
         (1) Glucagon produces rescue from hypoglycemic crisis. Glucagon rapidly increases blood glucose in insulin-induced hypoglycemia if hepatic glycogen stores are adequate.
         (2) Glucagon provides intestinal relaxation prior to radiologic examination.
         (3) Glucagon causes β-cell stimulation of insulin secretion; it is used to assess pancreatic reserves.
      d. Adverse effects. The adverse effects of glucagon are minimal; there is a low incidence of nausea and vomiting.

2. *Diazoxide (Proglycem)*

 a. Diazoxide is a nondiuretic thiazide that promptly increases blood glucose levels **by direct inhibition of insulin secretion**.

 b. Diazoxide is useful in cases of insulinoma or leucine-sensitive hypoglycemia.

 c. Diazoxide may cause sodium retention, GI irritation, and changes in circulating white blood cells.

IX. THE CALCIUM HOMEOSTATIC SYSTEM

A. Calcium is the major extracellular divalent cation, primarily (40–50%) existing as free ionized Ca^{2+} (the biologically active fraction). Approximately 40% of serum Ca^{2+} is bound to plasma proteins, especially albumin, with the remaining 10% complexed to such anions as citrate.

B. Drugs Affecting Ca^{2+} Homeostasis

 1. *Parathyroid hormone (PTH)*

 a. Structure

 (1) PTH is an 84-amino acid peptide secreted by the parathyroid glands in response to low serum ionized Ca^{2+}.

 (2) Agents such as β-adrenoceptor agonists, which increase cAMP in the parathyroid gland, cause an increase in PTH secretion.

 b. Actions and pharmacologic properties

 (1) Activity in the kidney and in bone is mediated by specific PTH receptors, which are in turn coupled to an increase in cAMP. Significant quantities of cAMP are found in the urine after PTH stimulation.

 (2) In bone, PTH can increase both the rate of bone formation and bone resorption. This is mediated by cytokines such as **RANKL** (aka osteoprotegrin ligand) produced by osteoblasts that regulate the number and activity of osteoclasts.

 (a) Continuous exposure to PTH results in net bone resorption.

 (b) Pulsatile exposure results in net bone formation.

 (3) In the kidney, PTH increases the reabsorption of Ca^{2+} and Mg^{2+}, and it increases the production of $1,25\text{-}(OH)_2D_3$ from $25\text{-}(OH)D_3$ (1-hydroxylase step). PTH also **decreases reabsorption of phosphate**, bicarbonate, amino acids, sulfate, sodium, and chloride.

 (4) In the GI tract, PTH increases intestinal absorption of Ca^{2+} indirectly by increasing $1,25\text{-}(OH)_2D_3$.

 (5) PTH is rapidly degraded ($t_{1/2}$ is 2–5 min) by renal and hepatic metabolism.

 c. Teriparatide

 (1) Teriparatide is recombinant human PTH 1-34 which behaves as a full PTH agonist.

 (2) Teriparatide is administered parenterally once a day, and **this intermittent exposure results in net bone formation**.

 (3) Teriparatide is used in the treatment of osteoporosis.

 (4) Teriparatide is also used as a diagnostic agent to distinguish pseudohypoparathyroidism from true hypoparathyroidism.

 (5) Major adverse effects are hypercalcemia and hypercalciurea. Infrequent adverse effects include dizziness, depression, pain, headache, and leg cramps.

 2. *Calcitonin*

 a. Structure. Calcitonin is a 32-amino acid peptide secreted by perifollicular cells of the thyroid gland In response to elevated plasma Ca^{2+}. Gastrin, glucagon, cholecystokinin, and epinephrine can also increase calcitonin secretion.

 b. Actions. Calcitonin antagonizes the actions of PTH through an independent mechanism:

 (1) Calcitonin interacts with specific receptors on osteoclasts to **decrease net reabsorption of Ca^{2+}**. Calcitonin may also stimulate bone formation.

 (2) Calcitonin **increases renal excretion of Ca^{2+}**, Na^+, and phosphate.

c. Pharmacologic properties
   (1) Synthetic salmon calcitonin (Fortical, Miacalcin) differs from human calcitonin at 13 of 32 amino acids and has a longer half-life.
   (2) Currently approved products are administered parenterally or as a nasal spray.
   (3) Decreases in plasma Ca^{2+} are seen in 2 hours and persist for 6–8 hours.

d. Therapeutic uses
   (1) Calcitonin reduces hypercalcemia due to **Paget disease,** hyperparathyroidism, idiopathic juvenile hypercalcemia, vitamin D intoxication, osteolytic bone disorders, and osteoporosis.
   (2) Patients frequently (20%) become refractory to chronic administration, possibly because of the production of anticalcitonin antibodies.

3. ***Vitamin D and vitamin D metabolites*** (Table 10.4)
   a. Structure. The calciferols, vitamin D_3 (cholecalciferol) and vitamin D_2 (ergocalciferol), are secosteroid members of the steroid hormone family.
   b. Synthesis
      (1) **Vitamin D_3 is produced in the skin** from cholesterol; this synthesis requires exposure to **ultraviolet light**.
      (2) $25\text{-}(OH)D_3$ (calcifediol)
         (a) **Calcifediol is produced in the liver by hydroxylation of vitamin D_3.**
         (b) Calcifediol is the most abundant calciferol metabolite in the plasma.
      (3) $1,25\text{-}(OH)_2D_3$ (calcitriol)
         (a) **Calcitriol is produced in the kidney by further hydroxylation of $25\text{-}(OH)D_3$ by $1\text{-}\alpha$hydroxylase.** Regulation of 1α-hydroxylase activity determines the serum levels of **calcitriol.** Enzymatic activity is increased by PTH, estrogens, prolactin, and other agents, and it is decreased by $1,25\text{-}(OH)_2D_3$, FGF23, and phosphate (direct effect).
         (b) **Calcitriol is the most active metabolite of vitamin D**.
      (4) Vitamin D_2 (ergocalciferol)
         (a) Vitamin D_2 is derived from plant metabolism of ergosterol and has a slightly different side chain, which does not alter its biologic effects in humans.
         (b) In humans, vitamin D_2 is metabolized in the same manner as vitamin D_3 and appears to be bioequivalent.
      (5) **Paricalcitol** $(1,25\text{-}(OH)_2\text{-}19$ norvitamin $D_2)$ is a 1,25-hydroxylated vitamin D_2 derivative that reduces serum PTH levels without affecting serum Ca^{2+} or PO_4^{2-} levels. It is approved for the treatment of **hyperparathyroidism in patients with renal failure** who are on dialysis. It is administered by infusion.
      (6) 22-Oxacalcitrol (maxacalcitrol) is a $1,25\text{-}(OH)_2D_3$ derivative containing an oxygen instead of a carbon at position 22 in the side chain. Compared with $1,25\text{-}D_3$, it binds with low affinity to the serum vitamin D-binding globulin. It is a **potent suppressor of PTH** and is useful in patients with secondary (to renal failure) or primary hyperparathyroidism.

t a b l e **10.4**	Pharmacologic Properties of Vitamin D Preparations		
Agent	**Metabolic Route**	**Onset of Action**	**Half-life**
Ergocalciferol (D2)	Hepatic, renal	10–14 d	30 d
Cholecalciferol (D3)	Hepatic, renal	10–14 d	30 d
Calcifediol	Renal	8–10 d	20 d
Calcitriol	None	10 h	15 h
Calcipotriene	Hepatic, renal	10 d	30 d
Doxercalciferol	Hepatic	5–8 h	36 h
Paricalcitol	None	Minutes (IV)	15 h

(7) Doxercalciferol (1α-(OH) vitamin D_2) is administered orally or IV for hyperparathyroidism secondary to renal failure. It does not increase intestinal Ca^{2+} absorption and does not cause hypercalcemia.

(8) Calcipotriene

(a) Calcipotriene is a 1,24-$(OH)_2D_3$ derivative for topical administration for the treatment of skin disorders such as psoriasis.

(b) Calcipotriene has reduced effects on calcium homeostasis.

c. Actions and pharmacologic properties (Table 10.4)

(1) Calcitriol **increases plasma levels of both Ca^{2+} and phosphate** by acting on several organ systems:

(a) **Intestine:** Increases Ca^{2+} absorption from the GI tract

(b) **Bone:** Mobilizes Ca^{2+} and phosphate, probably by stimulation of calcium flux out of osteoblasts

(c) **Kidney:** Increases reabsorption of both Ca^{2+} and phosphate

(2) All vitamin D metabolites bind to a specific plasma-binding protein, vitamin D-binding protein.

(3) Vitamin D, calcifediol, and calcitriol are all administered orally; calcitriol may be administered parenterally.

d. Therapeutic uses

(1) Elevate serum Ca^{2+}. Vitamin D and vitamin D metabolites are used to treat hypocalcemia caused by a number of diseases, including vitamin D deficiency (nutritional rickets), hypoparathyroidism, renal disease, malabsorption, and osteoporosis.

(2) Reduce cellular proliferation

(a) Recent evidence has shown that 1,25-$(OH)_2D_3$ can block differentiation and proliferation of many cell types. For this reason, the drug has been successfully used in the treatment of certain **leukemias.**

(b) **Topical calcipotriene** has been approved for the treatment of **psoriasis;** it reduces fibroblast proliferation and induces differentiation of epidermal keratinocytes.

4. *Bisphosphonates*

a. Chemistry and pharmacokinetics. Bisphosphonates (P-C-P) are analogs of pyrophosphate (P-O-P) that bind directly to hydroxyapatite crystals in bone and impair reabsorption.

(1) First-generation bisphosphonate: etidronate disodium.

(2) Second-generation bisphosphonates contain a nitrogen, are called aminobisphosphonates, and include **alendronate, ibandronate, tiludronate, and pamidronate.** They are at least 10 times more potent than first-generation agents.

(3) Third-generation bisphosphonates, risedronate and zoldronic acid, have a nitrogen within a heterocyclic ring and are 10,000 times more potent than first-generation agents.

(4) After oral administration, all bisphosphonates have very poor (1–3%) oral absorption that is decreased by food. Etidronate, especially, is associated with esophageal irritation and erosion. Recommendation is to administer on an empty stomach with a full glass of water and remain standing for 30 minutes.

b. Etidronate, the first bisphosphonate discovered

(1) Mechanism of action. The non-nitrogenous bisphosphonates are internalized by osteoclasts and converted into an ATP analog that cannot be hydrolyzed. This metabolite impairs various functions and induces apoptosis in osteoclasts.

(2) Can be administered IV or orally.

c. Aminobisphosphonates

(1) The mechanism of action is inhibition of farnesyl diphosphate synthase, part of the cholesterol biosynthetic pathway. This impairs posttranslational modification of a number of regulator proteins critical for osteoclast function, including Ras,

Rho, and Rac. There is recent evidence that aminobisphosphonates also induce a unique ATP analog that induces osteoclast apoptosis.

(2) Poorly absorbed, can be given by infusion, zolandronate once per year.

(3) Aminobisphosphonates are not associated with the problems of reflux and osteomalacia.

d. Uses

(1) Paget disease—given orally, clinical symptoms improve relatively slowly (1–3 months)

(2) Effective in 60%–70% of cases; normalization of serum Ca^{2+} levels in 2–8 days

(3) Heterotopic ossification

(4) Aminobisphosphonates are approved for the prevention of osteoporosis

e. Adverse effects. GI disturbances include GI bleeding and diarrhea, arthralgia, and nonspecified chest pain. When used for prolonged periods (years), etidronate can interfere with mineralization of bone (osteomalacia). Rare instances of osteonecrosis of the jaw.

5. Denosumab

a. Denosumab is a monoclonal antibody that blocks the action of RANKL (osteoprotegrin ligand).

b. This reduces osteoclast proliferation and activation.

c. Approved for the treatment of post-menopausal osteoporosis and for reducing the risk of bone loss and bone metastasis in patients with solid tumors.

d. Efficacy at reducing bone loss is comparable to that of bisphosphonates.

6. Calcium sensor sensitizers—calcimimetics

a. The parathyroid gland senses Ca^{2+} via the action of the protein **CaSR**. Activation of CaSR reduces the amount of PTH synthesized and released by the gland.

b. Cinacalcet (Sensipar) is an oral agent that acts similar to Ca^{2+} on the CaSR; this reduces serum PTH.

c. Cinacalcet is approved for use in patients with hyperparathyroidism secondary to renal disease.

d. Hypocalcemia is the major adverse effect of cinacalcet.

7. Secondary agents affecting Ca^{2+} homeostasis

a. Thiazide diuretics reduce the renal excretion of Ca^{2+} and the incidence of kidney stone formation in patients with idiopathic hypercalciuria.

b. Loop diuretics. Agents such as furosemide increase renal excretion of Ca^{2+}.

c. Glucocorticoids increase bone resorption and reduce intestinal absorption of Ca^{2+} by interfering with $1,25\text{-}(OH)_2D_3$. The net effect is to reduce plasma Ca^{2+} levels.

d. Estrogens

(1) Estrogens indirectly impair the action of PTH on bone and in the kidney.

(2) Estrogens are used in the treatment of osteoporosis.

C. Calcium Supplements

1. Calcium supplements are available in a variety of Ca^{2+} concentrations and in parenteral and oral formulations.

2. Calcium supplements are useful as dietary supplements for the treatment or prevention of osteoporosis and for the immediate treatment of acute hypocalcemia and hypocalcemic tetany.

3. Calcium supplements may cause hypercalcemia with long-term use.

X. RETINOIC ACID AND DERIVATIVES

A. Structure. Retinol (vitamin A) is a prohormone that is converted by intracellular enzymes to activate the active agents **all-*trans*-retinoic acid** and **9-*cis*-retinoic acid.** Other retinol metabolites are biologically active.

B. **Action**
 1. **The actions of retinoids are mediated via intracellular receptors of two main classes: retinoic acid receptor (RAR) and retinoid X receptor (RXR). Rexinoids are ligands that interact specifically with the RXRs.**
    a. Each of these classes has at least three distinct isoforms (α, β, ϒ with unique biologic properties).
    b. The retinoid receptors are members of the nuclear receptor family and act by modulating transcription of specific genes.
 2. **Retinoids are morphogens, playing important roles during embryonic development,** including the regulation of cellular proliferation and differentiation, and the modulation of immune function and cytokine production. They **cause severe fetal malformations** and must be used with extreme caution in females of childbearing age.

C. **Tretinoin**
 1. *Tretinoin is all-trans-retinoic acid,* a naturally occurring metabolite of vitamin A. Tretinoin as a topical preparation used for the treatment of acne and photoaged skin, as an oral agent it is used in the treatment of acute promyelocytic leukemia, and may be used in the treatment of Kaposi sarcoma.
 2. Adverse effects of tretinoin include tenderness, erythema, and burning. There is also an increased risk of sunburn. Oral administration is associated with a syndrome of hypervitaminosis A, which includes headache, fever, bone pain, nausea, vomiting, and rash.

D. **Isotretinoin**
 1. Isotretinoin is an oral agent used for the treatment of severe cystic acne and the symptomatic management of keratinization disorders. It reversibly reduces the size of sebaceous glands and hence the production of sebum. It is the 13-*cis* isomer of tretinoin.
 2. Adverse effects of isotretinoin include inflammation of mucous membranes (most often the lips), rash, and alopecia. Less common adverse effects include arthralgia and myalgia. **Retinoids tend to inhibit lipoprotein lipase**, which leads to an increase in serum triglycerides.
 3. Isotretinoin is teratogenic.

E. **Acitretin (Soriatane)**
 1. Acitretin is an oral agent approved for the treatment of psoriasis and other disorders of keratinization. In addition, acitretin has been studied in cutaneous T-cell lymphoma and for the prevention of skin cancers following solid organ transplantation.
 2. Adverse effects of acitretin include **skin and nail abnormalities.**
 3. Acitretin is teratogenic.

F. **Alitretinoin (Panretin)** is a synthetic version of 9-*cis*-retinoic acid. It is a topical cream approved for use in the skin disorders associated with Kaposi syndrome.

G. **Tazarotene (Avage)**
 1. Following topical application, tazarotene undergoes esterase hydrolysis to the active form, tazarotenic acid, which binds to all three members of the RAR family, with some specificity for the β and ϒ subtypes.
 2. It is used to treat psoriasis, photoaging (fine wrinkles), and acne vulgaris.
 3. The most common adverse effects seen with tazarotene are skin related: rash, desquamation, and pruritus.

H. **Adapalene** is a topical retinoid-like drug for the treatment of mild-to-moderate acne vulgaris. It is a naphtholic acid derivative that binds to RARs.

I. **Bexarotene**
 1. Bexarotene is a synthetic oral and topical rexinoid with selectivity for the retinoid X-receptor.

2. It is used in the treatment of cutaneous T-cell lymphoma, Kaposi sarcoma, and breast and lung cancers. It has also been used to treat psoriasis.

3. Its major adverse effects are hyperlipidemias, both hypertriglyceridemia and hyper-cholesterolemia. Other serious adverse effects include acute pancreatitis and hepatic dysfunction.

▉ DRUG SUMMARY TABLE

Hypothalamic/Pituitary Agents
Octreotide (Sandostatin)
Gonadorelin (Factrel, Leutrepulse)
Nafarelin acetate (Synarel)
Triptorelin (Trelstar Depot)
Goserelin (Zoladex)
Leuprolide acetate (Lupron, Eligard)
Histrelin (Vantas)
Cetrorelix (Cetrotide)
Ganirelix (Antagon)
Abarelix (Plenax)
Bromocriptine (Parlodel)
Cabergoline (Dostinex)
Pergolide (Permax)
Corticorelin (Acthrel)
Somatotropin, rhGH, (Humatrope, others)
Somatrem (Protropin)
Pegvisomant (Somavert)
Thyrotropin α (Thyrogen)
Corticotrophin, ACTH (H.P. Acthar)
Cosyntropin (Cortrosyn)
Oxytocin (Pitocin, Syntocinon)
Vasopressin (Pitressin)
Desmopressin acetate (DDAVP, Stimate)
Conivaptan (Vaprisol)
Tolvaptan ((Samsca)

Gonadotropins
Menotropins (Pergonal, Repronex)
Urofollitropin (Bravelle)
hCG (Pregnyl, Novarel, others)
Follitropin α (Gonal F)
Follitropin β (Puregon, Follistim)

Estrogens
17β-estradiol (generic)
Estrone (Primestrin, Estra AQ)
Equilin (Premarin)
Ethinyl estradiol (Estinyl, Feminone, others)
Mestranol
Diethylstilbestrol (Stilphostrol)
Dienestrol (DV, Estraguard)

Anti-Estrogens
Clomiphene (Clomid, Milophene, Serophene)
Fulvestrant (Faslodex)
Danazol (Danocrine)

SERMs
Tamoxifen (Novaldex, generic)
Raloxifene (Evista)
Toremifene (Fareston)

Regular (Humulin R, Novilin-R, others)
Lente (Humulin L, Novilin-L)
Isophane (Humulin N, Novilin-N
Insulin Glargine (Lantus)
Insulin Detemir (Levemir)
Ultralente (Humulin U)
Protamine-zinc (Humalog Mix 75/25, others)

Oral Hypoglycemics
Sulfonylureas
Tolbutamide (Orinase, Tol-Tab, generic)
Acetohexamide (Dymelor, generic)
Tolazamide (Tolinase, generic)
Glipizide (Glucotrol, generic)
Glyburide (Dibeta, Micronase, generic)
Glimepiride (Amaryl, generic)
Chlorpropamide (Diabinase, generic)

Biguanines
Metformin (Fotamet, generic)

Meglitinides
Repaglinide (Prandin)
Nateglinide (Starlix)

α-Glucosidase Inhibitors
Acarbose (Precose)
Miglitol (Glyset)

Thiazolidinediones
Pioglitazone (Actes)
Rosaglitazone (Avandia)
Incretins
Exenatide (Byetta)
Glucagon (Glucagen, generic)

DPP-IV Inhibitors
Sitagliptin (Januvia)
Saxagliptin (Onglyza)
Linagliptin (Tradjenta)

Aromatase Inhibitors
Exemestane (Aromasin)
Anastrazole (Arimidex)
Letrozole (Femara)

Progestins
Hydroxyprogesterone caproate (Delalu-tin, others)
Megestrol (Megace)
medroxyprogesterone acetate (Amen, Provera, others)
Norethindrone (Norlutin, Micronor, others)

Nandrolone (Hybolin, Deca-Durabolin)
Oxandrolone (Oxandrine)

Anti-Androgens
Flutamide (Eulexin)
Bicalutamide (Casodex)
Nilutamide (Niladron)
Finasteride (Proscar)
Dutasteride (Avodart)
Ketoconazole (Nizoral)
Spironolactone (Aldactone)

Corticosteroids
Cortisol (hydrocortisone) (generic)
Cortisone (Cortone)
Prednisone (Deltason, Predone, others)
Prednisolone (Prelone, generic)
Dexamethasone (Decadron, Corta-stat, others)
Betamethasone (Betastat)
Triamcinolone (Triamcot, others)
Aldosterone
Fludrocortisone (Florenif)
Clobetasol (Clobevate, Clovex, others)
Halobetasol (Ultravate)
Amcinonide (Cyclocort, generic)
Fluocinonide (Lidex, Vanos)
Beclomethasone (Beconase, Qvar)
Fluticasone (Cutivate, Flonase)
Desonide (Desowen, LoKara)

Adrenocortical Antagonists
Mitotane (Lysodren)
Aminoglutethimide (Cytadren)
Metyrapone (Metopirone)

Agents Affecting Ca²⁺ Homeostasis
Teriparatide (Forteo)
Calcitonin (salmon) (Fortical, Miacalcin)
Denosumab (Prolia, Xgeva)
Ergocalciferol (Calciferol, Ergo G, generic)
Calcifediol (Calderol)
Dihydrotachysterol (DHT)
Calcitriol (Rocaltrol, Calcijex, generic)
Calcipotriene (Dovonex)
Doxercalciferol (Hectorol)
Alfacalcidol (One-Alpha)
Paricalcitol (Zemplar)
Maxacalcitol (Oxarol)

Bisphosphonates
Etidronate disodium (Didronel)
Alendronate (Fosamax)
Ibandronate (Boniva)

Thyroid Hormones
Thyroid USP (Armour Thyroid, Dathroid)
Liotrix (Thyrolar)
Liothyronine sodium (Cytomel)
Levothyroxine sodium (Levothroid,
    Synthroid, others)

Antithyroid Preparations
Methimazole (Tapazole)
Propylthiouracil (PTU)
Iodine (Lugol's Solution)
Sodium Iodide (I^{131}) (Iodotope,
    Megatope)

Insulin Preparations
Insulin glulisine (Apidra)
Insulin aspart (NovoLog)
Insulin lispro (Humalog)

Norgestrel (Ovrette)
Norgestimate
Levonorgestrel (Mirena, Plan B)

Anti-Progestins
Mifepristone (RU-486) (Mifeprex)

Androgens
Testosterone (generic, Testoderm)
Testosterone propionate (Testex)
Testosterone enanthate (Andryl, Dela-
    testryl, others)
Testosterone cypionate (Depo-
    Testosterone)
Methyltestosterone (Metandren,
    Android, others)
Fluoxymesterone (Halotestin, others)
Oxymetholone (Anadrol, Anapolon)

Pamidronate (Aredia)
Risedronate (Actonel)
Zoldronic acid (Zolmeta)
Tiludronate (Skelid)

Calcimimetics
Cinacalcet (Sensipar)

Retinoids
Tretinoin (Retin A, Renova, ATRA)
Isotretinoin (Accutane)
Acitretin (Soriatane)
Alitretinoin (Panretin)
Tazarotene (Avage)
Adapalene (Differin)

Rexinoids
Bexarotene (Targretin)

Review Test

Directions: Each of the numbered items or incomplete statements in this section is followed by answers or by completions of the statement. Select the ONE lettered answer or completion that is BEST in each case.

1. A 49-year-old woman complains of sweating profusely nearly every night. She had a transvaginal hysterectomy 5 years ago but has intact ovaries. Upon physical examination, you note that she has a BMI of 22, but all her vital signs are normal. Which of the following would best treat her condition?

(A) Conjugated estrogens
(B) Levonorgestrel
(C) Raloxifene
(D) Calcitriol

2. A patient who has recently undergone a kidney transplant is immunosuppressed with dexamethasone and sirolimus. He is involved in a serious car accident. Besides the necessary treatment of the trauma, which of the following actions would be necessary?

(A) Begin low-dose fludrocortisone therapy
(B) Increase the dose of dexamethasone
(C) Discontinue use of sacrolimus
(D) Begin treatment with methyltestosterone

3. A male patient is diagnosed with a large, benign prostatic mass, and he has the urge to urinate frequently. He is begun on leuprolide acetate therapy. He returns to your office 3 days later complaining that his urge to urinate has increased, not decreased. What accounts for this action?

(A) Direct effect of leuprolide on the prostate
(B) Reduction of the conversion of testosterone to dihydrotachysterol (DHT)
(C) Transient agonist action ("flare") of leuprolide causing a temporary increase in androgen production
(D) Prostatic resistance to leuprolide

4. A 16-year-old female patient enters your dermatology clinic complaining of a rash. She is not taking any medications and is well dressed and groomed. You diagnose a mild case of acne vulgaris and notice that the girl's skin and hair appear unusually oily. Which of the following would be the best treatment for the acne?

(A) Calcipotriene
(B) Topical dexamethasone
(C) Isotretinoin
(D) Bexarotene

5. A 36-year-old woman complains of hot flashes, feelings of weakness, and increased appetite. You observe that she is tachycardic and has a prominent pulse pressure. Results of a test for anti-TSH antibodies are positive. Which of the following would be the most appropriate treatment for this patient?

(A) Methimazole
(B) Liotrix
(C) Thyrotropin α
(D) Ketoconazole

6. A 45-year-old female patient has fasting glucose levels of 147 mg/dL, and with a glucose tolerance test, you have confirmed the diagnosis of type II diabetes. You begin therapy with metformin, but her fasting glucose levels remain above 100 mg/dL. You elect to change her therapy to glyburide. This drug acts to

(A) Increase insulin secretion
(B) Decrease glucocorticoid levels
(C) Decrease tissue sensitivity to insulin
(D) Decrease insulin half-life

7. A 55-year-old woman complains of worsening pain in her back that is not alleviated by NSAIDs. You suspect a bone-related condition and order a series of x-rays and a magnetic resonance image of the spine. These studies indicate an advanced case of osteosarcoma. You admit the patient, and later that evening she becomes unresponsive and moribund. Her electrolytes are normal except for Ca^{2+}, which is elevated at 4.2 mM. Which of the following would be most appropriate choice for treating this condition?

(A) Furosemide
(B) Thiazides
(C) Vitamin D
(D) Parathyroid hormone

8. A cab driver with a 10-year history of alcoholism presents with ictarus and yellow sclera; serum bilirubin levels are elevated and liver function tests are all abnormal. In addition, his serum calcium at 2.0 mM is abnormally low. You elect to use a vitamin D derivative to correct his calcium level. Which of the following would be most appropriate for his patient?

(A) Ergosterol
(B) Dihydrotachysterol
(C) Calcitriol
(D) Cholecalciferol

9. A 59-year-old female nurse practitioner with a BMI of 30 and who has been diagnosed with type 2 diabetes is admitted to the emergency room. She is tachycardic, tachypneic, and appears very disoriented; she does not remember the day of the week or her address or any emergency contact numbers. She vaguely remembers taking her "sugar medicine" earlier in the day. Which of the following drugs is most likely responsible for her condition?

(A) Metformin
(B) Acarbose
(C) Glipizide
(D) Glucagon

10. A 60-year-old male with type II diabetes is taking glyburide for his disease but is not maintaining adequate glycemic control with an HbA1c level of 7.3%. You elect to add rosiglitazone to his medications. This drug acts to

(A) Increase insulin sensitivity in adipose and muscle
(B) Increase insulin secretion from β-cells
(C) Decrease somatostatin release from δ-cells
(D) Decrease glucose absorption in the small intestine

Answers and Explanations

1. **The answer is A.** Vasomotor symptoms are the most common complaint of perimeno-pausal women. Estrogen is the only effective treatment of these symptoms. Since there is no concern of endometrial cancer, a progestin is not indicated. Raloxifene makes hot flashes worse; and while a vitamin D analog might help maintain Ca^{2+}, it would not have any effect on the vasomotor symptoms.

2. **The answer is B.** Patients taking glucocorticoids long term have suppressed pituitary-adrenal function and do not respond to trauma with increased cortisol biosynthesis. It is necessary to increase the dose of glucocorticoid in this circumstance. A mineralocorticoid would not be beneficial.

3. **The answer is C.** Leuprolide and the other GnRH agonists typically cause a transient increase in gonadal steroid production before down-regulation of receptors occurs. This is called a "flare."

4. **The answer is C.** Isotretinoin is a retinoid that is especially useful in treating acne; it reduces oil production in the skin. Calcipotriene is used to treat psoriasis. Bexarotene is a rexinoid used to treat skin disorders, but not acne.

5. **The answer is B.** The patient has hyperthyroidism due to activating anti-TSH antibodies. Methimazole blocks the initial oxidation of iodine as well as the coupling of monoiodoty-rosine and diiodotyrosine into the mature T_4. Liotrix is a thyroid hormone preparation and would be contraindicated. Ketoconazole inhibits a number of P-450-catalyzed reactions but not the production of thyroid hormone.

6. **The answer is A.** Sulfonylureas such as glyburide increase the release of insulin from the pancreas. They also may cause an increase in insulin receptors, which increases tissue sensitivity to insulin. They do not slow insulin clearance, and they do not decrease gluco-corticoid levels.

7. **The answer is A.** Thiazides and loop diuretics have opposite effects on Ca^{2+} excretion; loop diuretics such as furosemide increase Ca^{2+} excretion and hence reduce hypercalcemia. Vitamin D and parathyroid hormone both increase serum Ca^{2+}.

8. **The answer is C.** Calcitriol would be the most effective agent for hypocalcemia in a patient with impaired liver function. The liver provides the required 25-hydroxylation of dihydro-tachysterol, cholecalciferol, and ergosterol.

9. **The answer is C.** Any of the sulfonylureas can cause hypoglycemia which can produce shock-like symptoms. Metformin and the α-glycosidase inhibitors such as acarbose rarely cause hypoglycemia. Glucagon would raise plasma glucose.

10. **The answer is A.** The major mechanism of action of thiazolidinediones is increasing sensitivity to insulin in adipose, skeletal muscle, and liver. Several classes of hypoglycemic drugs act to increase insulin release from the pancreas including the sulfonylureas, incre-tins, and DPP-IV antagonists. The α-glucosidase inhibitors inhibit intestinal hydrolysis of complex saccharides and thereby reduce glucose absorption.

chapter 11

Drugs Used in Treatment of Infectious Diseases

I. INFECTIOUS DISEASE THERAPY

Infectious disease therapy is based on the principle of selective toxicity: Destroy the infecting organism without damage to the host by exploiting basic biochemical and physical differences between the two organisms.

A. Choice of Appropriate Antibacterial Agent
1. The drug of choice is usually the most active drug against the pathogen or the least toxic of several alternative drugs.
2. An antibacterial agent is often used prophylactically against single microorganisms (e.g., to prevent endocarditis in patients undergoing procedures that lead to bacteremia, such as dental work).
3. The choice of drug depends on the effectiveness of host defense mechanisms in controlling the infection. The drug selected for use may be either a **bactericidal** agent (causing the death of the microorganism) or a **bacteriostatic** agent (temporarily inhibiting the growth of the microorganism).
4. Drug choice is related to the mechanism of drug action in one of the following general categories:
   a. Inhibits bacterial cell wall biosynthesis
   b. Inhibits bacterial protein synthesis
   c. Inhibits bacterial metabolism
   d. Inhibits bacterial nucleic acid synthesis

B. Host determinants include history of drug reactions; site of infection; renal, hepatic, and immune status; age; pregnancy and lactation; metabolic abnormalities; pharmacokinetic factors; preexisting organ dysfunction; and genetic factors.

C. Bacterial determinants include **intrinsic resistance**, escape from antibiotic effect, and **acquired resistance**, which can occur as a result of the following:
1. *Spontaneous, random chromosomal mutations,* which occur at a frequency of 10^{-2} to 10^{-5}. These mutations are commonly due to a change in either a structural protein receptor for an antibiotic or a protein involved in drug transport.
2. Extrachromosomal transfer of drug-resistant genes
   a. **Transformation** is transfer of naked DNA between cells of the same species.
   b. **Transduction via R plasmids** is asexual transfer of plasmid DNA in a bacterial virus between bacteria of the same species.
   c. **Conjugation** is the passage of genes from bacteria to bacteria via direct contact through a sex pilus or bridge. Conjugation occurs primarily in gram-negative bacilli, and it is the principal mechanism of acquired resistance among enterobacteria.
   d. **Transpositions** occur as a result of movement or "jumping" of **transposons** (stretches of DNA containing insertion sequences at each end) from plasmid to plasmid or from plasmid to chromosome and back; this process is independent of bacterial recombination.

II. ANTIBACTERIALS

A. **Inhibitors of Bacterial Cell Wall Biosynthesis**
 1. *Penicillins*
  a. **Structure and mechanism of action** (Fig. 11.1).
   (1) Penicillins have a β-**lactam ring** the integrity of which is required for antibacterial activity. Modifications of the R-group side-chain (attached to the β-lactam ring) alter the pharmacologic properties and resistance to β-lactamase.
   (2) Penicillins **inactivate bacterial transpeptidases** and prevent the cross-linking of peptidoglycan polymers that is essential for bacterial cell wall integrity. This results in **loss of rigidity and a susceptibility to rupture.** Penicillins also bind to, and **inactivate, penicillin-binding proteins (PBPs)** involved in cell wall synthesis. The action of autolysin in the presence of penicillin further weakens the cell wall.
   (3) Penicillins are **bactericidal** for growing cells. **Gram-positive bacteria** with thick external cell walls are particularly susceptible.
   (4) The major cause of **resistance** is the production of β-lactamases (penicillinases). The genes for β-lactamases can be transmitted during conjugation or as small

Penicillin nucleus

Cephalosporin nucleus

Clavulanic acid

FIGURE 11.1. Structures of penicillin, cephalosporin, and clavulanic acid nuclei. *Arrows* indicate bond attacked by β-lactamases.

plasmids (minus conjugation genes) via transduction. Common organisms capable of producing penicillinase include *Staphylococcus aureus, Escherichia coli, Pseudomonas aeruginosa, Neisseria gonorrhoeae,* and *Bacillus, Proteus,* and *Bacteroides* species.

(5) Resistance may also occur because bacteria lack receptors or other PBPs, are impermeable to penicillins, lack cell walls, or are metabolically inactive.

b. Pharmacologic properties

(1) Penicillins are absorbed rapidly after enteral administration, although erratically, and parenteral administration, and are distributed throughout body fluids; they penetrate the cerebrospinal fluid (CSF) and ocular fluid to a significant extent only during inflammation.

(2) Gastrointestinal (GI) absorption of penicillins may be decreased in the presence of food.

c. Selected drugs and their therapeutic uses (Table 11.1)

(1) **Penicillin G** is mainly used to treat infections with the following organisms (resistant strains of bacteria are being isolated more frequently):

(a) **Gram-positive cocci** (aerobic): Pneumococci, streptococci (except *S. faecalis*), and non-penicillinase-producing staphylococci.

(b) **Gram-positive rods** (aerobic): *Bacillus* species, also *Clostridium perfringens, C. diphtheriae,* and *Listeria* spp., although the use of these agents is declining due to the availability of better drugs.

(c) **Gram-negative aerobes:** Gonococci (non-penicillinase-producing) and meningococci

(d) **Gram-negative rods** (aerobic): None

(e) **Anaerobes:** Most, except *Bacteroides fragilis.* This agent is used against oral anaerobes.

(f) **Other:** *Treponema pallidum* (syphilis) and *Leptospira* spp. These are common pathogens for which first-generation penicillins are used today.

(2) **Penicillin V**, an oral form of penicillin G with poor bioavailability, has a narrower spectrum of activity.

t a b l e 11.1 Spectrum of Activity of Penicillins

Classification and Drugs	Gram-positive Cocci	Gram-positive Rods	Gram-negative Cocci	Gram-negative Rods	Anaerobes
Prototype Penicillin G, penicillin V	**Most**	*Bacillus*	Gonococci and meningococci[a]	None	Most (except *B. fragilis*)
Penicillinase resistant Nafcillin, oxacillin, dicloxacillin	**Staphylococci**[b]	—	—	—	—
Extended spectrum Ampicillin, amoxicillin, ampicillin/ sulbactam, amoxicillin/clavulanic acid	Most penicillinase-producing staphylococci[b]	*Bacillus*	Gonococci and meningococci[c]	*Salmonella, H. influenzae, Protons,* and *enterococci*	—
Antipseudomonal Ticarcillin/clavulanic acid, piperacillin	Less potent than prototypes	Less potent than prototypes	Less potent than prototypes	*Proteus, E. coli Salmonella, Pseudomonas, Enterobacter,* and *Klebsiella*	—

[a]Non-penicillinase-producing.
[b]Not effective against methicillin-resistant staphylococcal infections.
[c]Penicillinase producing.

(3) **Penicillin G benzathine and Penicillin G procaine** are suspensions of penicillin G that prolong its half-life (30 min) allowing a reduced frequency of injections. **Probenecid,** a uricosuric agent that blocks renal secretion of penicillin, is used for this purpose, but only rarely.

(4) **Penicillinase-resistant penicillins** (**oxacillin, dicloxacillin, methicillin,** and **nafcillin**) are used predominantly for penicillinase-producing **staphylococcal infections.** The use of these agents, which are administered orally, is declining due to the increased incidence of **methicillin-resistant S. aureus (MRSA)** that also confers resistance to cephalosporins.

(5) **Extended-spectrum penicillins**

(a) Extended-spectrum penicillins are inactivated by β-lactamases.

(b) These agents have a broadened **gram-negative** coverage. Resistance has become a more common problem.

(i) **Ampicillin.** Ampicillin is useful for infections caused by *Haemophilus influenzae, Streptococcus pneumonia, Streptococcus pyrogenes, Neisseria meningitidis, Proteus mirabilis,* and *Enterococcus faecalis.*

(ii) **Amoxicillin** (Amoxil) is similar to **ampicillin,** but has **better oral absorption.** Amoxicillin is commonly used for endocarditis prophylaxis before major procedures.

(iii) **Piperacillin** has good activity against *Pseudomonas* spp. and *Enterobacter* spp.

(6) **Clavulanic acid**

(a) Clavulanic acid is structurally related to **penicillin** (see Fig. 11.1), but has **no antimicrobial properties** of its own.

(b) Clavulanic acid **irreversibly inhibits β-lactamase;** when administered with penicillins, clavulanic acid exposes penicillinase-producing organisms to therapeutic concentrations of penicillin.

(c) Clavulanic acid is used in combination products **amoxicillin/clavulanic acid** (Augmentin) and **ticarcillin/clavulanic acid** (Timentin) for oral and parenteral administration, respectively.

(7) **Sulbactam, tazobactam**

(a) These agents are **β-lactamase inhibitors** structurally related to **penicillin.**

(b) Sulbactam is marketed in the combination product **ampicillin/sulbactam** (Unasyn). **Tazobactam** is used in combination with **piperacillin** under the name Zosyn.

(c) **Ampicillin/sulbactam** is used parenterally and provides coverage similar to that provided by amoxicillin/clavulanic acid. It is most commonly used for **gram-negative** bacteria as well as most **anaerobes. Piperacillin/tazobactam** is effective against most **gram-negative** organisms, including ***Pseudomonas*** spp.

d. **Adverse effects**

(1) Penicillins cause **hypersensitivity** reactions in nearly 10% of the patients. All types of reactions, from a simple rash to anaphylaxis, can be observed within 2 minutes or up to 3 days following administration.

(2) Other adverse effects result from direct irritation or pain on injection, GI upset, or superinfection.

e. **Endocarditis prophylaxis**

(1) Endocarditis prophylaxis is indicated for patients with **prosthetic heart valves;** those who have **previously been diagnosed with endocarditis;** patients **born with cyanotic heart disease;** and **patients with surgically constructed systemic pulmonary shunts.** Patients with intermediate risk for endocarditis are those who were born with other congenital cardiac abnormalities; those with acquired valvular dysfunction; and patients with hypertrophic cardiomyopathy.

(2) Endocarditis prophylaxis is recommended for the above patients who are planning to undergo **major dental procedures; procedures involving the respiratory tract,** such as bronchoscopy and tonsillectomy; and **operations and procedures involving the GI and genitourinary tracts.**

(3) Agents most commonly used for endocarditis prophylaxis are **amoxicillin or ampicillin.** Those who are allergic to penicillins can take **clindamycin or azithromycin.**

table **11.2** Properties of Cephalosporins

Drugs and Route of Administration[a]	Spectrum of Activity	Enters CNS	Resistance to β-Lactamase	
			Plasmid	*Chromosomal*
First generation				
Cephalexin (O)	Gram-positive and some gram-negative organisms	No	Yes	No
Cefadroxil (O)				
Cefazolin (P)	Use: *Escherichia coli, Klebsiella, Proteus mirabilis,* penicillin- and sulfonamide-resistant **UTI, surgical prophylaxis**			
Second generation				
Cefaclor (O)	Spectrum extends to indole-positive **Proteus,** and **anaerobes**	No	Yes	Relatively
Cefotetan (P)				
Cefoxitin (P)	Use: **UTI, respiratory tract infections, surgical prophylaxis**			
Cefuroxime (P,D)				
Third and fourth generation				
Ceftizoxime (P)	Reduced gram-positive activity; **Pseudomonas** (cefoperazone and ceftazidime only), *N. gonorrhoeae, N. meningitidis, H. influenza, Enterobacter, Salmonella,* indole-positive *Proteus, Serratia, E. coli;* moderate **anaerobe** activity	Yes, especially ceftriaxone (but not cefoperazone)	Yes	Relatively (most)
Cefotaxime (P)				
Ceftriaxone (P)				
Cefdinir (P)				
Ceftazidime (P)				
Cefixime (O)	Use: Serious **nosocomial infections, gonorrhea, meningitis**			
Cefepime (P)				
Other agents				
Aztreonam	**Gram-negative** organisms (no cross-sensitivity)	Yes	Yes	Yes
Imipenem/cilastatin	Use: **Broad-spectrum**			

[a]O, oral administration; P, parenteral administration.

2. *Cephalosporins* (Table 11.2)
   a. **Structure and mechanism of action**
      (1) Cephalosporins also have a β-lactam ring (see Fig. 11.1). Substitutions at R_1 determine antibacterial activity. Substitutions at R_2 determine pharmacokinetics.
      (2) Cephalosporins have the same mechanisms of action as penicillins.
   b. **Pharmacologic properties**
      (1) Cephalosporins are widely distributed in body fluids; selected agents (**cefuroxime** [Ceftin, Zinacef], **cefotaxime** [Claforan], and **ceftizoxime** [Cefizox]) penetrate CSF.
      (2) **Probenecid** slows the secretion of cephalosporins.
      (3) Each newer generation of cephalosporins is increasingly **resistant to penicillinases.** Third-generation cephalosporins are sensitive to another class of β-lactamase, the **cephalosporinases** (genes are generally located on chromosomes as opposed to plasmids).
   c. **Selected drugs and their therapeutic uses.** Cephalosporins are categorized by their antibacterial spectrum. All are inactive against enterococci and methicillin-resistant staphylococci.
      (1) **First-generation cephalosporins**
         (a) First-generation cephalosporins include **cephalexin** (Keflex), **cefazolin** (Ancef, Kefzol), and **cefadroxil** (Duricef).
         (b) These agents have good activity against **some gram-positive organisms** (streptococci) **and some gram-negative** organisms. First-generation cephalosporins are used mainly for *E. coil, Klebsiella* infections, and penicillin- and sulfonamide-resistant **urinary tract infections.** They are also used **prophylactically in various surgical procedures.**
         (c) These agents **do not penetrate CSF.**

    (2) Second-generation cephalosporins

      (a) Second-generation cephalosporins include **cefoxitin** (Mefoxin), **cefaclor** (Ceclor), **cefuroxime** (Zinacef, Ceftin), **cefotetan** (Cefotan), and **cefprozil** (Cefzil).

      (b) These agents have a somewhat broader spectrum of activity than first-generation drugs. They are used in the treatment of **streptococcal** infections as well as infections caused by *E. coli, Klebsiella,* and *Proteus* spp. Most **anaerobes** (with exception of *Clostridium difficile*) are covered as well.

      (c) Second-generation cephalosporins are used primarily in the management of **urinary and respiratory tract, bone, and soft-tissue infections** and prophylactically in various **surgical procedures.**

      (d) Second-generation agents have, to a great extent, been supplanted by third-generation agents.

      (e) With the exception of cefuroxime, these agents do not penetrate the CSF.

    (3) Third-generation cephalosporins

      (a) Third-generation cephalosporins include **cefdinir** (Omnicef), **cefixime** (Suprax), **cefotaxime** (Clarofan), **ceftizoxime** (Cefizox), **ceftazidime** (Fortaz, Tazicef), and **ceftriaxone** (Rocephin).

      (b) These agents have **enhanced activity against gram-negative** organisms. They demonstrate high potency against *H. influenzae, N. gonorrhoeae, N. meningitides, Enterobacter, Salmonella,* indole-positive *Proteus,* and *Serratia* spp., and *E. coli;* and **moderate activity against anaerobes. Cefoperazone** and **ceftazidime** have excellent activity against *P. aeruginosa.* **Ceftriaxone** is used for sexually transmitted infections caused by **gonorrhea,** as well as in empiric therapy for community-acquired **meningitis.**

      (c) With the exception of cefoperazone, third-generation cephalosporins **penetrate the CSF.**

      (d) These agents are excreted by the kidney, except **cefoperazone** and **ceftriaxone,** which are excreted through the biliary tract, thus enabling the use of these agents for **infections of the biliary tree.**

      (e) Third-generation cephalosporins are used to treat gonorrhea, Lyme disease, meningitis, and serious **hospital-acquired gram-negative infections,** alone or in combination with an aminoglycoside.

    (4) Fourth-generation cephalosporins.

      (a) Cefepime (Maxipime) has a powerful coverage against *Pseudomonas* spp., as well as other **gram-negative** bacteria.

      (b) Ceftaroline fosamil (Teflaro) is a prodrug that is active against methicillin-resistant staphylococci used to treat skin infections and community-acquired pneumonia. It has limited activity against β-lactamase producing bacteria.

  d. Adverse effects and drug interactions

    (1) Cephalosporins most commonly cause **hypersensitivity reactions** (2–5%); 5%–10% of penicillin-sensitive persons are also hypersensitive to cephalosporins.

    (2) Alcohol intolerance (**disulfiram-like**) is seen with **cefamandole and ceftriaxone.**

    (3) Cephalosporins may cause **bleeding disorders;** these disorders can be prevented by vitamin K administration.

    (4) Cephalosporins may be **nephrotoxic** when administered with diuretics.

    (5) These agents may cause **superinfection with gram-positive organisms or fungi.** Cephalosporins are the number one cause of **hospital-acquired *C. difficile* colitis,** a potentially life-threatening infection.

3. *Other Beta-lactam drugs*

  a. Aztreonam (Azactam)

    (1) Aztreonam is a naturally occurring monobactam lacking the thiazolidine ring that is **highly resistant to β-lactamases.**

    (2) Aztreonam has **good activity against gram-negative** organisms, but it lacks activity against anaerobes and gram-positive organisms.

    (3) This agent demonstrates **no cross-reactivity with penicillins or cephalosporins** for hypersensitivity reactions.

(4) Aztreonam is administered parenterally.

(5) Aztreonam is useful for various types of infections caused by *E. coli, Klebsiella pneumoniae, H. influenzae, P. aeruginosa, Enterobacter* spp., *Citrobacter* spp., and *P. mirabilis.*

b. Carbapenems (**imipenem-cilastatin** [Primaxin], **ertapenem** [Invanz], **meropenem** [Merrem IV], **doripenem** [Doribax])

(1) Carbapenems are relatively **resistant to β-lactamases.**

(2) Carbapenems demonstrate **no cross-resistance** with other antibiotics.

(3) Imipenem is marketed in the combination product **imipenem/cilastatin** (Primaxin); cilastatin is an inhibitor of renal dehydropeptidase I (which inactivates imipenem).

(4) These agents are useful for infections caused by **penicillinase-producing *S. aureus, E. coli, Klebsiella* spp., *Enterobacter* spp.,** and *H. influenzae,* among others. They are powerful agents used for *Pseudomonas* infections.

(5) Nausea, vomiting, diarrhea, and skin rashes, and at higher doses, seizures, are their most common adverse effects, particularly for **imipenem.**

4. *Other inhibitors of bacterial cell wall biosynthesis*

   a. Vancomycin (Vancocin, Vancoled), **telavancin** (Vibativ)

   (1) Vancomycin **binds to the terminal end of the growing peptidoglycan to prevent further elongation and cross-linking due to inhibition of transglycosylase;** this results in decreased cell membrane activity and increased cell lysis. Telavancin has actions similar to that of vancomycin, and also daptomycin (see below).

   (2) Vancomycin is active against **gram-positive organisms;** resistant strains have been reported.

   (3) Vancomycin is used in **serious MRSA infections,** in patients allergic to penicillins and cephalosporins, and to treat **antibiotic-associated enterocolitis** (*C. difficile* colitis). Telavancin is used to treat skin infections.

   (4) Vancomycin penetrates CSF only during inflammation.

   (5) Vancomycin is administered by slow intravenous (IV) infusion, except in the treatment of enterocolitis, when it is given orally.

   (6) Rapid infusion of vancomycin may cause anaphylactoid reactions and **"red neck" syndrome** (flushing caused by release of histamine).

   (7) Rarely, high levels of vancomycin may cause **ototoxicity** with permanent auditory impairment, and also nephrotoxicity.

   (8) Telavancin is potentially teratogenic.

   b. Bacitracin

   (1) Bacitracin inhibits dephosphorylation and reuse of the phospholipid required for acceptance of *N*-acetylmuramic acid pentapeptide, the building block of the peptidoglycan complex.

   (2) Bacitracin is most active against **gram-positive** bacteria.

   (3) Bacitracin is **used only topically** in combination with **neomycin or polymyxin** for minor infections (Neosporin).

   c. Cycloserine (Seromycin)

   (1) Cycloserine inhibits alanine racemase and the incorporation of alanine into the peptidoglycan pentapeptide.

   (2) Cycloserine is active against **mycobacteria and gram-negative bacteria.**

   (3) This agent is used only as a second-line drug for the treatment of urinary tract infection and tuberculosis (TB).

   (4) At high doses, cycloserine may cause severe central nervous system (CNS) toxicity, including seizures and acute psychosis.

   d. Daptomycin (Cubicin)

   (1) Daptomycin is a bactericidal agent that binds to and depolarizes the cell membrane resulting in loss of membrane potential and rapid cell death.

   (2) Daptomycin has antibacterial actions similar to that of vancomycin.

   (3) It is active against vancomycin-resistant strains.

   (4) Daptomycin may cause myopathy.

e. **Fosfomycin** (Monural)

   (1) Fosfomycin inhibits the enzyme **enolpyruvate transferase** and thereby interferes downstream with the formation of bacterial cell wall specific *N*-acetylmuramic acid.

   (2) This oral agent is active against both gram-positive and gram-negative organisms. It is used to treat simple lower **urinary tract infection**.

B. Inhibitors of Bacterial Protein Synthesis

1. ***Aminoglycosides*** (Fig. 11.2)

   a. **Structure and mechanism of action**

      (1) Aminoglycosides **inhibit bacterial protein synthesis;** they are **bacteriocidal** against most **gram-negative aerobic bacteria.**

      (2) Aminoglycosides passively diffuse via **porin channels** through the outer membrane of gram-negative aerobic bacteria. Transport across the inner membrane requires active uptake that is dependent on electron transport (**gram-negative aerobes only**), the so-called **energy dependent phase I transport.**

      (3) Inside the cell, these agents interact with receptor proteins on the **30S ribosomal subunit.** This "freezes" the initiation complex and leads to a buildup of monosomes; it also causes translation errors.

      (4) Resistance generally results from bacterial enzymes that inactivate the drugs. The resistance contained on plasmids is transmitted by conjugation.

   b. **Pharmacologic properties.** These agents do not penetrate the CSF.

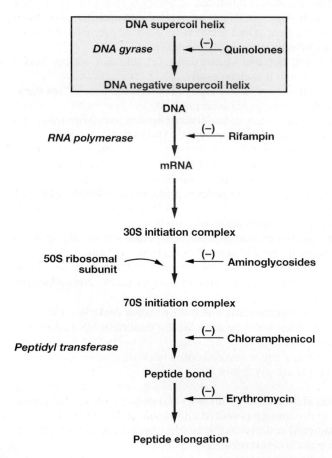

FIGURE 11.2. Antimicrobial action on bacterial nucleic acid and protein synthesis.

c. **Selected drugs and their therapeutic uses**
  (1) The role for aminoglycosides has decreased substantially due to their **narrow spectrum of activity and toxicity,** and the availability of other agents.
  (2) **Streptomycin** is currently used only for **plague** *(Yersinia pestis),* for **severe cases of brucellosis,** and as an adjunct to the treatment of recalcitrant **mycobacterial infections.**
  (3) **Gentamicin** (Garamycin), **tobramycin** (Nebcin)
    (a) Gentamicin and tobramycin are active against *Enterobacter,* **indole-positive** *Proteus, Pseudomonas, Klebsiella,* **and** *Serratia* spp., among other gram-negative organisms.
    (b) These agents are often **used synergistically in combination with** β-lactam **antibiotics or vancomycin** for serious infections that require broad coverage.
  (4) **Amikacin** (Amikin) is used in the treatment of **severe gram-negative infections,** especially those resistant to gentamicin or tobramycin.
  (5) **Neomycin** (Mycifradin) **and kanamycin** (Kantrex, Klebcil) are **administered topically for minor soft-tissue infections** (often in combination with **bacitracin** and **polymyxin)** or orally (neomycin) for **hepatic encephalopathy** (GI bacteria by-products result in large amounts of ammonia, which is normally cleared by liver; use of neomycin temporarily inactivates the intestinal flora).
  (6) **Spectinomycin** (Tobicin) is structurally related to aminoglycosides and is administered intramuscularly as an **alternative for the treatment of acute gonorrhea** or in patients hypersensitive to penicillin or for gonococci resistant to penicillin.

d. **Adverse effects**
  (1) Aminoglycosides have a **narrow therapeutic index;** it may be necessary to monitor serum concentrations and individualize the dose.
  (2) Aminoglycosides are ototoxic, affecting either vestibular (**streptomycin, gentamicin,** and **tobramycin**) or cochlear auditory (**neomycin, kanamycin, amikacin** [Amikin], **gentamicin,** and **tobramycin**) function.
  (3) Aminoglycosides, particularly **gentamycin, neomycin, and tobramycin,** are **nephrotoxic;** they produce acute tubular necrosis that leads to a reduction in the glomerular filtration rate and a rise in serum creatinine and blood urea nitrogen. Damage is usually reversible.
  (4) At high doses, these agents produce a curare-like neuromuscular blockade with respiratory paralysis. Calcium gluconate and neostigmine are antidotes.
  (5) Aminoglycosides rarely cause hypersensitivity reactions, except **spectinomycin** and **neomycin,** which, when applied topically, can cause contact dermatitis in as many as 8% of the patients.

2. *Tetracyclines (tetracycline [Sumycin],* **oxytetracycline** *[Terramycin],* **demeclocycline** *[Declomycin],* **doxycycline** *[Vibramycin],* **minocycline** *[Minocin],* **tigecycline** *[Tygacil])*
  a. **Structure and mechanism of action**
    (1) Tetracyclines are derivatives of naphthacene carboxamide.
    (2) Tetracyclines bind reversibly to the **30S subunit** of bacterial ribosomes. This prevents the binding of aminoacyl tRNA to the acceptor site on the mRNA–ribosome complex and addition of amino acids to the growing peptide, thus **inhibiting bacterial protein synthesis;** these agents are **bacteriostatic.**
    (3) Resistance is plasmid-mediated and results primarily from a decreased ability to accumulate in the bacteria and from the production of an inhibitor of the binding site for tetracyclines. Resistance to one tetracycline confers resistance to some, but not all, congeners.
  b. **Pharmacologic properties**
    (1) Tetracyclines are variably, but adequately, absorbed from the GI tract; they can also be administered parenterally; **tigecycline,** an exception, is only administered IV. Absorption is impaired by stomach contents, especially milk and antacids.
    (2) Tetracyclines are distributed throughout body fluids; therapeutic concentrations in the brain and CSF can be achieved with minocycline.

(3) The primary route of elimination for most tetracyclines is the kidney. **Doxycycline and tigecycline do not accumulate** and hence are the **safest tetracycline** to administer to individuals **with impaired renal function.**

(4) Many tetracyclines undergo **enterohepatic recirculation.**

c. **Spectrum and therapeutic uses**

(1) Tetracyclines are active against **both gram-negative and gram-positive organisms,** but the use of these agents is declining because of increased resistance and the development of safer drugs.

(2) Tetracyclines are used predominantly for the treatment of **rickettsial infections,** including Rocky Mountain spotted fever, **cholera, Lyme disease, and infections caused by *Chlamydia* spp. and *Mycoplasma pneumoniae.*** These agents may be useful for the treatment of **inflammatory acne vulgaris.** They are also used in combination regimens for the elimination of infections caused by *Helicobacter pylori.*

(3) **Demeclocycline** is used in refractory cases of **"syndrome of inappropriate secretion of antidiuretic hormone".** It interferes with the action of ADH at the renal collecting duct by impairing the generation and action of cyclic AMP.

(4) **Tigecycline** has a broad spectrum of activity and has activity against many tetracycline-resistant organisms.

d. **Adverse effects**

(1) Tetracyclines produce GI upset, including nausea, vomiting, and diarrhea.

(2) At high doses, most tetracyclines can cause **hepatic damage,** particularly in pregnant women.

(3) When exposed to strong ultraviolet light, as in sunlight, these agents, **demeclocycline** in particular, can cause **dermatologic reactions.**

(4) Tetracyclines can complex with calcium in bone. Children aged 6 months to 5 years receiving tetracycline therapy can develop **tooth discolorations.** These agents can also **retard bone growth in neonates.**

(5) Tetracyclines can cause superinfection by resistant staphylococci or clostridia as a result of altered GI ecology; this condition can be life-threatening.

3. *Chloramphenicol*

a. **Structure and mechanism of action** (see Fig. 11.2)

(1) Chloramphenicol **inhibits bacterial protein synthesis** by binding to the bacterial **50S ribosomal subunit** to block the action of peptidyl transferase and thus prevents amino acid incorporation into newly formed peptides. High concentrations inhibit eukaryote mitochondrial protein synthesis.

(2) Resistance results from the production of a plasmid-encoded **acetyltransferase** capable of inactivating the drug.

b. **Pharmacologic properties**

(1) Chloramphenicol is absorbed rapidly and distributed throughout body fluids.

(2) Therapeutic levels can be obtained in the CSF.

(3) An inactive pro-drug, **chloramphenicol succinate,** is used for parenteral administration. On absorption, it is hydrolyzed by plasma esterases.

(4) Chloramphenicol inhibits cytochrome P-450 isozymes (CYP).

c. **Therapeutic uses**

(1) Chloramphenicol is a broad-spectrum, bacteriostatic, antibiotic that is active against most **gram-negative organisms,** many **anaerobes, clostridia, chlamydia, mycoplasma, and rickettsia.** However, because of the potential for **severe and sometimes fatal adverse effects,** use of this agent is limited to the treatment of infections that cannot be treated with other drugs; these infections include **typhoid fever** (although resistance is increasingly a problem), **meningitis** due to *H. influenzae* in patients allergic to penicillins and the newer cephalosporins, and some instances of infections caused by **ampicillin-resistant strains.**

(2) Chloramphenicol may also be used for the treatment of certain **anaerobic infections of the brain** (especially *B. fragilis*) in combination with **penicillin,** and as an alternative to **tetracycline** in the treatment of **rickettsial** disease, and topically for **infections of the eye.**

d. Adverse effects

(1) Chloramphenicol causes dose-related **bone marrow suppression,** resulting in pancytopenia that may lead to **irreversible aplastic anemia.** This effect has low incidence (1:30,000) but a **high mortality rate.** Also, chloramphenicol causes **hemolytic anemia** in patients with low levels of **glucose 6-phosphate dehydrogenase.**

(2) Chloramphenicol causes **reticulocytopenia,** perhaps as a result of the inhibition of mitochondrial protein synthesis.

(3) Neonates given large doses of chloramphenicol develop **gray baby syndrome.** This syndrome results from the inadequacy of both cytochrome P-450 and glucuronic acid conjugation systems to detoxify the drug. Elevated plasma chloramphenicol levels cause a shock-like syndrome and a reduction in peripheral circulation; the incidence of fatalities is high (40%).

(4) Chloramphenicol inhibition of cytochrome P-450 isozymes can result in elevated and toxic levels of other drugs.

4. *Erythromycin, clarithromycin (Biaxin), azithromycin (Zithromax), telithromycin (Ketek)*

a. Structure and mechanism of action (see Fig. 11.2)

(1) Erythromycin **inhibits protein synthesis** by binding irreversibly to the bacterial **50S ribosomal subunit.** It inhibits aminoacyl translocation and the formation of initiation complexes. It is usually bacteriostatic, but at higher concentrations can be bactericidal.

(2) Resistance is plasmid-encoded and is prevalent in most strains of staphylococci and, to some extent, in streptococci. It is due primarily to increased **active efflux** or **ribosomal protection** by increased methylase production.

b. Pharmacologic properties

(1) Erythromycin is inactivated by stomach acid and is therefore administered as an **enteric-coated tablet.**

(2) Erythromycin distributes into all body fluids except the brain and CSF.

c. Therapeutic uses

(1) Erythromycin is active against **gram-positive organisms.**

(2) This agent is useful as a penicillin substitute in **penicillin-hypersensitive patients.**

(3) Erythromycin is the most effective drug for **Legionnaires disease** *(Legionella pneumophila);* it is also useful for the treatment of **syphilis, *M. pneumoniae,* corynebacterial infections (e.g., diphtheria),** and *Bordetella pertussis* **disease (whooping cough).** Azithromycin is commonly used for **community-acquired "walking" pneumonia and sinusitis.**

(4) Clarithromycin or azithromycin is effective in the multidrug-regimen treatment of disseminated *Mycobacterium avium–intracellulare* **complex infections in AIDS patients.**

d. Adverse effects

(1) Erythromycin and other macrolides cause GI dysfunction (clarithromycin less so) but rarely produce serious adverse effects; the oral form of erythromycin may cause **allergic cholestatic hepatitis,** which is readily reversible by cessation of the drug.

(2) Erythromycin has a high incidence of **thrombophlebitis** when administered IV.

(3) Erythromycin and clarithromycin inhibit hepatic **cytochrome P-450–mediated metabolism** of **warfarin, phenytoin,** and others, possibly leading to toxic accumulation. Azithromycin is devoid of this action.

5. *Clindamycin (Cleocin)*

a. Clindamycin acts similar to erythromycin.

b. Clindamycin can be administered orally and is well distributed throughout body fluids, except for the CNS.

c. Use of clindamycin is limited to alternative therapy for abscesses associated with infections caused by anaerobes, such as *B. fragilis.* It is used in dental patients with valvular heart disease for **prophylaxis of endocarditis.** Topical preparations of the drug are used for the treatment of acne.

d. Clindamycin produces **diarrhea,** which is observed in up to 20% of individuals. Potential severe **pseudomembranous colitis** occurs as a result of superinfection by resistant clostridia.

C. Inhibitors of Bacterial Metabolism

1.   *Sulfonamides: sulfisoxazole, sulfacetamide, sulfadiazine, silver sulfadiazine* (Silvadene), *sulfasalazine* (Azulfidine), *mafenide* (Sulfamylon), *pyrimethamine* (Daraprim), *pyrimethamine/sulfadoxine* (Fansidar), *trimethoprim* (Proloprim), *and trimethoprim/sulfamethoxazole* (Bactrim)

   a.   Structure and mechanism of action (Fig. 11.3)

   (1) Sulfonamides are structural analogs of *para*-aminobenzoic acid (PABA). As such, they compete with endogenous bacterial PABA to **inhibit the activity of dihydropteroate synthase** and prevent the synthesis of **dihydrofolic acid** that is essential for the production of nucleic acid (purines and pyrimidines) and amino acids, and thus bacterial growth. Sulfonamides are **bacteriostatic.**

   (2) The sulfonamides are infrequently used as monotherapy due to the development of resistant strains of bacteria. However, **sulfadoxine** and **sulfamethoxazole** in combination respectively with **pyrimethamine** and **trimethoprim**, agents which inhibit downstream **dihydrofolate reductase** (Fig. 11.3), result in synergistic inhibitory **bactericidal** activity that is clinically useful.

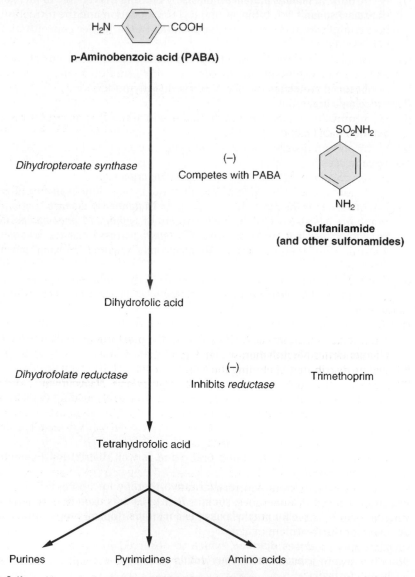

FIGURE 11.3. Sulfonamides and trimethoprim inhibition of tetrahydrofolic acid synthesis.

b. **Pharmacologic properties.** Most sulfonamides are well absorbed from the GI tract and readily penetrate the CSF.

c. **Spectrum and therapeutic uses**

(1) Sulfonamides inhibit both **gram-negative and gram-positive** organisms. They are used in combination with trimethoprim or pyrimethamine to treat **urinary tract infections (*E. coli*), nocardiosis (*Actinomyces* spp.),** and **toxoplasmosis** and as bacterial prophylaxis for **recurrent otitis media.**

(2) Trimethoprim alone, or in combination with sulfamethazole (Bactrim), is used to treat **uncomplicated urinary tract infections,** especially those associated with the use of indwelling catheters; bacterial **prostatitis; GI infections (particularly shigellosis); and traveler's diarrhea.**

(3) Bactrim is also used for **prophylaxis of PCP** (*Pneumocystis jirovecii)* in patients with HIV/AIDS, and in patients who are on immune-suppressive therapy. It is also used for actual **treatment of PCP** at higher doses.

(4) The combination agent **sulfadoxine/pyrimethamine** (Fansidar) is used as an alternative in the **treatment of malaria** caused by chloroquine-resistant *Plasmodium falciparum.*

(5) **Poorly absorbed sulfonamides** such as **sulfasalazine** (Azaline, Azulfidine) are used to treat **ulcerative colitis** and **regional enteritis.**

(6) **Topically used sulfonamides** such as **silver sulfadiazine** (Silvadene) are used for the treatment of **wound and burn infections.**

d. **Adverse effects**

(1) Sulfonamides produce **hypersensitivity** reactions (rashes, fever, eosinophilia) in approximately 3% of the individuals receiving oral doses.

(2) Sulfonamides rarely cause **Stevens-Johnson syndrome,** an infrequent but fatal form of erythema multiforme associated with lesions of the skin and mucous membranes.

(3) Sulfonamides produce nausea and vomiting; also, they occasionally produce photosensitivity and serum sickness reactions.

(4) Patients with glucose-6-phosphate dehydrogenase deficiency are more susceptible to adverse effects, manifested primarily as **hemolytic aplastic anemia**.

(5) Sulfonamides may produce **kernicterus** in neonates because of the displacement of bilirubin from serum albumin-binding sites.

(6) Sulfonamides may potentiate the effects of other drugs, such as oral anticoagulants, sulfonylureas, and hydantoin anticonvulsants, possibly by displacement from albumin.

D. **Inhibitors of Bacterial Nucleic Acid Synthesis**

1. *Rifampin (Rifadin)*

a. Rifampin **inhibits RNA synthesis** by binding selectively to the β-subunit of bacterial DNA-dependent RNA polymerase (see Fig. 11.2).

b. It is widely distributed, including the CSF.

c. Rifampin is active against **most gram-positive organisms, *Neisseria* spp.,** and **mycobacteria,** including *M. tuberculosis* (in combination with other drugs such as **isoniazid**). It is also used in combination with other drugs for the treatment of most **atypical mycobacteria,** including *M. leprae.* Rifampin is also **used prophylactically for meningitis** from meningococci or *H. influenzae.*

d. Resistance develops rapidly because of decreased affinity of RNA polymerase.

e. Adverse effects of rifampin include nausea and vomiting, dermatitis, and **red-orange discoloration of feces, urine, tears, and sweat.**

f. Rifampin induces liver microsomal enzymes and **enhances the metabolism of other drugs** such as anticoagulants, contraceptives, and corticosteroids.

2. *DNA-binding agents*

a. **Nitrofurantoin** (Furadantin)

(1) Nitrofurantoin causes **bacterial DNA damage** by an unknown mechanism; it is **bacteriostatic.**

(2) **Nitrofurantoin** is concentrated in urine and is used solely as a **urinary tract antiseptic** against *E. coli*. Other urinary tract gram-negative bacteria are often resistant.

(3) Adverse effects of nitrofurantoin include nausea and vomiting, headache, **hemolytic anemia** in glucose-6-phosphatase-deficient patients, and acute pneumonitis; this agent **turns urine brown**.

b. Fluoroquinolones

(1) These agents, ***ciprofloxacin** (Cipro)*, ***norfloxacin** (Noroxin)*, ***ofloxacin** (Floxin)*, ***levofloxacin** (Levaquin)*, ***moxifloxacin** (Avelox)*, ***lomefloxacin** (Maxaquin)*, *and* ***gemifloxacin** (Factive)*, are fluorinated analogs of ***nalidixic acid** (NegGram)*, which is now used infrequently.

(2) Fluoroquinolones inhibit bacterial **DNA gyrase (topoisomerase II),** and therefore, DNA supercooling in **gram-negative bacteria.** They also inhibit **topoisomerase IV** in **gram-positive organisms** and thereby interfere with separation of replicated chromosomal DNA. They are bactericidal.

(3) **Ciprofloxacin, ofloxacin, levofloxacin,** and **lomefloxacin** are highly active against gram-negative bacteria and moderately active against gram-positive bacteria. **Moxifloxacin and gemifloxacin** have even greater activity against gram-positive organisms.

(4) Quinolones are concentrated in urine; they are useful against urinary tract infections and against infections caused by ***N. gonorrhoeae*** (except **ciprofloxacin** and **levofloxacin**) or **methicillin-resistant staphylococci,** as well as for upper and lower respiratory tract infections (**levofloxacin, moxifloxacin,** and **gemifloxacin**) resulting from infections with **mycoplasma, legionella,** and **chlamydia,** among others. **Ofloxacin** is used for **otitis media** in a topical (otic drop) form. **Ciprofloxacin** is used against ***Bacillus anthracis.***

(5) Resistance and cross-resistance is due to point mutations in the target enzyme or to changes in the organism's permeability to the drugs.

(6) Adverse effects include nausea and vomiting, GI pain, rashes, and fever. **Cartilage toxicity** has been reported, and thus these agents should not be used in children and young adults.

E. Polymyxins, Mupirocin (Bactroban)

1. Polymyxin is a polypeptide that acts as a deterrent to **disrupt the cell membrane** functions of **gram-negative** bacteria (bactericidal).

2. Polymyxin has substantial **nephrotoxicity** and **neurotoxicity** and is therefore only for ophthalmic, otic, or topical use.

3. Polymyxin B often is applied as a topical ointment in mixture with bacitracin or neomycin, or both (Neosporin).

4. *Mupirocin* is used topically and prophylactically for *S. aureus* infections such as **impetigo**.

F. Metronidazole (Flagyl)

1. Metronidazole, a prodrug, is **bactericidal** against most **anaerobic bacteria,** as well as other organisms, including **anaerobic protozoal parasites.**

2. It has been proposed that an intermediate in the reduction of metronidazole, produced only in anaerobic bacteria and protozoa, is bound to DNA and electron-transport proteins, thus **inhibiting nucleic acid synthesis.**

3. This agent is used for many anaerobic infections (e.g., ***Trichomonas vaginalis, C. difficile* colitis**), alone, or as part of a multicoverage regimen.

4. Metronidazole has a **disulfiram-like effect;** therefore, alcohol should be avoided. Neuropathy is seen with long-term use.

G. Agents Used against Vancomycin-resistant Organisms

1. *Daptomycin (Cubicin)* is a bactericidal agent that has a spectrum of activity similar to that of vancomycin. It is used to treat complicated infections caused by **MRSA, VRE** (vancomycin-resistant *enterococci)*, **MRSE (*S. epidermidis*),** and ***Streptococcus pyogenes.*** It can cause **myopathy**.

2. **Linezolid** *(Zyvox)*, which uniquely binds to the 23S ribosomal RNA of the 50S subunit to inhibit protein synthesis, is used to treat severe infections caused by **MRSA and VRE,** as well as **multidrug-resistant *S. pneumoniae.*** It has been successfully used for **staphylococcal osteomyelitis. Thrombocytopenia** can occur with the use of this agent. In combination with selective serotonin reuptake inhibitors, it may precipitate the **serotonin syndrome**.

3. A combination product *(Synercid)* of **quinupristin** and **dalfopristin** is administered IV to treat severe infections caused by **VRE, MRSA,** and **multidrug-resistant streptococci. As with clindamycin and erythromycin,** it **binds the 50S ribosomal subunit** and is **bactericidal** for most organisms. It inhibit CYP 3A4 and may influence the metabolism of a wide variety of drugs. Adverse effects include a complex arthralgia-myalgia.

III. ANTIMYCOBACTERIAL AGENTS (TABLE 11.3)

A. **First-line Drugs Used in the Treatment of TB**
   1. **Isoniazid (INH)**
      a. **Structure and mechanism of action**
         (1) INH is an analog of pyridoxine (vitamin B_6).
         (2) INH is a **prodrug** that is activated in *M. tuberculosis* by KatG, a catalase-peroxidase. The active metabolite inhibits synthesis of the **mycobacterial cell wall.** It does so by inhibiting the enzyme enoyl-ACP reductase required for the synthesis of mycolic acid which is unique to mycobacteria.
      b. **Pharmacologic properties**
         (1) INH **penetrates most body fluids and accumulates in caseated lesions.** It enters host cells and has access to intracellular forms of mycobacteria.
         (2) INH is active against *Mycobacterium tuberculosis*, but is not active against most atypical mycobacteria.
         (3) INH demonstrates no cross-resistance with other first-line antitubercular drugs.
         (4) INH is acetylated in the liver; acetylisoniazid is eliminated faster than isoniazid. The rate of acetylation of INH is genetically determined (**"rapid acetylators"** and **"slow acetylators"**).
      c. **Therapeutic uses**
         (1) INH is **administered in combination** with one (rifampin) and sometimes two (rifampin, pyrazinamide) or more other first-line drugs to counter the development of resistance (see below) most often due to mutations that result in its decreased conversion of INH to the active metabolite.
         (2) For **prophylaxis,** INH is used alone.
      d. **Adverse effects**
         (1) INH may produce allergic reactions, including rash or fever, in up to 2% of the patients.
         (2) The metabolites of INH may be hepatotoxic; fast acetylators are more susceptible. **Hepatotoxicity** with jaundice is observed in up to 3% of the individuals over age 35.
         (3) INH can inhibit mammalian pyridoxal kinase. High serum concentrations of this agent may result in **peripheral neuropathy;** slow acetylators are more susceptible. This effect is minimized by the coadministration of **pyridoxine.**
         (4) Isoniazid inhibits the metabolism of other drugs, especially diphenylhydantoin.
   2. **Rifampin** *(Rifadin)*, **rifapentine** *(Priftin)*, **rifabutin** *(Ansamycin)*
      a. **Structure and mechanism of action**
         (1) Rifampin selectively **inhibits the β-subunit of the DNA-dependent RNA polymerase** of microorganisms to **suppress the initiation of RNA synthesis.** Most atypical mycobacteria are sensitive. Resistance, a change in affinity of the polymerase, develops rapidly when the drug is used alone.
         (2) **Rifampin** is used in combination with **isoniazid** and **pyrazinamide** (see below) and also **prophylactically** for exposure to **meningococci and *H. influenzae.***
         (3) **Rifapentine** and **rifabutin** are analogs of rifampin. Their pharmacology is similar to that of rifampin.

table **11.3** Major Uses of Antibacterial and Antifungal Drugs

Drug	Major Organisms	Alternative Drugs
Penicillin	All aerobic gram-positive cocci (except penicillinase-producing and methicillin-resistant staphylococci, penicillinase-producing gonococci, and *Streptococcus faecalis*); *Leptospira;* **Treponema** (syphilis, yaws); all gram-positive anaerobes (peptococci, peptostreptococci, clostridia) and gram-negative anaerobes (except *B. fragilis*)	Ampicillin or tetracycline, amoxicillin/ clavulanic acid, ticarcillin/clavulanic acid, chloramphenicol, or erythromycin[a]
Penicillinase-resistant penicillins	Penicillinase-producing staphylococci	Vancomycin or cephalosporin
Vancomycin	Methicillin-resistant staphylococci	Daptomycin
Ampicillin	Penicillinase-producing staphylococci, *N meningitides, H influenzae*	Penicillin and aminoglycoside or vancomycin
Aminoglycosides	Coliforms (*E. coli, Klebsiella, Enterobacter, Serratia, Proteus*)	Third-generation cephalosporin, trimethoprim/ sulfamethoxazole, or extended-spectrum penicillin[a]
Aminoglycoside and extended-spectrum penicillin (**double coverage**)	*Pseudomonas aeruginosa*	Third-generation cephalosporin
Tetracycline	*Brucella, Campylobacter, Yersinia pestis* (plague), *Francisella tularensis* (tularemia), *Vibrio, Pseudomonas pseudomallei* and *mallei, Borrelia* (relapsing fever), *Mycoplasma pneumoniae,* chlamydiae, and rickettsiae	Streptomycin, erythromycin, chloramphenicol, or trimethoprim/sulfamethoxazole
Chloramphenicol	*Salmonella, Haemophilus* spp.	Trimethoprim/sulfamethoxazole, ampicillin, or third-generation cephalosporin
Erythromycin	*Legionella* spp.	
Trimethoprim/sulfamethoxazole	*E coli,* PCP	
Sulfonamides	*Nocardia*	
Metronidazole	*B. fragilis, C. difficile*	
Isoniazid (and rifampin and/or ethambutol)	*M. tuberculosis* and atypical *Mycobacterium* spp.	
Dapsone (and rifampin)	*M. leprae*	
Amphotericin B	*Candida, Torulopsis,* coccidioidomycosis, histoplasmosis, aspergillosis, and mucormycosis	
Amphotericin B and flucytosine	*Cryptococcus neoformans*	
Ketoconazole	Blastomycosis, paracoccidioidomycosis, and sporotrichosis	

[a]Choice of particular drug depends on sensitivity of the individual organism.

b. **Pharmacologic properties**
   (1) **Rifampin** is absorbed orally. It enters enterohepatic circulation and induces hepatic microsomes **to decrease the half-lives of other drugs** such as **anticonvulsants.**
   (2) Adverse effects are minor; they include nausea and vomiting, fever, jaundice, and an orange color to urine and other excretions.

3. ***Ethambutol*** *(Myambutol)*
    a. **Structure and mechanism of action**
        (1) Ethambutol inhibits **arabinosyl transferases** involved in cell wall biosynthesis.
        (2) Ethambutol is specific for ***M. tuberculosis*** and *M. kansasii.*
    b. **Therapeutic use.** Ethambutol is administered orally in **combination with isoniazid** to limit the development of resistance.
    c. **Adverse effects**
        (1) Ethambutol produces **visual disturbances,** resulting from reversible retrobulbar neuritis, and minor GI disturbances. Dose adjustment may be necessary in cases of renal failure.
        (2) Ethambutol decreases urate secretion and may precipitate gout.
4. ***Streptomycin*** on occasion is administered parenterally in **combination with other antimycobacterial agents;** it may be a part of multidrug regimens to treat resistant strains of TB.
5. ***Pyrazinamide***
    a. Pyrazinamide is a **prodrug** that is converted to pyrazinoic acid which **inhibits mycobacterial cell function.**
    b. Pyrazinamide is inactive at neutral pH, but it inhibits tubercle bacilli in the acidic (pH 5) phagosomes of macrophages.
    c. **Hepatotoxicity** is the major adverse effect, with occasional jaundice and (rarely) death. Pyrazinamide inhibits urate excretion and can precipitate acute episodes of gout.
    d. Pyrazinamide primarily acts on **extracellular tubercle bacilli.**

B. **Second-line Drugs Used in the Treatment of Tuberculosis**
    1. ***Aminosalicylic acid (PAS)***
        a. Aminosalicylic acid is an analog of PABA; it works similar to sulfonamides but only **penetrates mycobacteria.**
        b. Aminosalicylic acid produces GI disturbances.
    2. ***Ethionamide*** *(Trecator-SC)*
        a. Ethionamide, like isoniazid, blocks the **synthesis of mycolic acids.** Resistance develops rapidly, but there is no cross-resistance to INH.
        b. Ethionamide is **poorly tolerated;** it commonly produces severe GI disturbances. Without concomitant pyridoxine peripheral, neuropathies may occur. Hepatotoxicity is not uncommon.
    3. ***Cycloserine (Seromycin)***
        a. Cycloserine is an analog of D-alanine that **inhibits cell wall biosynthesis.**
        b. Cycloserine causes **CNS toxicity,** including seizures and peripheral neuropathy; alcohol increases the possibility of seizures. Pyridoxine administered with cycloserine reduces the incidence of neuropathies.
    4. ***Other agents.*** Parenterally and/or orally administered agents include **fluoroquinolones, amikacin,** and **capreomycin** (Capastat), protein synthesis inhibitors. These agents, used in combination with other active drugs, are used to treat multi-drug resistant TB.
    5. ***Commonly used drug regimens for TB.*** In general, **6-month regimens** are used for patients with culture-positive TB. The regimen consists of **INH, rifampin, pyrazinamide, and ethambutol.** All four agents are used for the initial 2 months. The continuation phase is 4 months and consists of the first two agents only. This phase is extended for an additional 3 months in patients who had cavitary lesions at presentation or on a follow-up chest x-ray, or are culture positive at the 2-month point. **Second-line agents** (e.g., fluoroquinolones, cycloserine, and amikacin) can be used when there is resistance to first-line agents.

C. **Drugs Used in the Treatment of Infections Caused by** *Mycobacterium leprae* **(Leprosy)**
    1. Dapsone
        a. Dapsone is structurally related to sulfonamides; it competitively **inhibits dihydropteroate synthase to prevent folic acid biosynthesis.**
        b. Dapsone is more effective against ***M. leprae*** than against *M. tuberculosis;* it is also used as a **second-line** agent to treat ***Pneumocystis*** **pneumonia** in AIDS patients.

    c. Treatment may require several years to life; dapsone is often used initially in **combination with rifampin and clofazimine** *(Lamprene)*, to delay the development of resistance. **Clofazimine,** a dye, may discolor the skin.

    d. Dapsone produces hemolysis, methemoglobinemia, nausea, rash, and headache.

D. Drugs Used against Atypical Mycobacteria

  1. Atypical, non-communicable, mycobacteria include *M. kansasii, M. marinum, M. avium complex, M. scrofulaceum,* and **others.** These account for about 10% of mycobacterial infections in the United States.

  2. A combination of *rifampin, ethambutol, and isoniazid is used to treat M. kanasii.*

  3. *MAC (M. avium complex)* includes *M. avium* and *M. intracellulare* that cause disseminated disease in the **late stages of AIDS**. A combination of agents, e.g., **clarithromycin, ethambutol, and ciprofloxacin**, is used to prevent the emergence of resistance. The treatment for this infection is usually **life-long.**

IV. ANTIFUNGAL AGENTS (SEE TABLE 11.3)

A. Drugs that Affect Fungal Membranes

  1. *Amphotericin B*

    a. Structure and mechanism of action. Amphotericin B is an antibiotic that binds to ergosterol, a major component of fungal cell membranes. It forms "amphotericin pores" that alter membrane stability and allow **leakage of cellular contents.** Bacteria are not susceptible because they lack ergosterol. Amphotericin B binds to mammalian cholesterol with much lower affinity, but this action may explain some adverse effects.

    b. Pharmacologic properties. Amphotericin B is poorly absorbed from the GI tract; it is effective by this route only on GI fungal infections. Amphotericin B is usually administered IV as a lipid formulation; it has poor penetration into the CNS but can be administered intrathecally for CNS infections that do not respond to other agents.

    c. Therapeutic uses

      (1) Amphotericin B has the broadest spectrum of activity. It is used to treat **topical infections,** and before switching to a less toxic agent, it is used for the **initial treatment for severe systemic fungal infections,** including those caused by *Candida albicans, Histoplasma capsulatum, Cryptococcus neoformans, Coccidioides immitis, Blastomyces dermatitidis, Aspergillus* spp., and *Sporothrix schenckii*.

      (2) In some cases, combination therapy with **flucytosine** (Ancoban) is advantageous for the treatment of cryptococcal meningitis.

    d. Adverse effects

      (1) The adverse effects of amphotericin B are significant; this agent causes **chills and fever** in 50% of the patients and **impaired renal function** in 80% that may be irreversible.

      (2) Amphotericin B may also produce anaphylaxis, thrombocytopenia, severe pain, and seizures.

  2. *Itraconazole, ketoconazole, miconazole, fluconazole, clotrimazole, voriconazole, and others*

    a. General properties

      (1) These agents are azoles that selectively **inhibit the cytochrome P–450-mediated sterol demethylation of lanosterol to ergosterol** in fungal membranes. The affinity of the mammalian P-450-dependent enzyme is significantly lower.

      (2) These agents are **broad-spectrum** antifungals; they also inhibit many gram-positive bacteria and some protozoa.

    b. Itraconazole (Sporonox)

      (1) Itraconazole has replaced **ketaconazole** (Nizoral) for the treatment of all mycoses except when cost is a factor. It is used **topically for dermatophyte infections** and mucocutaneous candidiasis and as a shampoo for **seborrheic dermatitis.**

(2) Itraconazole can be administered orally or topically. It is also used systemically for certain mycoses. It does not penetrate the CSF.

(3) Itraconazole is the drug of choice for **disseminated blastomycosis;** it is very useful for the treatment of **histoplasmosis** and also for paracoccidioidomycosis.

(4) **Inhibition of cytochrome P-450 metabolism (CYP3A4)** increases or decreases the metabolism of many drugs, which may lead to serious toxicities.

(5) Itraconazole most commonly causes **gastric upset** (3%–20% of patients). Itching, rashes, and headaches are observed in 1% of the patients.

c. **Miconazole** (Micatin), **clotrimazole** (Lotrimin), **nystatin** *(Mycostatin)*, **econazole** (Spectazole), **oxiconazole** (Oxistat), **sulconazole** (Exelderm), **sertaconazole** (Ertaczo), **butoconazole** (Gynazole-1), **terconazole** (terazol-3).

    (1) **Miconazole and clotrimazole** (and others) are available for **topical** application. They are useful for many **dermatophyte infections**, including **tinea pedis, ringworm, and cutaneous and vulvovaginal candidiasis.**

    (2) **Nystatin** is used topically for *Candida* **infections of the skin, mucous membranes, and intestinal tract.**

d. **Fluconazole** (Diflucan)

    (1) Fluconazole is available for IV or oral administration.

    (2) Fluconazole is useful for oropharyngeal, isopharyngeal, and systemic **candidiasis.** Fluconazole also penetrates the CSF and is the drug of choice for short-term and maintenance therapy of **cryptococcal meningitis** and for the treatment of disseminated **histoplasmosis** and **coccidioidomycosis.**

    (3) Adverse effects include nausea and vomiting, diarrhea, and reversible alopecia.

    (4) Fluconazole **inhibits CYP34A and CYP2C9** to increase plasma levels of numerous other drugs.

e. **Voriconazole** (Vfend), **Posaconazole** (Noxafil)

    (1) Among other activities, voriconazole and posaconazole are approved for **invasive aspergillosis.**

    (2) They **inhibit** several **cytochrome P-450 liver enzymes** to significantly decrease the clearance of numerous drugs.

    (3) Short-lived visual disturbance is reported for voriconazole but not posconazole. Dermatitis is common with voriconazole.

B. Other Antifungal Agents

1. Griseofulvin *(Fulvicin, Grisactin)*

    a. Griseofulvin binds to microtubules and **prevents spindle formation and mitosis in fungi.** It also binds filament proteins such as keratin. The drug **accumulates in skin, hair, and nails.**

    b. Griseofulvin is administered as oral therapy for **dermatophyte infections.**

    c. Griseofulvin is used for long-term therapy of **hair and nail infections.**

    d. Griseofulvin is generally well tolerated (GI distress and rash); rare CNS effects and hepatotoxicity occur (blood checks should be conducted during therapy).

2. Flucytosine *(Ancobon)*

    a. Flucytosine is actively transported into fungal cells and is converted to **5-fluorouracil** and subsequently to **5-fluorodeoxyuridylic acid,** which inhibits thymidylate synthetase and thus pyrimidine and **nucleic acid synthesis.** Human cells lack the ability to convert large amounts of flucytosine to the uracil form.

    b. Resistance develops rapidly and limits its use; flucytosine is rarely used as a single drug, but it is often used in **combination with other antifungal agents.**

    c. Flucytosine is relatively nontoxic; the major adverse effects of this agent are **depression of bone marrow function** at high doses and hair loss. **Uracil** administration can limit bone marrow effects.

3. Tolnaftate *(Tinactin)*, **naftifine** *(Naftin)*, **terbinefine** *(Lamisil)*, **butenafine** *(Lotrimin)*. These drugs are used topically for **dermatophyte infections.**

4. **Caspofungin** *(Cancidas),* **micafungin** *(Mycamine),* **anidulafungin** *(Eraxis)*
   a. These agents are large cyclic peptides that disrupt the fungal cell wall resulting in cell death.
   b. They are useful in **systemic candidal infections**. **Caspofungin** is used for salvage therapy in patients with **severe invasive aspergillosis** who failed therapy with amphotericin B.

V. ANTIPARASITIC DRUGS

A. Agents Active against Protozoal Infections
   1. *Antimalarials*
      a. **Malaria**
         (1) In the primary state of infection, sporozoites are injected into the host by the female mosquito (or a contaminated needle). In this **preerythrocytic stage,** the sporozoites are resistant to drug therapy. The sporozoites migrate to the liver (**primary exoerythrocytic stage**) and then sporulate (*Plasmodium vivax* and *P. ovale* may not develop to mature liver stages for up to 2 years [**hypnozoites**]). The merozoites that emerge infect erythrocytes (**erythrocytic stage**), where asexual division leads to cell lysis and causes clinical symptoms. In *P. vivax* and *P. ovale,* the merozoites released can reinfect other red blood cells (secondary erythrocytic stage), reinfect the liver, or differentiate into sexual forms (gametocytes) that can reproduce in the gut of another female mosquito. Elimination of parasites from erythrocytes and the liver requires multi-drug therapy effect as cure.
         (2) *P. malariae* and *P. falciparum* differ from the other plasmodia in that the merozoites cannot reinfect the liver to produce a secondary exoerythrocytic stage. The lack of a tissue reservoir makes therapy somewhat easier.
      b. **Therapy rationale** (see www.cdc.gov/travel)
         (1) **Chloroquine** (Aralen)
            (a) Chloroquine concentrates in acidic parasite vacuoles, raising their pH and **inhibiting the activity of heme polymerase,** which converts host hemoglobin toxic by-products to nontoxic polymerized material.
            (b) Chloroquine is used for the control of **acute, recurrent attacks,** but it is not radically curative. **Chloroquine** is effective against all plasmodia (*P. falciparum, P. vivax, P. malariae,* and *P. ovale*). For chloroquine-resistant plasmodia, **quinine sulfate is** used. **Pyrimethamine/sulfadoxine, doxycycline, quinidine,** or **clindamycin** may be used as adjunctive therapy.
            (c) **In prophylaxis, chloroquine** is used to suppress erythrocytic forms either before or during exposure; **primaquine** is added after exposure to treat exoerythrocytic forms. In regions with chloroquine-resistant strains, **mefloquine** or **atovaquone/proguanil** (Malarone) is used for prophylaxis. Doxycycline, an antibiotic, is used when multidrug resistance to *P. falciparum* is prevalent.
            (d) Chloroquine is also occasionally used in **rheumatoid arthritis** for anti-inflammatory action and as an alternative with emetine for amebiasis.
            (e) **Many species of *P. falciparum* are resistant to chloroquine. Artemisinin analogs are now widely used instead**.
            (f) Rarely, **hemolysis** can develop in glucose-6-phosphate dehydrogenase-deficient persons. **Pruritus** is common.
            (g) **Rapid parenteral administration or a single high dose (~30 mg/kg) may be fatal.**
         (2) **Primaquine (8-aminoquinoline)**
            (a) In combination with chloroquine, Primaquine is used specifically to **eliminate liver hypnozoites after exposure to *P. vivax* or *P. ovale* for terminal prophylaxis and (radical) cure** from malaria. It can be also be used for prophylaxis before exposure (casual prophylaxis) when other drugs are ineffective or unavailable.

(b) Primaquine is not given parenterally because of **severe hypotension. Blood dycrasias** or **arrhythmias** may rarely occur.

(c) Primaquine may result in **intravascular hemolysis or methemoglobinemia** in African Americans and dark-skinned Caucasians with glucose-6-phosphate dehydrogenase deficiency. Due to the relative deficiency of glucose-6-phosphate dehydrogenase, use of this agent is not advised during the first trimester of **pregnancy.**

(3) Quinine, quinidine

(a) Quinine is active against the **erythrocytic stage.** It is primarily used to treat **chloroquine-resistant *P. falciparum,*** often in combination with **doxycycline.**

(b) Quinine has a **low therapeutic index.** This agent produces **curare-like effects** on the skeletal muscle, and it can cause headache, nausea, visual disturbances, dizziness, and tinnitus **(cinchonism). Hypoglycemia, which can be fatal,** and (rarely) **hypotension** may also occur.

(c) Quinine is associated with **"blackwater fever"** in previously sensitized patients; although rare, blackwater fever has a **fatality rate of 25%** due to intravascular coagulation and renal failure.

(d) Intravenous administration of quinidine should include cardiac monitoring (parenteral quinine is unavailable in the United States).

(4) Mefloquine (Lariam)

(a) Mefloquine is useful for **prophylaxis and the treatment of chloroquine-resistant *P. falciparum*** and with chloroquine for **prophylaxis against *P. vivax* and *P. ovale.*** It acts specifically on the **erythocytic stage** of infection. For eradication of *P. falciparum*, it is used with artesunate. For eradication of *P. ovale* and *P. vivax*, it is used with primaquine.

(b) Mefloquinine causes GI disturbances at therapeutic doses. Seizures and other CNS manifestations are also seen.

(c) Use of mefloquine is **contraindicated** in patients with epilepsy or psychiatric disorders, and in patients using drugs that alter cardiac conduction.

(5) Atovaquone (Mepron), **atovaquone/proguanil** (Malarone)

(a) Atovaquone inhibits electron transport to reduce the membrane potential of mitochondria. Resistance develops rapidly.

(b) Co-administration of **atovaquone with proguanil** (Malarone) is effective for the **treatment and prophylaxis of *P. falciparum.*** The mechanism of antimalarial action of proguanil is uncertain. Its metabolite, cycloguanil, selectively inhibits plasmodia **dihydrofolate reductase/thymidylate synthetase** to inhibit DNA synthesis.

(c) These drugs are generally well tolerated. Adverse effects include GI dysfunction, headache, and rash.

(d) Atovaquone is used as an alternative treatment for *P. jirovici* pneumonia.

(6) Pyrimethamine (Daraprim)

(a) Pyrimethamine, and its prodrug analog **proguanil, inhibit dihydrofolate reductase** of plasmodia at concentrations less than that needed to inhibit the host enzyme.

(b) Pyrimethamine is used in combination with **sulfadoxine,** a sulfonamide with similar pharmacologic properties, in the combination product **Fansidar**.

(c) Pyrimethamine is associated with **megaloblastic anemia and folate deficiency** (at high doses).

c. Antibacterial agents

(1) Sulfonamides and sulfones are particularly important in the **prophylaxis of chloroquine-resistant strains.**

(2) Tetracyclines and **doxycycline** are used as short-term prophylactic agents in areas with multiresistant strains of plasmodia.

d. Artemisinins

(1) Artemisin (quinghaosu) is the active agent of a herbal medicine. It, and its major synthetic analogs, **artensuate and artemether,** are now widely used in a variety of combination treatments depending on the region of the world (mefloquine; amodia-quine; piperaquine; sulfadoxine + pyimethamine; lumefantrine) as standard therapy to treat *P. falciparum.*

(2) These agents are rapidly metabolized to **dihydroartemisinin** (also available as a drug) which has good activity for the initial treatment of the erythrocytic stage of *P. falciparum* infections.

(3) Adverse effects include GI disturbances and, rarely, allergic reactions and anemia.

e. **Lumefantrine,** the mechanism of which is unclear, is used as first-line therapy to treat the erythrocytic stage of *P. falciparum,* but only in a combination preparation (Coartem) **with artemether**. Its adverse effect profile is relatively unremarkable.

2. ***Agents active against amebiasis*** (Fig. 11.4)

a. **Amebiasis.** The major infecting organism is *Entamoeba histolytica,* which is ingested in cyst form, divides in the colon, and can invade the intestinal wall to cause severe dysentery.

b. **General drug characteristics.** The tissue amebicides **metronidazole and tindazole** are active against organisms in the intestinal wall, liver, and other **extraintestinal tissues**. The luminal amebicides, **iodoquinol, paromomycin,** and **nitazoxanide** act effectively in the **intestinal lumen.**

c. **Metronidazole** (Flagyl), **tindazole** (Tindamax)

(1) Metronidazole and tindazole are used for **intestinal amebiasis** as well as for **amebic liver abscesses,** generally in combination with a luminal amebicide **iodoquinol** or **paromycin** to eradicate luminal disease. These agents are also active against ***Giardia intestinalis*** (formerly G. *lamblia*) and ***T. vaginalis.*** Metronidazole shows activity against many **anaerobic bacteria.**

(2) **Metronidazole** has a **disulfiram-like action;** therefore, alcohol should be avoided. Tindazole appears to be better tolerated.

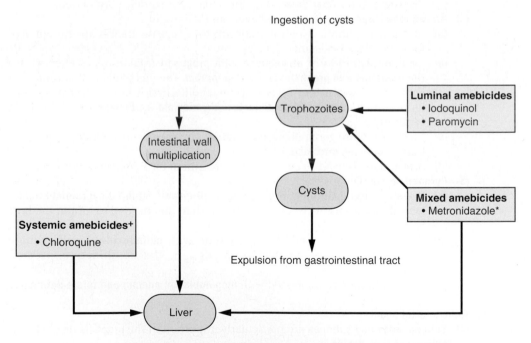

* Partially effective against luminal trophozoites; used with other luminal amebicides.
+ Rarely used

FIGURE 11.4. Agents active against amebiasis.

(3) **Metronidazole** should be avoided in the **first trimester of pregnancy** due to possible teratogenic effects.

   d. **Iodoquinol (Yodoxin)**
   (1) Iodoquinol is active against both **trophozoite and cyst forms in the intestinal lumen** but not in the intestinal wall or extraintestinal tissues.
   (2) Iodoquinol produces GI disturbances and changes in iodine levels that may cause toxicity.

   e. **Paromomycin** (Humatin) is a broad-spectrum antibiotic related to neomycin and streptomycin that is useful as an alternative treatment for **mild-to-moderate luminal infections** or in **asymptomatic carriers** in place of iodoquinol.

3. *Agents active against leishmaniasis*
   a. **Stibogluconate sodium** (Pentostam). This antimonial agent, the mechanism of which is unknown, is effective against all *Leishmania* (cutaneous, visceral); GI disturbances are common and ECG changes occur with continued therapy.

   b. **Pentamidine (Pentam)**
   (1) It is administered intramuscularly to treat *L. donovani* **infections** when antimonials have failed or are contraindicated.
   (2) It is the drug of choice to treat *T. brucei gambiense* (see below).
   (3) Adverse effects are numerous and include severe and dangerous **nephrotoxicity** and **hypoglycemia.**

   c. **Nitazoxanide (Alinia)** is used to treat *G. lamblia and C. parvum.* It inhibits the pyruvate-ferredoxin metabolic pathway. It is well tolerated.

4. *Agents used in the treatment of trypanosomiasis*
   a. **Nifurtimox** is used to treat South American trypanosomiasis caused by *Trypanosoma cruzi* **(Chagas disease).**

   b. **Suramin**, the mechanism of which is unknown, is useful for the treatment of early-stage **African trypanosomiasis,** or **sleeping sickness,** caused by *T. brucei rhodesiense.* Adverse effects include GI disturbances and rarely rash, among others.

   c. **Eflornithine** (Ornidyl), an alternative for late-stage West African trypanosomiasis, is an ornithine decarboxylase inhibitor.

   d. **Melarsoprol (mel B)**
   (1) Melarsoprol is an **arsenical** that reacts with the sulfhydryl groups in proteins. It is useful in the late-stage treatment of the **meningoencephalitic stage of East- and West-African trypanosomiasis,** especially that caused by *T. brucei.*
   (2) A potentially fatal effect is **reactive encephalopathy** (seen in 1–5% of patients).

   e. **Pentamidine** is standard therapy for the disease caused by *T. rhodesiense;* it can be used as an alternative to **suramin** in the early stage of the disease.

5. *Drug therapy for other protozoal infections*
   a. **Giardiasis. Metronidazole** and **tindazole** are the drugs of choice. **Nitazoxanide** (Alinia) is also used.

   b. **Toxoplasmosis** is treated with a combination of **pyrimethamine** and **sulfadiazine** (or **clindamycin**). This is a common opportunistic infection in immune-compromised patients.

B. Agents Active against Metazoan Infections (Anthelmintics)
   1. *Agents effective against nematode (roundworm) infections*
      a. **Albendazole** (Albenza) and **mebendazole** (Vermox)
      (1) Albendazole and mebendazole **bind with high affinity to parasite free B-tubulin** to inhibit its polymerization and microtubule assembly. These agents also irreversibly **inhibit glucose uptake by nematodes;** the resulting glycogen depletion and decreased ATP production **immobilize the intestinal parasite,** which is then cleared from the GI tract.
      (2) Albendazole is used to treat **cysticercosis and cystic hydatid disease,** for which it is the drug of choice.

(3) Mebendazole and albendazole are used to treat **roundworm infections** caused by *Ascaris lumbricoides, Capillaria philippinensis, Enterobius vermicularis* (**pinworm),** *Necator americanus* (**hookworm),** and *Trichuris trichiura* (**whipworm).** It is also recommended for infections caused by the **cestodes** *E. granulosus* **and** *E. multilocularis.*

(4) Mebendazole and albendazole cause GI distress during short-term therapy. They are potentially **teratogenic.**

(5) Thiabendazole (Mintezol) has been used to treat a wide variety of nematodes but, due to its toxicity, its clinical use has declined sharply.

b. Pyrantel pamoate (Antiminth)

(1) Pyrantel pamoate selectively produces **depolarizing neuromuscular blockade and inhibition of acetylcholinesterase (AChE)** of the worm, resulting in **paralysis;** intestinal nematodes are flushed from the system.

(2) Pyrantel pamoate is useful for the treatment of infections caused by **roundworm, hookworm, and pinworm.**

c. Piperazine (Vermizine)

(1) Piperazine citrate **blocks the response to ACh,** which results in altered parasite membrane permeability and **paralysis.**

(2) Piperazine citrate is absorbed from the GI tract; adverse effects are minimal.

(3) Piperazine citrate provides effective treatment of **ascariasis** and **enterobiasis.**

d. Diethylcarbamazine (Hetrazan)

(1) This agent decreases microfilariae **muscular activity,** causing their dislocation, and it also **disrupts their membranes,** making them susceptible to host defense mechanisms.

(2) Diethylcarbamazine is the drug of choice to treat **loiasis,** despite host response-induced toxicity, and it is a first-line agent for the treatment of **lymphatic filariasis and tropical pulmonary eosinophilia caused by** *Wuchereria bancrofti* and *Brugia malayi.*

(3) Its plasma half-life of 2 hours may increase up to fivefold if the urine is alkaline.

(4) Host destruction of parasites results, depending on the parasite, in **severe but reversible reactions,** including leukocytosis, retinal hemorrhages and ocular complications, tachycardia, rash, fever, encephalitis, and lymph node enlargement and swelling.

e. Ivermectin (Mectizan)

(1) Ivermectin causes **paralysis of the organism's musculature** by activation of **invertebrate-specific glutamate-gated Cl⁻ channels.**

(2) This agent is the drug of choice for the oral treatment of **onchocerciasis,** and it is a first-line agent for the treatment of **lymphatic filariasis** and **tropical pulmonary eosinophilia** caused by *W. bancrofti* and *B. malayi.*

(3) In onchocerciasis, the destruction of the microfilariae can cause mild or moderate reactions. In up to 0.1% of the patients, the reactions may be severe and include bronchospasm, hypotension, and high fever.

2. *Agents effective against cestode (tapeworm) and trematode (fluke) infections*

a. Praziquantel (Biltricide)

(1) Praziquantel causes **paralysis** of the worm due to increased cell membrane permeability of calcium.

(2) Praziquantel is the most effective drug against all types of **fluke infections,** including blood fluke infections **(schistosomiasis),** intestinal and liver fluke infections, and lung fluke infections **(paragonimiasis).** It is also useful in the treatment of **tapeworm infections.**

(3) It causes mild, but common, adverse reactions that include fever and rashes. Use of this agent is contraindicated in ocular cysticercosis because of host-defense-induced **irreversible eye damage.**

b. Bithionol inhibits parasite respiration. It is an alternative for *Fasciola hepatica* (sheep liver fluke infection) and as an alternative to **praziquantel** for **acute pulmonary paragonimiasis.**

VI. ANTIVIRAL DRUGS

A. **Antiherpesvirus Drugs**

1. **Acyclovir** (*Zovirax*)

   a. **Acyclovir** is a **purine analog** that needs to be converted to nucleoside triphosphate for activity.

   b. **Acyclovir requires viral thymidine kinase** to be selectively converted to monophosphate; it then uses cellular enzymes to be converted to a triphosphate form that competitively **inhibits the activity of viral DNA polymerase;** acyclovir triphosphate is also incorporated into viral DNA, where it acts to compete with deoxy GTP for viral DNA polymerase and as a chain terminator. Acyclovir **does not eradicate latent virus;** it has good CSF penetration. It can be administered orally and intravenously.

   c. **Valacyclovir** (Valtrex), a prodrug administered orally, is converted rapidly and completely in the intestine and liver to acyclovir with **increased oral bioavailability** (~15% to ~60%).

   d. These agents are active against **herpes simplex virus (HSV)** types I and II, and to a lesser extent against **Epstein–Barr virus, varicella-zoster virus,** and cytomegalovirus (**CMV**). Chronic oral administration provides suppression and **shortening of duration of symptoms** in recurrent genital herpes. It is also used in herpes zoster in immunocompromised patients; ophthalmic application is used to treat **herpes simplex dendritic keratitis;** and topical application is used for **mucocutaneous herpetic infections** in immunosuppressed patients. The agent is also used in immune-compromised patients for **prevention of reactivation of HSV** infection.

   e. Reversible **renal insufficiency** (crystalline nephropathy) or **neurotoxicity,** including tremor, delirium, and seizures, may develop without adequate patient hydration.

   f. Resistance generally develops due to decreased viral thymidine kinase activity or an alteration in DNA polymerase.

   g. **Famciclovir** (*Famvir*) is a prodrug that is well absorbed and then converted by deacetylation to **penciclovir,** which has activity similar to that of acyclovir except that it does not cause chain termination.

2. **Penciclovir** (*Denavir*), **docosanol** (*Abreva*), and **trifluridine** (*Viroptic*) are used as topical creams to treat herpes infection. **Docosanol prevents fusion of the HSV envelope with cell plasma membranes,** thereby inhibiting viral penetration. Host cell phosphorylated **trifluridine inhibits viral DNA polymerase** with inhibition of DNA synthesis.

3. **Ganciclovir** (*Cytovene*)

   a. Ganciclovir is a deoxyguanosine analog that, as the triphosphate (like acyclovir), **inhibits replication of CMV** (also HSV but not as well); monophosphorylation in CMV is catalyzed by a viral phosphotransferase (in HSV by a viral thymidine kinase).

   b. Ganciclovir is used intravenously or orally to treat **CMV retinitis** (also intraocularly), **colitis,** or **esophagitis** in immunocompromised patients and in patients with **AIDS;** it is also used for the **prevention or suppression of CMV infection in transplant patients.** It can also be used in combination therapy with **Foscarnet,** which is shown to be more effective. Ganciclovir is also used for **CMV pneumonitis** in combination with CMV antibody.

   c. **Resistance** is primarily the result of impaired phosphorylation due to a point mutation or a deletion in the **viral phosphotransferase.**

   d. The dose-limiting toxicity is **reversible neutropenia** and **thrombocytopenia.**

   e. **Valganciclovir** (*Valcyte*) is an ester prodrug that is converted to ganciclovir by intestinal and liver enzymes. Its uses are similar to those of ganciclovir.

4. **Foscarnet** (*Foscavir*)

   a. **Foscarnet inhibits viral DNA and RNA polymerase and HIV reverse transcriptase** directly by binding to the pyrophosphate binding site.

   b. **Resistance** is due to point mutations in **viral DNA polymerase and HIV reverse transcriptase;** foscarnet is **not cross-resistant** with most other antivirals.

c. Foscarnet is approved for use in the treatment of **CMV infections** and **acyclovir-resistant HSV infections.**

d. The therapeutic efficacy of foscarnet is limited by nephrotoxicity and hypocalcemia-related symptoms, including paresthesia, arrhythmias, and seizures.

5. *Cidofovir (Vistide)* is a **cytosine analog active against CMV.** It does not require viral enzymes for phosphorylation and subsequent **inhibition of DNA polymerase** and DNA synthesis. This agent is used for **CMV retinitis.** It must be **administered IV with probenecid and hydration** to reduce **nephrotoxicity. Neutropenia** is also common.

B. Anti-influenza Agents

1. *Amantadine (Symmetrel) and rimantadine (Flumadine)*

   a. Amantadine and rimantadine **interact with the M2 protein of the proton channel of the virus to inhibit the uncoating and replication of the viral RNA in infected cells.** The point-mutation development of resistance is common.

   b. Amantadine and rimantadine are used to treat orthomyxovirus (**influenza A**) infections when **administered within the first 48 hours of symptoms,** and as **prophylaxis during flu season.** These agents do not suppress the immune response to the influenza A vaccine.

   c. **Dose reductions** for both are necessary in the elderly and in patients with renal dysfunction and for rimantadine in patients with liver dysfunction.

   d. These agents cause mild CNS effects (insomnia, nervousness) and some GI dysfunction. Patients with a history of **seizures** require close monitoring. **Teratogenic** effects have been noted.

2. *Ribavirin (Virazole, Rebetol)*

   a. Ribavirin, a guanosine analog that alters the synthesis of guanosine triphosphate, appears to inhibit capping of the viral messenger RNA and inhibit viral RNA polymerases; the mechanism of action is not clear.

   b. Ribavirin is administered as an aerosol to treat **respiratory syncytial virus (RSV).** Oral formulations are used to treat **influenza A and B.**

   c. **Hemolytic anemia and teratogenicity** are major adverse effects to monitor.

3. *Zanamivir (Relenza) and Oseltamivir (Tamiflu)*

   a. Zanamivir, administered by inhalation, and oseltamivir, administered orally, are **neuraminidase inhibitors.**

   b. They are used for the treatment and prophylaxis of **acute uncomplicated influenza infection.** The agents are effective against both **influenza A and B.**

   c. **Oseltamivir** is a prodrug activated by liver esterases. Dose adjustment is made with reduced renal function.

   d. **Abdominal pain and GI dysfunction** are common with **oseltamivir. Zanamivir** may cause **bronchospasm.**

C. Antiretroviral Drugs (Fig. 11.5)—**Nucleoside Reverse Transcriptase Inhibitors (NRTIs)**

1. NRTIs act by competitively **inhibiting HIV-encoded RNA-dependent DNA polymerase (reverse transcriptase)** to cause chain termination that decreases viral DNA synthesis and virus replication. They prevent infection but do not clear cells already infected.

2. NRTIs must first **undergo intracellular phosphorylation** to be active.

3. **Combination therapy** of NRTIs with drugs from the other classes of antiretroviral agents that reduce or prevent replication, and have different modes of action, is most effective, both for treatment and to **reduce the likelihood of the development of resistance.** However, there are **significant drug–drug interactions** that must be taken into account.

4. NRTIs may cause metabolic acidosis and **hepatic toxicity** that can be fatal.

5. *Zidovudine (AZT) (Retrovir)*

   a. The major adverse effects of zidovudine, a pyrimidine analog, include **granulocytopenia, anemia,** and dyslipidemia and insulin resistance; other common effects are headache, fever, and GI disturbances.

   b. **Drug interactions** that increase blood levels of zidovudine are common.

   c. Zidovudine reduces the **rate of progression of HIV.** When given to pregnant women starting in the second trimester, then during labor, and then to the newborn, the

HIV attachment to cell

(−) ⟵ Enfuvirtide

Penetration of cell by pinocytosis and uncoating

Reverse transcriptase   (−) ⟵ Zidovudine, didanosine
stavudine, zalcitabine

DNA copy of viral RNA

Integration of viral DNA into host genome

Transcription of viral DNA

Translation of viral mRNA

Viral coat protein and viral RNA assembly

HIV-1 protease   (−) ⟵ Saquinavir, ritonavir, indinavir,
nelfinavir

Budding and release of virus particles from host cell

FIGURE 11.5. Sites of action of anti-AIDS drugs.

    vertical transmission of HIV is reduced by up to 25%. This agent is also used for **postexposure prophylaxis.**
6. **Didanosine (ddI)** *(Videx)*
    a. Didanosine, a purine analog, requires administration on an empty stomach.
    b. Toxicities include **pancreatitis, sensory peripheral neuropathy, optic neuritis,** and reports of myocardial infarction.
7. **Stavudine** *(Zerit)*. Except for acid lability and hepatic dysfunction, stavudine, a thymidine nucleoside analog, is **similar to didanosine** in pharmacokinetics, therapeutic use, and adverse effects that typically resolve with discontinuation.
8. **Zalcitabine (ddC)** *(Hivid)*. **Reversible peripheral neuropathy** may limit the use of this agent in up to 30% of the patients. **Oral ulceration** has been noted.
9. **Lamivudine (3TC) (Epivir),** emtricitabine (Emtriva), **abacavir (ABC), (Ziagen)**
    a. Side effects of **lamivudine,** a **cytosine analog,** include headache and GI upset. **Emtricitabine** is a fluorinated analog of lamivudine with a long half-life that allows for once-daily dosing. Its adverse effect profile includes **hyperpigmentation,** but otherwise is **similar to lamivudine.**
    b. **Abacavir** is a **guanosine analog.** Occasional **fatal hypersensitivity reactions** have been reported. **Skin rashes** and **respiratory distress** are common.

10. *Tenofovir (TDF)* *(Viread)* is an **analog of adenosine.** This agent is more convenient than older antiretroviral agents in that it has a **once-daily** dosing schedule. Most common side effects are GI. **Renal dysfunction** has been occasionally noted.

D. **Antiretroviral Agents—Non-nucleoside Reverse Transcriptase Inhibitors (NNRTIs)**
   1. NNRTIs act in a manner similar to NRTIs (see above).
   2. These agents **do not require phosphorylation** for their activity but rather act directly.
   3. Common adverse reactions of this class include **GI dysfunction** and **skin rash** that may be severe **(Steven-Johnson syndrome and toxic epidermal necrolysis).**
   4. **Drug–drug interactions** are numerous.
   5. *Nevirapine (NVP) (Viramune)*
      a. **Nevirapine** is used in combination regimens. It has been shown to **reduce vertical transmission** of HIV from the mother to the newborn when used as monotherapy.
      b. **Skin rash** is very common. **Hepatitis** has been noted.
   6. *Delavirdine (DLV)* *(Rescriptor)*, *Efavirenz (EFV)* *(Sustiva)*, *Etravirine* *(Intelence)*, **Raltegravir** *(Isentress)*, **Rilpivirin** *(Edurant)*,
      a. These agents are used in combination regimens.
      b. **Delaviridine** adverse effects include **skin rash** and **GI upset**. The drug is metabolized by **CYP enzyme systems. Drug interaction** should be monitored.
      c. **Efavirenz** is dosed **once daily.** It is also metabolized by **CYP enzyme systems.** Main side effects of this agent are dizziness, insomnia, confusion, amnesia, nightmares, and other **CNS effects.** These are observed in up to 50% of the patients and usually abate with time. **Teratogenicity** in animals has been noted.
      d. **Etravirine** causes **rash** and **GI dysfunction**. Its metabolism by CYP enzyme systems results in significant **drug–drug interactions**.
      e. **Raltegravir** is a newer non-nucleoside reverse transcription inhibitor that unlike others **binds the viral enzyme integrase** to prevent HIV replication and viral integration into the host cell. Thus far, drug–drug interactions have been few. Adverse effects may include depression and suicide ideation.
      f. **Rilpivirine** is a new agent in this class of drugs.

E. **HIV-1 Protease Inhibitors (PIs;** see Fig. 11.5)
   1. *HIV-1 protease inhibitors* competitively **inhibit viral-induced Gag-Pol polyprotein cleavage by HIV-1 protease,** a step necessary for virion maturation; this leads to clearance of the immature virion.
   2. *These agents are* used in combination **with nucleoside analogs to delay and possibly reverse the clinical progression of AIDS.**
   3. Bioavailability of most PIs is increased with a high-fat meal.
   4. These drugs, with the possible exception of **atazanavir**, are frequently associated with a significant **redistribution of body fat and obesity.** Significant **drug–drug interactions** have been noted that are due to inhibition or induction of CYP isoforms and that require dosage adjustments.
   5. *Resistance* due to changes in the protease gene has been described; different modifications may be responsible for resistance to some protease inhibitors. Resistance is more common when patients are noncompliant or take drug "holidays" or when inhibitors are used as monotherapy or are given at subtherapeutic doses.
   6. HIV-1 protease inhibitors include the following:
      a. **Saquinavir** (Invirase)
         (1) Saquinavir is administered as a hard capsule, which has limited bioavailability due to extensive first-pass metabolism, or as tablets with improved bioavailability. For greater efficacy, it is often **co-administered with ritonavir,** another protease inhibitor (see below).
         (2) Drug–drug interactions due to inhibition of CYP3A4 are common.
         (3) The most important adverse effects are GI disturbances and dyslipidemia that are reduced with the use of tablets and by co-administration of ritonavir. However, the latter combination may increase the possibility of arrhythmia.

b. **Ritonavir** (Norvir)
   (1) Ritonavir extensively **inhibits many liver CYP enzymes,** leading to accumulation of many drugs that are metabolized by this system (including saquinavir). It also **induces** some forms of **cytochrome P-450 enzymes,** leading to reduced bioavailability of other drugs. Close monitoring of other agents patients are using is recommended.
   (2) Ritonavir has an adverse effect profile that includes moderate GI disturbances, headache, fatigue, taste disturbances, and perioral paresthesia.
   (3) **Lopinavir–ritonavir** (Kaletra) combination is shown to enhance the efficacy of both drugs while reducing toxicity.

c. **Indinavir** (Crixivan)
   (1) As with ritonavir, it **interferes with liver microsomal enzyme metabolism,** but not to the same extent, and it inhibits the metabolism of some drugs and vice versa.
   (2) Indinavir is well tolerated. Mild GI symptoms and reversible **nephrolithiasis** can develop due to precipitation in the renal collecting duct system; these effects can be prevented with attention to hydration. Indirect **hyperbilirubinemia** is also common. Insulin resistance has been reported.

d. **Nelfinavir** (Viracept), **Fosamprenavir** (Lexiva)
   (1) These agents exhibit numerous drug–drug interactions similar to those of **indinavir.**
   (2) **Nefinavir** commonly causes **GI disturbances**.
   (3) **Fosamprenavir** is a prodrug, converted in the intestine to amprenavir, that is often administered with **ritonavir**. It may cause severe **rashes,** including, rarely, Steven-Johnson syndrome, that may require termination of therapy. The more common adverse effects include GI dysfunction and paresthesias.

e. **Atazanavir** (Reataz)
   (1) Common adverse effects of atazanavir include GI disturbances and indirect hyperbilirubinemia with jaundice. Unlike other PIs, atazanavir does not appear to cause dyslipidemia and fat redistribution.
   (2) **Atazanavir,** similar to other PIs, inhibits CYP isoforms with a great likelihood of **drug–drug interactions**.

f. **Tipranavir** (Aptivus), **Darunavir** (Prezista)
   (1) Tipranavir and darunavir are used to treat patients resistant to other PIs. They are co-administered with **ritonavir** to increase their bioavailability.
   (2) Their most common adverse effects are **GI disturbances. Rash** is seen with **tipranavir** and **darunavir** (they have a sulfonamide component). Their use is also associated with the development of **hepatic dysfunction** (black box warning). **Drug–drug interactions** are numerous.

F. **Anti-HIV Agents—Fusion Inhibitors**
   1. **Enfuvirtide** *(Fuzeon)* **binds to the gp41 subunit of** the HIV-1 viral envelope gp160 glycoprotein complex (gp41 and gp120) to **block the conformational change in the glycoprotein that is necessary for interaction with CD4 receptors and viral membrane fusion with the host cell membrane**. This drug is administered **subcutaneously,** with injection site reactions being the most common side effect. It is used in **combination** therapies.
   2. **Maraviroc** *(Seizentry)* binds with high selectivity to those host cells with CCR5 chemokine receptors to prevent the conformational change in the viral envelope gp120 subunit that is also necessary for HIV entry. It is used to treat R5 HIV infection that has shown resistance to other antiretroviral drugs. Drug–drug interactions are numerous, due to CYP3A metabolism, requiring dosage adjustments. Adverse effects include allergy, joint and muscle pain, and GI disturbances. Hepatotoxicity has been reported.

G. **Antihepatitis agents.** These drugs suppress viral DNA replication.
   1. **Lamivudine** *(Epivir)* is a NRTI (see above) used for **HBV** infections, providing effective and rapid response in most patients. It is a cytosine analog that competes with deoxycytidine triphosphate to subsequently **inhibit HBV DNA polymerase.** This agent **slows progression to liver fibrosis.** It has only minor adverse effects at doses used for HBV infections.

2. **Adefovir** *(Hepsera)* is also used for the treatment of **HBV.** This agent is a nucleotide analog that is **phosphorylated to its active metabolite.** Adefovir is relatively well tolerated. However, dose-related **nephrotoxicity** has been documented.

3. **Interferon alpha** *(Intron A, Roferon-A, Rebetron, Alferon N),* **peginterferon alfa** *(pegylated interferon alpha, PEG-Intron, Pegasys),* and **Interferon alfacon-1** (Infergen) are agents that bind to cell membrane receptors to initiate a series of complex reactions that lead to inhibition of viral activity, including viral replication. These agents are used for both **HBV** and **HCV.** Combination with **ribavirin** leads to synergistic effects. Pegylated agents allow for once-weekly dosing. Adverse effects include an **influenza-like syndrome** after injection, **thrombocytopenia and granulocytopenia,** as well as **neuropsychiatric effects.**

4. **Telbivudine** *(Tyzeka),* **Entecavir** *(Baraclude).*
   a. **Telbivudine and Entecavir inhibit HBV DNA polymerase.** They are nucleoside analogs that are phosphorylated to their active metabolites. They are generally well tolerated with headache and fatigue being the most common effects.
   b. **Entecavir inhibits HBV DNA polymerase.**
   c. **Tenofovir** *(Viread),* in addition to being used to treat HIV infection (see above), is also used to treat HBV infection.

H. Other Antivirals

1. **Palivizumab (Synagis)** is a humanized **monoclonal antibody** directed against the F glycoprotein on the surface of RSV. It is used for the prevention of **RSV** in children and premature infants and children. Adverse effects include respiratory infection rash, and GI dysfunction.

2. **Imiquimod (Aldara)** is a topical cream used for **anal and genital warts** caused by human papilloma virus. The exact mechanism of action is not well elucidated. Skin reactions are a common effect.

DRUG SUMMARY TABLE

Penicillins
Penicillin G (Pentids, generic)
Penicillin V (Pen-Vee K, generic)
Penicillin G benzathine (Bicillin)
Penicillin G procaine (generic)
Oxacillin (generic)
Dicloxacillin (generic)
Nafcillin (generic)
Ampicillin (generic)
Amoxicillin (Amoxil, generic)
Piperacillin (Pipracid)
Carbenicillin (Geocillin)
Amoxicillin/clavulanic acid
  (Augmentin)
Ticarcillin/clavulanic acid (Timentin)
Ampicillin/sulbactam (Unasyn)
Piperacillin/tazobactam (Zosyn)
Ticarcillin (Ticar)

Cephalosporins
First-generation
Cephalexin (Keflex, generic)
Cefazolin (Kefzol, generic)
Cefadroxil (Duricef, generic)
Second-generation
Cefoxitin (Mefoxin)
Cefaclor (Ceclor, generic)
Cefmetazole (Zefazone)
Cefuroxime (Ceftin, generic)
Cefotetan (Cefotan)
Cefprozil (Cefzil)
Third- and fourth-generation

Aminoglycosides
Streptomycin (generic)
Gentamicin (Garamycin, generic)
Tobramycin (Nebcin, generic)
Amikacin (Amikin, generic)
Neomycin (Mycifradin, generic)
Kanamycin (Kantrex)
Paromomycin (Humatin)

Tetracyclines
Tetracycline (Sumycin, generic)
Demeclocycline (Declomycin)
Doxycycline (Vibramycin, generic)
Minocycline (Minocin, generic)
Oxytetracycline (Terramycin)
Tigecycline (Tygacil)

Chloramphenicol
Macrolides
Erythromycin (generic)
Clarithromycin (Biaxin, generic)
Azithromycin (Zithromax)
Telithromycin (Ketek)
Clindamycin (Cleocin, generic)

Sulfonamides
Sulfisoxazole (generic)
Sulfadiazine, Silver sulfadiazine
  (Silvadene, generic)
Sulfasalazine (Azulfidine)
Sulfacetamide (generic)
Mafenide (Sulfamylon)

Rilpivirin (Edurant)
Saquinavir (Invirase)
Darunavir (Prezista)
Etravirine (Intelence)
Lopinavir/ritonavir (Kaletra)
Maraviroc (Selzentry)
Raltegravir (Isentress)
Rilpivirine (Edurant)
Atazanavir (Reataz)
Tipranavir (Aptivus)
Ritonavir (Norvir)
Indinavir (Crixivan)
Nelfinavir (Viracept)
Fosamprenavir (Lexiva)
Enfuvirtide (Fuzeon)

Miscellaneous Antimicrobials
Polymyxin B
Mupirocin (Bactroban)
Nitrofurantoin (Macrodantin,
  generic)
Metronidazole (Flagyl, generic)
Fidaxomicin (Dificid)
Linezolid (Zyvox)
Quinupristin/dalfopristin (Synercid)

Antimycobacterial Agents
Isoniazid (generic)
Rifampin (Rifadin, generic)
Rifapentine (Priftin)
Rifabutin (Mycobutin)
Ethambutol (Myambutol)

Cefdinir (Omnicef)
Cefixime (Suprax)
Cefotaxime (Clarofan)
Ceftizoxime (Cefizox)
Ceftazidime (Fortaz, generic)
Ceftriaxone (Rocephin)
Ceftaroline fosamil (Teflaro)
Cefepime (Maxipime)
Cefditoren (Spectracef)
Cefpodoxime proxetil (Vantin)
Ceftibutin (Cedax)

Other Beta-lactams
Aztreonam (Azactam)
Imipenem-cilastatin (Primaxin)
Ertapenem (Invanz)
Meropenem (Merrem IV)
Doripenem (Doribax)

Antiparasitic Agents
Chloroquine (Aralen, generic)
Primaquine (generic)
Quinine, Quinidine (generic)
Mefloquine (Lariam, generic)
Atovaquone (Mepron), Atavaquone/
    Proguanil (Malarone)
Pyrimethamine/sulfadoxine (Fansidar)
Doxycycline (Vibramycin, generic)
Metronidazole (Flagyl, generic)
Tindazole (Tindamax)
Nitazoxanide (Alinia)
Iodoquinol (Yodoxin)
Paromomycin (Humatin)
Pentamidine (Pentam)
*Sodium Stibogluconate
Eflornithine (Ornidyl)
*Melarsoprol (Mel B)
*Artesunate
Mebendazole (Vermox, generic)
Albendazole (Albenza)
Artemether/lumefatrine (Coartem)
Thiabendazole (Mintezol)
Pyrantel pamoate (Antiminth)
Piperazine (Vermizine, generic)
Diethylcarbamazine (Hertazan)
Ivermectin (Mectizan)
Praziquantel (Biltricide)
Bithionol (Bitin)
*Nifurtimox
*Available from the CDC.

Other Cell Wall Inhibitors
Vancomycin (Vancocin, generic)
Bacitracin (generic)
Cycloserine (Seromycin)
Daptomycin (Cubicin)
Fosfomycin (Monurol)

Pyrimethamine
Pyrimethamine (Daraprim, generic)
Pyrimethamine/sulfadoxine
    (Fansidar)

Trimethoprim
Trimethoprim (Proloprim, generic)
Trimethoprim/Sulfamethoxazole
    (Bactrim, generic)

Nucleic Acid Inhibitors
Rifampin (Rifadin, generic)
Nitrofurantoin (Furadantin,
    generic)

Quinolones
Nalidixic acid (NegGram)
Norfloxacin (Noroxin)
Ciprofloxacin (Cipro, generic)
Ofloxacin (Floxin)
Levofloxacin (Levaquin)
Moxifloxacin (Avelox)
Gemifloxacin (Factive)
Lomefloxacin (Maxaquin)

Antivirals—antiherpetic
Acyclovir (Zovirax)
Valacyclovir (Valtrex)
Famciclovir (Famvir)
Ganciclovir (Cytovene)
Idoxuridine (Herplex)
Valganciclovir (Valcyte)
Foscarnet (Foscavir)
Trifluridine (Viroptic)
Cidofovir (Vistide)
Penciclovir (Denavir)
Docosanol (Abreva)

Antivirals—anti-influenza
Amantadine (Symmetrel)
Rimantadine (Flumadine)
Ribavirin (Virazole)
Zanamivir (Relenza)
Oseltamivir (Tamiflu)

Antivirals—antiretroviral
Zidovudine (Retrovir)
Didanosine (Videx)
Stavudine (Zerit)
Zalcitabine (Hivid)
Lamivudine (Epivir)
Abacavir (Ziagen)
Tenofovir (Viread)
Emtrictabine (Emtriva)
Nevirapine (Viramune)
Delavirdine (Rescriptor)
Efavirenz (Sustiva)

Streptomycin (generic)
Capreomycin (Capstat)
Rifaximin (Xifaxan)
Pyrazinamide (generic)
Aminosalicylic acid (PAS)
Ethionamide (Trecator-SC)
Cycloserine (Seromycin)

Drugs for *Mycobacteria leprae*
Dapsone (generic)
Clofazimine (Lamprene)

Antifungal Agents
Amphotericin B (Fungizone,
    others)
Ketoconazole (Nizoral, generic)
Miconazole (Micatin, generic)
Clotrimazole (Lotrimin, generic)
Econazole (Spectazole, generic)
Oxiconazole (Oxistat)
Fluconazole (Diflucan)
Voriconazole (Vfend)
Itraconazole (Sporonox)
Sertaconazole (Ertaczo)
Butoconazole (Gynazole-1)
Terconazole (terazol-3)
Nystatin (Mycostatin, generic)
Griseofulvin (Fulvicin, Grisactin)
Flucytosine (Ancobon)
Tolnaftate (Tinactin, generic)
Naftifine (Naftin),
Terbinefine (Lamisil)
Butenafine (Lotrimin)
Mycafungin (Mycamine)
Caspofungin (Cancidas)
Posaconazole (Noxafil)
Sulconazole (Exelderm)
Tioconazole (Monistat 1)

Antivirals—antihepatitis
Lamivudine (Epivir)
Adefovir (Hepsera)
Interferon alpha (Intron A,
    Rebetron, Alferon-N, Roferon-A)
Interferon alphacon1 (Infergen)
Pegylated interferon alfa (*pegylated
    interferon alpha*, Pegasys,
    PEG-Intron)
Entecavir (Baraclude)
Telbivudine (Tyzeka)
Boceprivir (Victrelis)
Telaprevir (Incivek)
Ribavirin (Isentress)

Antivirals—other
Palivizumab (Synagis)
Imiquimod (Aldera)

Review Test

Directions: Each of the numbered items or incomplete statements in this section is followed by answers or by completions of the statement. Select the ONE lettered answer or completion that is BEST in each case.

1. A 27-year-old man presents with complaints of a painless ulcer on his penis. He admits to having unprotected intercourse with a woman he met in a bar during a conference 2 weeks ago. A scraping of the lesion, visualized by dark field microscopy, demonstrates spirochetes, and a diagnosis of syphilis is made. Which of the following is the treatment of choice assuming the patient has no known allergies?

(A) Benzathine penicillin G
(B) Penicillin G
(C) Penicillin V
(D) Doxycycline
(E) Bacitracin

2. A 19-year-old military recruit living in the army barracks develops a severe headache, photophobia, and a stiff neck, prompting a visit to the emergency room. A lumbar puncture reveals a diagnosis of bacterial meningitis. Which of the following cephalosporins is likely to be given to this patient?

(A) Cefazolin
(B) Cefuroxime axetil
(C) Ceftriaxone
(D) Cefepime

3. A 27-year-old intravenous drug abuser is admitted for fever and shortness of breath. Multiple blood cultures drawn demonstrate *S. aureus*. The cultures further suggest resistance to methicillin. The attending physician also orders a transesophageal echocardiogram that shows tricuspid vegetations consistent with endocarditis. Which of the following is an appropriate antibiotic?

(A) Aztreonam
(B) Imipenem
(C) Gentamicin
(D) Vancomycin
(E) Ceftriaxone

4. A 57-year-old chronic alcoholic develops hepatic encephalopathy. In an attempt to decrease his ammonia levels, you decide to sterilize his intestines, knowing that the gastrointestinal flora is responsible for the ammonia that his liver can no longer detoxify. Which antibiotic, given orally, will accomplish this?

(A) Neomycin
(B) Vancomycin
(C) Erythromycin
(D) Ciprofloxacin
(E) Nitrofurantoin

5. A 12-year-old boy presents with a rash on the palms and soles of his feet as well as fever and headache. He was camping last weekend and admits to being bitten by a tick. His Weil-Felix test result is positive, suggesting Rocky Mountain spotted fever. What antibiotic should be given?

(A) Streptomycin
(B) Bacitracin
(C) Ciprofloxacin
(D) Doxycycline
(E) Erythromycin

6. A 27-year-old African American woman is seen in the emergency room with complaints of urinary frequency, urgency, and dysuria. A urinary analysis demonstrates bacteria and white blood cells, and she is given trimethoprim/sulfamethoxazole. She now returns with sores and blisters around her mouth and on the inside of her mouth. Given her history and findings, what should you include in the differential of her current complaint?

(A) Glucose-6-phosphate dehydrogenase deficiency
(B) Steven-Johnson syndrome
(C) Red man syndrome
(D) Aplastic anemia
(E) Disseminated *M. avium–intracellulare* infection

7. A 43-year-old HIV-positive woman with a CD4$^+$ count of 150 presents with shortness of breath. An arterial blood gas determination indicates hypoxia, and a chest x-ray shows bilateral interstitial infiltrates. A suspected diagnosis of *Pneumocystis jirovesi* pneumonia is confirmed with bronchoscopy and silver staining of bronchial washings. Which of the following therapies should be started?

(A) Isoniazid
(B) Clindamycin
(C) Azithromycin
(D) Miconazole
(E) Trimethoprim/sulfamethoxazole

8. A 35-year-old diabetic woman presents to the emergency room with signs and symptoms of urinary tract infection, including fever, dysuria, and bacteriuria. Given that she is diabetic, she is admitted for treatment with intravenous ciprofloxacin. What is the mechanism of action of this drug?

(A) Inhibition of the 30s ribosome
(B) Inhibition of the 50s ribosome
(C) Inhibition of bacterial cell wall synthesis
(D) Inhibition of RNA synthesis
(E) Inhibition of DNA gyrase

9. A 35-year-old Mexican-American man presents to his family physician because his mother has been visiting from Mexico and was found to have tuberculosis (TB). The family physician places a purified protein derivative (PPD), which has negative results, but recommends prophylaxis against TB. Which of the following is indicated for TB prophylaxis in exposed adult patients?

(A) Rifampin
(B) Ethambutol
(C) Isoniazid
(D) Streptomycin
(E) Pyrazinamide

10. A 19-year-old woman has been under the care of an allergist and immunologist since she learned she had a deficiency of C5-9 (the membrane attack complex) of the complement cascade. Her roommate at college recently developed meningitis due to *Neisseria meningitidis*. Upon learning this, her physician recommends that she begin taking what antibiotic for prophylaxis?

(A) Ceftriaxone
(B) Isoniazid Rifampin
(C) Dapsone
(D) *para*-Aminosalicylic acid (PAS)

11. A 12-year-old girl has undergone a bone marrow transplant for the treatment of acute lymphoblastic leukemia. Five days later, she develops fever, and blood cultures reveal *Candida albicans* in her blood. Which of the following antifungals would be appropriate to use immediately?

(A) Nystatin
(B) Miconazole
(C) Clotrimazole
(D) Ketoconazole
(E) Amphotericin

12. A 23-year-old AIDS patient develops fever, neck pain, and photophobia. He is seen in the emergency room, where a lumbar puncture is performed. The cerebrospinal fluid reveals *Cryptococcus neoformans* on India ink stain. Which of the following agents is preferred for the treatment of cryptococcal meningitis?

(A) Tolnaftate
(B) Fluconazole
(C) Griseofulvin
(D) Cycloserine
(E) Flucytosine

13. A 23-year-old recent college graduate has plans to go to Africa to work for a year in the Peace Corps before returning to start medical school. He visits his family physician for a prescription for appropriate malarial prophylaxis. He brings a map from the Centers for Disease Control that shows that the area he will be in has a high incidence of chloroquine resistance. Which antimalarial should he take?

(A) Primaquine
(B) Doxycycline
(C) Mefloquine
(D) Pyrimethamine
(E) Quinine

14. A 14-year-old boy returns from a Boy Scout backpack trip with foul-smelling watery diarrhea. On further questioning, he admits to drinking water from a mountain brook without first boiling it. Stool is sent for ova and parasites, confirming the diagnosis of *Giardia lamblia* infection. Which of the following drugs is appropriate treatment?

(A) Metronidazole
(B) Nifurtimox
(C) Suramin
(D) Mebendazole
(E) Thiabendazole

15. A 42-year-old MDS patient presents to the emergency room with mental status changes and a headache. A computed tomography scan is ordered and demonstrates a ring-enhancing lesion. You decide to treat him empirically due to the possibility of *Toxoplasmosis gondii* abscess. Which agent should be included in his treatment?

(A) Ivermectin
(B) Praziquantel
(C) Pyrimethamine
(D) Niclosamide
(E) Pyrantel pamoate

16. A 23-year-old immunocompetent woman sees her family physician with painful "bumps" on her labia and vulva. On examination, there are vesicles in the described region. You suspect herpes simplex infection on clinical grounds and recommend which of the following?

(A) Amantadine
(B) Valacyclovir
(C) Vidarabine
(D) Foscarnet
(E) Rimantadine

17. A 23-year-old HIV-positive woman presents to the obstetrician. The patient admits to missing her last two menstrual periods, and a urinary human chorionic gonadotropin indicates that she is indeed pregnant. Which agent is used to decrease the risk of transmission of HIV to the unborn child?

(A) Idoxuridine
(B) Didanosine
(C) Saquinavir
(D) Zidovudine
(E) Interferon α

18. A 37-year-old woman presents with fever, malaise, and right upper quadrant pain. Blood tests reveal that she has an increase in her liver enzymes. In addition, hepatitis serology indicates that she has hepatitis B virus. Which of the following agents can be used in the management of this virus?

(A) Lamivudine
(B) Zidovudine
(C) Ribavirin
(D) Interferon α
(E) Acyclovir

Answers and Explanations

1. **The answer is A.** Patients with primary syphilis require a single intramuscular dose of benzathine penicillin G. Oral preparations of Pen G or Pen V are insufficient. Doxycycline for 14 days is an alternative treatment in penicillin-allergic patients. Bacitracin is only topical and insufficient for syphilis.

2. **The answer is C.** Ceftriaxone is a third-generation cephalosporin that has excellent CNS penetration. All the third-generation cephalosporins enter the CNS. The first-and second-generation agents, cefazolin and cefuroxime, respectively, do not enter the CNS. There are limited data on the effectiveness of the fourth-generation agent, cefepime, in meningitis.

3. **The answer is D.** Vancomycin is the drug of choice for serious infections due to methicillin-resistant *S. aureus* (MRSA). In the case of endocarditis, the treatment is usually 6 weeks. The resistance of MRSA is often due to altered penicillin-binding proteins, not β-lactamases, so aztreonam, imipenem, and ceftriaxone would not be useful. Gentamicin is often used in conjunction with penicillins in a non-MRSA setting.

4. **The answer is A.** Neomycin is used to sterilize the bowel, as it is not well absorbed from the gut. It is potentially nephrotoxic and ototoxic due to low (1%–3%) absorption. Vancomycin is typically used intravenously, although orally available, and does not provide adequate coverage for bowel sterilization. Although orally available, erythromycin, nitrofurantoin, and ciprofloxacin also do not have adequate coverage.

5. **The answer is D.** Doxycycline, a tetracycline (30S ribosome inhibitor), is the antibiotic of choice to treat Rocky Mountain spotted fever, a rickettsial disease. Streptomycin can be used to treat plague and brucellosis. Bacitracin is only used topically. Ciprofloxacin can be used to treat anthrax, and erythromycin is the most effective drug for the treatment of Legionnaires disease.

6. **The answer is B.** Steven-Johnson syndrome is a form of erythema multiforme, rarely associated with sulfonamide use. Patients with glucose-6-phosphate dehydrogenase deficiency are at risk of developing hemolytic anemia. Red man syndrome is associated with vancomycin. Aplastic anemia is a rare complication of clindamycin use. Disseminated *Mycobacterium avium–intracellulare* infection, more common in AIDS patients, is treated with macrolides.

7. **The answer is E.** Trimethoprim/sulfamoxazole is not only the treatment for *Pneumocystis jirovecii* pneumonia but also should be considered for prophylaxis in patients undergoing immunosuppressive therapy or with HIV. Azithromycin can be use in *Mycobacterium avium–intracellulare* (MAC complex) in AIDS patients. Isoniazid is used for tuberculosis (TB), yet another illness more common in AIDS patients. Miconazole is an antifungal used for vulvovaginal candidiasis.

8. **The answer is E.** Ciprofloxacin is a quinolone, a group of antibiotics that inhibit bacterial topoisomerase II (DNA gyrase). The antibiotic classes that inhibit the 30S ribosome include aminoglycosides and tetracycline. Inhibitors of the 50S ribosome include chloramphenicol, erythromycin, and clindamycin. Bacterial cell wall inhibitors include penicillins, cephalosporins, and vancomycin. Rifampin inhibits DNA-dependent RNA polymerase (RNA synthesis).

9. **The answer is C.** Isoniazid can be used alone for the prophylaxis of tuberculosis (TB) in the case of such exposure. All the other agents are important in the treatment of known TB infection and are often used in combination with isoniazid. Often rifampin, ethambutol, streptomycin, isoniazid, and pyrazinamide are used for months together, as many strains are multidrug resistant.

10. **The answer is A.** Patients with increased risk of *Neisseria meningitidis* infection can be given rifampin for prophylaxis. Ceftriaxone is often used in the case of confirmed meningitis. Isoniazid is used for single-agent prophylaxis in the case of tuberculosis exposure. Dapsone and *para*-aminosalicylic acid are used in the treatment of leprosy.

11. **The answer is E.** Amphotericin is used in the treatment of severe disseminated candidiasis, sometimes in conjunction with flucytosine. It is often toxic and causes fevers and chills on infusion, the "shake and bake." Toxicity has been decreased with liposomal preparations. Nystatin is used as a "swish and swallow" treatment for oral candidiasis. Miconazole and clotrimazole are topical antifungals. Ketoconazole is good for mucocutaneous candidiasis.

12. **The answer is B.** Fluconazole is the best agent to treat cryptococcal meningitis and has good central nervous system (CNS) penetration. Flucytosine penetrates the CNS and is often used with other antifungals, as resistance to flucytosine commonly develops. Tolnaftate and griseofulvin are topical agents used in dermatophyte infections. Cycloserine is an alternative drug used for mycobacterial infections and is both nephrotoxic and causes seizures.

13. **The answer is C.** Mefloquine is the primary agent used for prophylaxis in chloroquine-resistant areas. Primaquine is not used for prophylaxis before exposure. Doxycycline is used with quinine for acute malarial attacks due to multiresistant strains. Pyrimethamine is used for suppressive care and not for acute attacks.

14. **The answer is A.** Metronidazole is used to treat protozoal infections due to *Giardia*, *Entamoeba,* and *Trichomonas* spp. Nifurtimox is used to treat Chagas disease (due to *Trypanosoma cruzii*). Suramin is used to treat African trypanosomiasis. Mebendazole is used to treat round worm infections, and thiabendazole is used to treat *Strongyloides* infection.

15. **The answer is C.** Toxoplasmosis is treated with a combination of pyrimethamine and sulfadiazine. Ivermectin is used to treat filariasis, whereas praziquantel is used to treat schistosomiasis. Niclosamide can be used to treat tapeworm infections, and pyrantel pamoate is used to treat many helminth infections.

16. **The answer is B.** Valacyclovir is related to acyclovir, both of which are used for the treatment of oral and genital herpes in immunocompetent individuals. Vidarabine is used in more severe infections in neonates as well as in the treatment of zoster. Both amantadine and rimantadine are used in the treatment of influenza. Foscarnet is used in the treatment of cytomegalovirus retinitis and acyclovir-resistant herpes simplex virus infection.

17. **The answer is D.** Zidovudine is the only agent approved to prevent fetal transmission of HIV as it crosses the placenta. Idoxuridine is used in the treatment of herpes simplex virus (HSV) keratitis. Didanosine is used to treat HIV in children as young as 6 months. Saquinavir is used to treat HIV and is a protease inhibitor. Interferon a works best against single-stranded RNA viruses.

18. **The answer is A.** Lamivudine, a reverse transcriptase inhibitor of the HIV reverse transcriptase, also has activity against the reverse transcriptase of hepatitis B virus. Zidovudine does not display such cross-activity. Ribavirin and interferon-a can be used in the treatment of hepatitis C, an RNA virus. Acyclovir is only effective against the herpes family DNA polymerase.

chapter 12

Cancer Chemotherapy

I. PRINCIPLES OF CANCER CHEMOTHERAPY

A. Therapeutic Effect of Anticancer Agents

1. Since cancer may potentially arise from a single malignant cell, the therapeutic goal of cancer chemotherapy may require **total tumor cell kill,** which is the elimination of all neoplastic cells.

2. Early treatment is critical because the greater the tumor burden, the more difficult it is to treat the disease.

3. Achievement of a **therapeutic effect** often involves drugs that have a narrow **therapeutic index** (TI); it may require combinations of several drugs with different mechanisms of action, dose-limiting toxicities, or cross-resistance to minimize the adverse effects on nonneoplastic cells (Fig. 12.1).

4. A therapeutic effect is usually achieved by killing **actively growing cells,** which are most sensitive to this class of agents. Since normal cells and cancer cells have similar sensitivity to chemotherapeutic agents, adverse effects are mostly seen in normally dividing nonneoplastic cells, such as **bone marrow stem cells, gastric and intestinal mucosa, and hair follicles.**

5. Achievement of a therapeutic effect may involve the use of drugs, sometimes sequentially, that act only at **specific stages in the cell cycle** (e.g., the S phase and the M phase; Fig. 12.2).

B. Resistance

1. *Primary resistance*

   a. Primary resistance is seen in tumor cells that **do not respond to initial therapy** using currently available drugs.

   b. Primary resistance is related to the **frequency of spontaneous mutation** (10^{-5}–10^{-10}). There is a less likelihood that a small tumor burden has resistant cells. The probability that any tumor population has primary resistance to two noncross-resistant drugs is even less likely (approximately the product of the two individual probabilities).

2. *Acquired resistance*

   a. Acquired resistance **develops or appears during therapy.**

   b. Acquired resistance can result from the **amplification of target genes** (e.g., the gene for dihydrofolate reductase, which is the target for **methotrexate**). Gene amplification also occurs in the **multidrug resistance phenotype** (*MDR1* gene). In this case, cells overproduce cell surface glycoproteins (*P*-glycoproteins) that actively transport bulky, natural product agents out of cells (Table 12.1). As a result, the cell fails to accumulate toxic concentrations of several different types of drugs.

3. *Pharmacologic sanctuaries.* Resistance may occur due to the inability of chemotherapeutic agents to reach sufficient "kill" levels in certain tissues (e.g., brain, ovaries, testes).

FIGURE 12.1. Sites of action for cancer chemotherapeutic drugs.

II. ALKYLATING AGENTS (selected)

A. General Characteristics

1. Clinically useful alkylating agents have an **electrophilic center** that becomes covalently linked to the nucleophilic centers of target molecules.

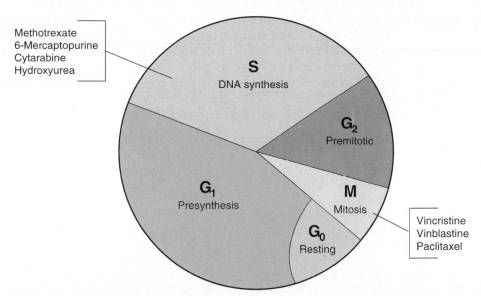

FIGURE 12.2. Cell-cycle specificity of some antitumor drugs. *S* is the phase of DNA synthesis; *G₂* is the premitotic phase for synthesis of essential components for mitosis; *M* is the phase of mitosis in which cell division occurs; *G₁* is the phase for synthesis of essential components for DNA synthesis; *G₀* is a "resting" phase that cells may enter when they do not divide.

2. Alkylating agents target the **nitrogens** and **oxygens of purines and pyrimidines** in DNA. This may lead to abnormal DNA strand crosslinks. These agents also target **other critical biologic moieties**—including carboxyl, imidazole, amino, sulfhydryl, and phosphate groups—which become alkylated.
3. These agents can act at all stages of the cell cycle, but the cells are more susceptible to alkylation in **late G₁ to S phases**.

t a b l e   12.1 The Multidrug Resistance (*MDR*) Gene: Drug Specificity and Tissue Distribution

Drugs Affected by *MDR*	Drugs Not Affected by *MDR*
Adriamycin	Methotrexate
Daunomycin	6-Thioguanine
Dactinomycin	Cytarabine
Plicamycin	Cyclophosphamide
Etoposide	BCNU
Vinblastine	Bleomycin
Vincristine	Cisplatin
VP-16	
Tissues with High *MDR* Expression	**Tissues with Low *MDR* Expression**
Colon	Bone marrow
Liver	Breast
Pancreas	Ovary
Kidney	Skin
Adrenal	Central nervous system

4. *Acquired resistance* can involve an increase in DNA repair processes, reduction in cellular permeability to the drug, increased metabolism, and the production of glutathione (and other molecules containing thiols), which neutralizes alkylating agents by a conjugation reaction that is enzymatically catalyzed by glutathione S-transferase.

5. With the exception of cyclophosphamide, parenterally administered alkylating agents are **direct vesicants** and can damage tissue at the injection site.

6. Some degree of **leucopenia** occurs at adequate therapeutic doses with all oral alkylating agents.

7. The dose-limiting toxicity is **bone marrow suppression**. Alkylating agents are also highly toxic to dividing **mucosal cells**, causing oral and gastrointestinal (GI) ulcers.

8. Most of these agents also cause nausea and vomiting, which can be minimized by pretreatment with **5-HT$_3$ antagonists**. Also, most of these alkylating agents can cause **sterility** and **alopecia**, which is common.

9. Patients with **xeroderma pigmentosa** are hypersensitive to alkylating agents.

10. Alkylating agents are **mutagenic** and can cause **secondary cancer** (e.g., leukemia) and sterility later in life.

B. *Cyclophosphamide (Cytoxan) and Ifosfamide (Ifex):* nitrogen mustards
1. *Mechanism of action:* Cyclophosphamide is metabolically activated to 4-hydroxycyclophosphamide, which in turn is nonenzymatically cleaved to aldophosphamide. In tumor cells aldophosphamide is cleaved to **phosphoramide mustard**, which is toxic to tumor cells, and **acrolein**, the agent suspected to cause sterile hemorrhagic cystitis.

2. *Pharmacologic properties:* Cyclophosphamide may be administered orally, intravenously (IV), or intramuscularly.

3. *Therapeutic uses:* Cyclophosphamide is used to treat non-Hodgkin's lymphomas, leukemias, mycosis fungoides, multiple myeloma, retinoblastoma, breast and ovarian carcinoma, and small cell lung cancer. It is a component of many combination treatments for a variety of cancers (Table 12.2). It is also used in some autoimmune conditions, such as lupus nephritis and arteritis.

4. *Adverse effects:* Cyclophosphamide has less incidence of thrombocytopenia than **mechlorethamine** (see below), but **immunosuppression** is still the most important toxic effect. Acrolein-induced **hemorrhagic cystitis** can be prevented by co-administration of the sulfhydryl compound 2-mercaptoethanesulfonate **(MESNA)**, which neutralizes acrolein at acidic pH in the urine, or acetylcysteine, or ample hydration. Reversible alopecia often occurs.

5. *Ifosfamide (Ifex)* is a cyclophosphamide analog with less potential to cause hemorrhagic cystitis. Central nervous system (CNS) and urinary tract toxicity limit its use to special applications (testicular cancer, stem cell rescue).

t a b l e **12.2** Common Combination Regimens		
ABVD	Adriamycin (doxorubicin), bleomycin, vinblastine, dacarbazine	Hodgkin' lymphoma
BEP	Bleomycin, etoposide, platinum (cisplatin)	Testicular
CHOP	Cyclophosphamide, hydroxydaunorubicin (doxorubicin), vincristine, prednisone	Non-Hodgkin lymphoma
CAF	Cyclophosphamide, adriamycin (doxorubicin), 5-FU	Breast
CMF	Cyclophosphamide, methotrexate, 5-FU	Breast
FOLFOX	5-FU, oxaliplatin, leucovorin	Colorectal
MOPP	Mechlorethamine, vincristine, prednisone, procarbazine	Hodgkin's lymphoma
MVAC	Methotrexate, vinblastin, adriamycin, cisplatin	Bladder
R-CHOP	Rituximab, cyclophosphamide, hydroxydaunorubicin (doxorubicin), vincristine, prednisone	Non-Hodgkin lymphoma
PVB	Platinum (cisplatin), vinblastine, bleomycin	Testicular
VAD	Vincristine, adriamycin (doxorubicin), dexamethasone	Multiple myeloma

C. *Mechlorethamine (Mustargen):* nitrogen mustard
1. *Pharmacologic properties:* Mechlorethamine is administered IV; it causes severe **local reactions**.
2. *Therapeutic uses:* This agent is used primarily in the **MOPP regimen** (Table 12.2) as a second-line therapy to treat **Hodgkin's lymphoma**.
3. *Adverse effects:* **Leukopenia** and **thrombocytopenia** are dose-limiting toxicities; repeated courses of treatment are given only after marrow function has recovered. Its use may reveal latent viral infections (e.g., herpes zoster).

D. *Melphalan (Alkeran) and chlorambucil (Leukeran):* nitrogen mustards
1. The pharmacology of melphalan and chlorambucil is similar to mechlorethamine. These agents are administered orally.
2. **Melphalan** is often used to treat **multiple myeloma** and **carcinoma of the ovary and breast**. It is the agent of choice for **chronic lymphocytic leukemia**. Its toxicity is related mostly to myelosuppression. Nausea and vomiting are infrequent; there is no alopecia.
3. **Chlorambucil** is used to treat **chronic lymphocytic leukemia, some lymphomas, and Hodgkin disease**. It produces less severe marrow suppression than other nitrogen mustards.

E. *Busulfan (Myleran): alkylsulfonate; **thiotepa** (triethylene thiophosphoramide):* ethylenimine
1. Busulfan is administered orally to treat **chronic myelogenous leukemia** and other myelo-proliferative disorders. It produces adverse effects related to **myelosuppression.** It only occasionally produces nausea and vomiting. In high doses, it produces a rare but some-times fatal **pulmonary fibrosis,** "busulfan lung." Its use is associated with adrenal insuf-ficiency and skin pigmentation.
2. **Thiotepa** is an ethylenimine that is converted rapidly by liver mixed-function oxidases to its active metabolite triethylenephosphoramide (TEPA); it is used in high-dose chemo-therapy regimens; it is active in ovarian cancer. Myelosuppression is a major toxicity.

F. *Carmustine (BiCNU), lomustine (CeeNU): nitrosoureas*
1. *Mechanism of action:* Carmustine and lomustine are highly lipophilic; they **cross the blood–brain barrier**. These nitrosoureas can alkylate DNA and can carbamylate intracel-lular proteins.
2. *Pharmacologic properties:* These agents are given orally except **carmustine**, which is administered IV.
3. *Therapeutic uses:* Carmustine, lomustine, and semustine are useful in the treatment of **Hodgkin's disease** and other lymphomas, as well as in **tumors of the brain**.
4. *Adverse effects:* These agents are markedly **myelosuppressive**, but with delayed effect, possibly up to 6 weeks. The use of these agents may also result in **renal failure**.

G. *Dacarbazine (DTIC-Dome):* triazine
1. *Mechanism of action:* Dacarbazine is activated in the liver to a metabolite that on decom-position produces alkylating cytotoxic carbonium ions.
2. *Pharmacologic properties:* Dacarbazine is administered IV (extravasation may cause tis-sue necrosis), and is a component of the **ABVD** regimen (adriamycin, bleomycin, vinblas-tine, and dacarbazine).
3. *Therapeutic uses:* Dacarbazine is used to treat **Hodgkin's lymphoma disease, malignant melanoma, and soft tissue sarcomas**.
4. *Adverse effects:* Dacarbazine is moderately **myelosuppressive**. Nausea and vomiting occur in 90% of patients. Flu-like symptoms also occur.

H. *Procarbazine (Matulane):* triazine
1. *Mechanism of action:* Procarbazine is a substituted hydrazine that needs to be activated metabolically. It produces **chromosomal breaks** and inhibits **DNA, RNA, and protein syntheses**.
2. *Pharmacologic properties:* Procarbazine is administered **orally**. It is lipophilic and enters most cells by diffusion; it is **found in the CSF**. It has no cross-resistance with other antican-cer drugs.

3. **Therapeutic uses:** Procarbazine is particularly useful in the treatment of **Hodgkin's disease** as part of the **MOPP regimen**; it is also active against **non-Hodgkin's lymphoma** and **brain tumors**.

4. **Adverse effects:** Procarbazine most commonly produces **leukopenia** and **thrombocytopenia**, along with GI disturbances. Myelosuppression is dose-dependent. This agent has a **10% risk of causing acute leukemia**. Procarbazine augments the effects of **sedatives**. It also causes **infertility**. Procarbazine is a weak **monoamine oxidase inhibitor** that may cause **hypertension**, particularly in the presence of sympathomimetic agents and **food with high tyramine content**.

I. *Mitomycin (Mutamycin)*
1. **Mechanism of action:** Mitomycin is a natural **antibiotic** that is activated intracellularly by an alkylating agent that causes single strand breaks by free radical mechanisms.
2. **Pharmacologic properties:** Mitomycin is administered IV. Extravasation may cause local injury.
3. **Therapeutic uses:** Mitomycin is used for the palliative treatment of gastric carcinomas.
4. **Adverse effects:** Its dose-limiting toxicity is myelosuppression.

J. *Cisplatin (Platinol), Carboplatin (CBDCA, JM-8) (Paraplatin), Oxaliplatin (Eloxatin)*
1. **Mechanism of action:** Cisplatin is a platinum compound that enters cells by diffusion and active transport. After intracellular replacement of its chloride atoms by water, it acts by **complexing with DNA to form crosslinks**. Adjacent **guanines** are the most frequently crosslinked, which leads to the **inhibition of DNA replication and transcription**. The effect of cisplatin is most prominent during the S phase of the cell cycle.
2. **Pharmacologic properties:** Cisplatin is administered **IV**.
3. **Therapeutic uses:** Cisplatin is used to treat **testicular tumors** (usually with **bleomycin** and either **vinblastine, the PVP regimen, or etoposide, the BEP regimen**), **ovarian carcinomas** (with **doxorubicin**), and **bladder carcinomas**. It is also used for several other carcinomas.
4. **Adverse effects:** The dose-limiting toxicity of cisplatin is **cumulative damage to the renal tubules** that may be irreversible following high or repeated doses, but which is routinely **prevented by hydration and diuresis** of the patient. This agent almost always produces **nausea and vomiting**. It is **ototoxic**, with tinnitus and hearing loss, and it also produces **peripheral neuropathy**. Cisplatin is only moderately myelosuppressive.
5. **Carboplatin** is a platinum compound administered IV for patients with **ovarian cancer**, as well as **non-Hodgkin's lymphoma, non-small-cell lung cancer, testicular cancer**, and **transitional cancers of the urinary tract**. This agent has similar but **less severe toxicities than cisplatin**; hence it has replaced cisplatin in some chemotherapy combinations. The dose-limiting toxicity of carboplatin is **myelosuppression**.
6. **Oxaliplatin**, another platinum compound, is used for the treatment of **metastatic colon cancer** in conjunction with **5-FU and leucovorin** (FOLFOX regimen). This agent can cause myelosuppression and **peripheral neuropathy**.

III. ANTIMETABOLITES (selected)

A. General Characteristics
1. Antimetabolites are **S-phase-specific** drugs that are structural analogs of essential metabolites and that interfere with DNA synthesis.
2. **Myelosuppression** is the dose-limiting toxicity for all drugs in this class.

B. Methotrexate (Trexall)
1. **Mechanism of action:** Methotrexate (MTX) is a **folic acid analog** that **inhibits dihydrofolate reductase (DHFR)**. This reduces the pool of tetrahydrofolate required for the conversion of deoxyuridylic acid (dUMP) to deoxythymidylic acid (dTMP), and consequently, N^5,N^{10}-methylenetetrahydrofolate is not formed. The net result is **indirect inhibition of DNA synthesis** (Fig. 12.3). Methotrexate also inhibits RNA and protein syntheses. This agent also inhibits enzymes involved in **folate metabolism**, including dihydrofolate reductase.

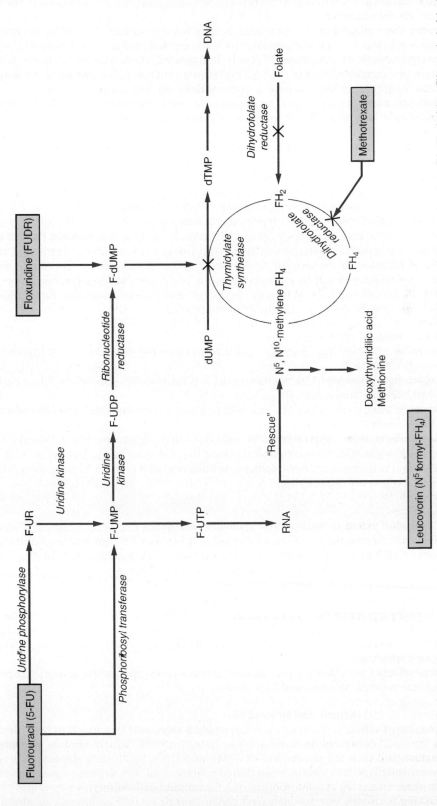

FIGURE 12.3. Mechanism of action of fluorouracil, floxuridine, methotrexate, and leucovorin (*5-FU, 5-fluorouracil; dUMP, deoxyuridine monophosphate; FH₂, dihydrofolate; FH₄, tetrahydrofolate*).

2. **Resistance** results from transport defects and also amplification or alterations in the gene for dihydrofolate reductase.

3. *Pharmacologic properties:* Methotrexate is administered orally, IV, intramuscularly, or intrathecally. It is transported into cells by folate carriers and activated to various forms of polyglutamate. Methotrexate is poorly transported across the blood–brain barrier. Therapeutic concentrations in the CNS occur only with high-dose therapy or by **intrathecal** administration, such as to treat or prevent leukemic meningitis.

4. *Therapeutic uses:* Methotrexate is an important agent in the treatment of **childhood acute lymphoblastic leukemia, choriocarcinoma in women**, and other trophoblastic tumors in women. It is also useful in combination with other drugs in the treatment of **Burkitt's lymphoma and other non-Hodgkin's lymphomas, osteogenic sarcoma**, lung carcinoma, and head and neck carcinomas. Methotrexate can be used for the treatment of **severe psoriasis** and has been used for immunosuppression following transplantation or in the management of a variety of **immune disorders**, including **refractory rheumatoid arthritis**, Crohn's disease, Takayasu arteritis, and Wegener granulomatosis.

5. *Adverse effects:* Methotrexate is **myelosuppressive**, producing severe leukopenia, bone marrow aplasia, and thrombocytopenia. Dose monitoring and **leucovorin (folinic acid) "rescue"** are important adjuncts to successful therapy (leucovorin is converted to an essential cofactor for thymidylate sythetase). This agent may produce **severe GI disturbances**. Other adverse effects can occur in most body systems; alopecia, headache, and mucositis are common. **Renal toxicity** may occur at high doses because of precipitation (crystalluria) of the 7-OH metabolite of methotrexate.

C. **Pemetrexed (Alimta)**

1. *Mechanism of action:* The primary action of pemetrexed is inhibition of thymidylate synthetase (Fig. 12.3).

2. *Pharmacologic properties:* Like methotrexate, it is transported into cell by folate carriers and activated to various forms of polyglutamate.

3. *Therapeutic uses:* It is approved for use **with cisplatin** to treat **mesothelioma and non-small-cell lung cancer.**

4. *Adverse effects:* **Myelosuppression** is its main dose-limiting adverse effect. Other notable adverse effects include mucositis and also swelling of the hands and feet (hand–foot syndrome) that is treated with dexamethasone. Folic acid and vitamin B_{12} supplementation reduces the severity of toxicities.

D. **Cytarabine** (ara-C)

1. *Mechanism of action:* Cytarabine is a **pyrimidine antagonist** that is an analog of 2'-deoxycytidine. The accumulation of one of its metabolites, Ara-CTP triphosphate, inhibits the activity of **DNA polymerases** and, if incorporated into DNA, results in altered function of newly replicated DNA. Cytarabine is most active in the **S phase** of the cell cycle.

2. *Resistance* can occur via changes in any of the **enzymes** required for conversion of the nucleoside to the various phosphorylated forms.

3. *Pharmacologic properties:* Cytarabine is administered **IV**, generally by continuous infusion, or intrathecally, because absorption after oral administration is poor and unpredictable.

4. *Therapeutic uses:* Cytarabine is used to treat **acute myelogenous leukemia** (AML) and **non-Hodgkin's lymphoma**.

5. *Adverse effects:* Cytarabine is highly **myelosuppressive** and can produce severe leukopenia, thrombocytopenia, anemia, and GI disturbances.

E. **5-Fluorouracil** (5-FU) **(Adrucil) and Floxuridine**

1. *Mechanism of action:* 5-Fluorouracil is a **pyrimidine antagonist** that needs to be converted to 5-fluoro-2'-deoxyuridine-5'-monophosphate, F-dUMP, which inhibits **thymidylate synthetase** and thus the production of dTMP and DNA, by forming a ternary complex between itself, N^5,N^{10}- methylenetetrahydrofolate, and the enzyme (see Fig. 12.3). **Floxuridine**, an analog of 5-fluorouracil, is a fluorinated pyrimidine.

2. *Resistance* is usually due to decreased conversion to F-UMP, or altered, or amplified thymidylate synthetase.

3. *Pharmacologic properties:* 5-Fluorouracil is administered IV; it is also used topically to treat skin cancers. It is very rapidly metabolized by dihydropyrimidine dehydrogenase (DPD) that may be lacking in up to 5% of patients who are more susceptible to the adverse effects of 5-FU.

4. *Therapeutic uses:* Fluorouracil is useful in certain types of solid carcinomas; the major use of this agent is in the treatment of **colorectal carcinomas**. It is also effective against **carcinomas of the breast, pancreas, liver, and others**. Applied **topically**, fluorouracil is used to treat **premalignant keratoses** and **superficial basal cell carcinomas**.

5. *Adverse effects:* This agent is markedly **myelosuppressive**. Fluorouracil produces GI disturbances, alopecia, and neurologic manifestations, along with other toxic effects.

F. **Capecitabine (Xeloda)** is a prodrug that is **converted to 5-FU** once ingested. It is an **oral** agent used for **metastatic breast cancer** and for **metastatic colorectal cancer**. **Myelosuppression** is common with the use of this agent, as is the **"hand–foot" syndrome**. Hepatic enzymes should be monitored, as capecitabine may elevate **bilirubin** levels.

G. **Gemcitabine** (Gemzar) is a **pyrimidine antagonist that inhibits DNA synthesis** via chain termination and other mechanisms. It is an **IV** agent used for treating **pancreatic cancer** as well as **non-small-cell lung cancer** and **bladder cancer**. Myelosuppression is the main limiting effect.

H. **6-Mercaptopurine (Purinethol) and 6-thioguanine**
1. *Mechanism of action:* 6-Mercaptopurine and 6-thioguanine are **purine antagonists (analogs of hypoxanthine and guanine,** respectively). They must be converted to ribonucleotides by the salvage pathway enzyme hypoxanthine-guanine phosphoribosyltransferase (**HGPRT**) to produce 6-thioguanosine-5′-phosphate (6-thioGMP) and 6-thioinosine-5′-phosphate (T-IMP). 6-thioGMP can be further phosphorylated and is incorporated into DNA. This appears to be its major site of action, although the precise mechanism of cytotoxicity is unknown. T-IMP accumulates and **inhibits nucleotide metabolism** at several steps. It can be converted into **thioguanine** derivatives and can also be incorporated into DNA.

2. *Resistance* is generally due to **deficiency in tumor cells of HGPRT**.

3. *Pharmacologic properties: 6-Mercaptopurine* and **6-thioguanine** can be administered orally. **6-Mercaptopurine** is inactivated by a reaction that is catalyzed by xanthine oxidase. In the presence of the xanthine oxidase inhibitor, allopurinol, the dose of 6-MP must be decreased significantly to avoid increased toxicity.

4. *Therapeutic uses: 6-Mercaptopurine* is useful in the treatment of **acute lymphoblastic leukemia (ALL)**. **6-Thioguanine** is used to treat ALL and **acute myelogenous leukemia (AML)**.

5. *Adverse effects:* **Bone marrow depression** is the dose-limiting toxicity. Hepatotoxicity is noted. GI disturbances occur, including anorexia, nausea, and vomiting (less with 6-MP).

I. **Cladribine (Leustatin)**, a purine **antagonist**, is an **adenosine analog** administered IV that is resistant to adenosine deaminase. Its phosphorylated form causes **DNA synthesis**. This agent is used for **hairy cell leukemia** and **non-Hodgkin lymphoma**. Cladribine is transiently myelosuppressive.

J. **Fludarabine (Fludara)**, a **purine antagonist** administered IV, interferes with **DNA synthesis** and induces cellular **apoptosis**. This agent is used for the treatment of **chronic lymphocytic leukemia (CLL)** and **non-Hodgkin lymphoma**. Its main side effect is **myelosuppression**.

IV. NATURAL PRODUCTS

A. **Vinca Alkaloids**
1. Vinca alkaloids interfere with microtubule assembly and block cells in mitosis. These agents are most active during mitosis at **metaphase**, blocking chromosomal migration and cell division.

2. **Resistance** is often accounted for by increased levels of the **MDR1** gene product **P-glycoprotein** that transports drugs out of the cell.

3. **Vinblastine (Velban)**
   a. Vinblastine, administered IV in combination with other agents, is used for treating **Hodgkin's and non-Hodgkin's lymphoma**, and several solid tumors.
   b. Although a marker for its therapeutic effect, **bone marrow suppression with leukopenia** is the dose-limiting toxicity; other adverse effects include **neurologic toxicity**, nausea and vomiting, alopecia, and ulceration from subcutaneous extravasation.

4. **Vincristine**: Vincristine, administered IV in combination with other agents, is used for the treatment of **acute lymphoblastic leukemia, Hodgkin and non-Hodgkin's lymphoma, and neuroblastoma**; it is **less toxic** to bone marrow than **vinblastine. Peripheral neuropathies** are the dose-limiting toxicities. This agent may also cause **severe constipation** and alopecia.

5. **Vinorelbine (Navelbine)**: Vinorelbine, administered orally, is used to treat **non-small-cell lung cancer** and **breast and ovarian cancer**. It has an intermediate toxicity profile relative to vinblastine and vincristine.

B. **Taxanes: Paclitaxel (Taxol), Docetaxel (Taxotere), and Cabazitaxel (Jevtana)**
   1. **Mechanism of action: Paclitaxel**, administered IV, binds to and **stabilizes microtubules by enhancing tubulin polymerization**. This results in **cell arrest in mitosis**.
   2. **Resistance** is associated with the expression of **P-glycoprotein**.
   3. **Therapeutic uses: Paclitaxel** shows its activity in **ovarian cancer** and in **breast** and **non-small-cell lung cancer**, and **Kaposi sarcoma**.
   4. **Adverse effects: Myelosuppression and peripheral neuropathies** are the dose-limiting toxicities. Paclitaxel also causes **hypersensitivity** specific to the vehicle (50% polyethoxylated castor oil and 50% ethanol) used for its administration. Co-administration of a histamine H_1-receptor antagonist (e.g., diphenhydramine), a histamine H_2-receptor antagonist (e.g., cimetidine), and dexamethasone reduces the impact of hypersensitivity.
   5. **Docetaxel** properties are similar to paclitaxel. It is used, primarily as an alternative agent, to treat **breast, prostate, non-small lung, gastric, and ovarian cancers**, among others. **Cabazitaxel** is similar in all respects to the other taxanes. However, it shows its activity in multi-drug-resistant tumors.

C. **Epipodophyllotoxins: Etoposide**: Etoposide, administered IV, blocks cells in the G_2 phase. It acts by forming a ternary complex with **topoisomerase II** and DNA, resulting in double-stranded DNA breaks. It is used for **testicular tumors** and, in combination with cisplatin, for **small-cell lung carcinoma. Leukopenia** is the dose-limiting toxicity.

D. **Antibiotics** (Selected Drugs)
   1. **Doxorubicin (Adriamycin), daunorubicin (daunomycin, [Cerubidine]), idarubicin (Idamycin), dactinomycin (actinomycin D), (Cosmegen), epirubicin (Ellence), valrubium (Valstar), and mitoxantrone (Novantrone).**
      a. **Mechanism of action: Doxorubicin** and the other antitumor antibiotics, isolated from *Streptomyces*, are **DNA-intercalating agents** that block the **synthesis of DNA and RNA**. They also fragment DNA by **inhibition of topoisomerase II** or the **generation of superoxide** anion radicals. They are active in all phases of the cell cycle.
      b. **Resistance** is due to decreased drug accumulation related to the generation of **P-glycoprotein**, and to **altered topoisomerase II**.
      c. **Pharmacologic properties:** All are administered IV.
      d. **Therapeutic uses:**
         (1) **Doxorubicin** is used in many standard combination regimens. It is used to treat **Hodgkin's and non-Hodgkin's lymphomas, and cancers of the breast, bladder, ovary, and lung**. The other uses of this agent include leukemias, multiple myeloma, and thyroid malignancies, among others.
         (2) **Daunorubicin and idarubicin** are used primarily in the treatment of **acute lymphocytic** and **myelogenous leukemias**.
         (3) **Dactinomycin** is used to treat rhabdomyosarcoma and Wilms tumor.

(4) **Epirubicin** is used to treat breast cancer. **Valrubicin** is used to treat refractory bladder cancer.

(5) **Mitoxantrone** is used to treat prostate and breast cancer and non-Hodgkin's lymphoma.

  e. *Adverse effects:* These agents produce dose-limiting **acute and chronic cardiomyopathies**. The acute form includes arrhythmias and myocarditis that are usually transient and clinically inconsequential. The **chronic form**, related to the generation of **free radicals,** may result in **heart failure**. They are also **myelosuppressive**. Mucositis is also noted.

2. *Bleomycin (Blenoxane)*

  a. *Mechanism of action:* Bleomycin is a mixture of copper-chelating glycopeptides isolated from *Streptomyces verticillus*. It binds to DNA with free radical formation, which results in **DNA chain scission and fragmentation.** Cells accumulate in the G_2 phase of the cell cycle.

  b. **Resistance** to bleomycin is mediated by increased levels of hydrolase or increased DNA repair activity.

  c. *Pharmacologic properties:* Bleomycin is administered parenterally. It is **inactivated by hydrolase** found in many tissues, **except lungs and skin** that have low hydrolase activity and are major sites of toxicity.

  d. *Therapeutic uses:* Bleomycin is used to treat testicular carcinoma, squamous cell carcinomas, Hodgkin's and other lymphomas, and head and neck cancer.

  e. *Adverse effects:* The most serious adverse effect is a cumulative **dose-related pulmonary toxicity with fibrosis** that may be fatal. Bleomycin also causes serious **cutaneous toxicity**. Acute reactions that can be fatal occur in 1% of patients with lymphoma; this reaction consists of the **anaphylactoid-like reactions** of profound hyperthermia, hypotension, and cardio-respiratory collapse. Bleomycin causes minimal myelosuppression.

E. **Camptothecins**

1. *Topotecan (Hycamtin)* inhibits **topoisomerase I** (an enzyme that allows relaxation and replication of specific regions of supercoiled DNA), thus resulting in **DNA damage.** Topotecan is used as an alternative therapy for **ovarian** and **small-cell lung cancer.** The main side effect of this drug is **myelosuppression.**

2. *Irinotecan (Camptosar)* also inhibits of **topoisomerase I**. This agent is used for treating **metastatic colorectal cancer** in combination with **5-FU and leucovorin.** Toxicity of this drug includes **diarrhea,** which can be severe, and **myelosuppression.**

V. MISCELLANEOUS AGENTS

A. **Hydroxyurea (Hydrea)**

1. *Mechanism of action:* Hydroxyurea inhibits **ribonucleoside diphosphate reductase** (during the S-phase of the cell cycle), which catalyzes the conversion of ribonucleotides to deoxyribonucleotides and is crucial for the **synthesis of DNA.**

2. *Therapeutic uses:* Hydroxyurea is primarily used in the management of **chronic granulocytic leukemia** and other myeloproliferative disorders. This agent is also used to treat **sickle cell crisis**.

3. *Adverse effects:* The major adverse effect of hydroxyurea is **hematopoietic depression and GI dysfunction.**

B. **L-asparaginase (Elspar)**

1. *Mechanism of action:* L-asparaginase is an enzyme that **reduces the levels of L-asparaginase**, an amino acid **not synthesized by some tumors**, to **inhibit protein synthesis** and cell division. This agent is **synergistic with methotrexate** when the folic acid analog is administered prior to L-asparaginase.

2. *Pharmacologic properties:* L-asparaginase is administered IV or intramuscularly.
3. *Therapeutic uses:* This agent is used in treating **lymphoblastic leukemia** and for the induction of remission in **ALL** (with **vincristine** and **prednisone**).
4. *Adverse effects:* L-asparaginase is **minimally marrow suppressive**; it is toxic to the **liver and pancreas. Hypersensitivity** and anaphylactic shock to the protein may develop. **Hemorrhaging** may occur due to the inhibition of clotting factor synthesis.

C. **Bortezomib (Velcade)**
1. Bortezomib **inhibits the 26S proteosome and down-regulates the nuclear factor kappa B signaling pathway** (**NF-KB**). Cancer cells rely on proteosomes for proliferation, as well as on metastases.
2. Bortezomib is approved for the treatment of **multiple myeloma**.
3. GI complaints are the most common side effects of bortezomib, but peripheral neuropathy has also been reported.

D. **Biologic Agents**
1. Biologic response modifiers are compounds that influence how an individual responds to the presence of a neoplasm.
2. Many biologic response modifiers have been produced using recombinant DNA technology, including **tumor necrosis factor, the interferons, and the interleukins**, among others.
3. *Cytokines and cytokine modifiers*
   a. **Interferon alfa-2b (Intron-A)** is approved for the treatment of hairy cell leukemia, and **Kaposi sarcoma.**
   b. **Interleukin-2 (aldesleukin) (Proleukin)** is approved for metastatic kidney cancer and **melanoma.**
   c. **Thalidomide (Thalomid) and lenalidomide (Revlimid)** are **tumor necrosis factor modifiers** with restricted distribution in the US. They assist in degradation of THF-α mRNA encoding protein. These agents are used in the treatment of **brain tumors, Kaposi sarcoma, multiple myeloma**, and many noncancerous conditions. Thalidomide's most common adverse effects are sedation, constipation, and peripheral neuropathy (30%). **Thalidomide** is also **highly teratogenic. Lenalidomide** is an analog of thalidomide with increased potency and an apparent decreased toxicity.
4. *Tyrosine kinase inhibitors*
   a. **Imatinib (Gleevec), Dasatinib (Sprycel)**
      (1) Imatinib and dasatinib are **tyrosine kinase inhibitors** that are specific for **Bcr–Abl** oncoprotein (dasatinib also inhibits several other kinases).
      (2) These agents are used for treating **chronic myelogenous leukemia**, which displays the Bcr–Abl chromosomal translocation (**Philadelphia chromosome**).
      (3) **Imatinib** has also been used for treating **GI stromal tumors** (GIST), which express another tyrosine kinase inhibited by Imatinib, **c-kit. Dasatinib** is also used for **ALL**.
      (4) These are oral agents, and their main toxicities are **edema**, nausea and vomiting.
   b. **Gefitinib (Iressa)**
      (1) Gefitinib is an inhibitor of **epidermal growth factor receptor tyrosine kinase** that is over-expressed in many cancers.
      (2) It is approved for use in non-small-cell lung cancer, where it is generally used with **gemcitabine and cisplatin.**
      (3) Side effects of this oral agent include severe diarrhea, acne, and other skin abnormalities.
   c. **Erlotinib (Tarceva)**
      (1) Erlotinib is another inhibitor of **epidermal growth factor receptor tyrosine kinase**.
      (2) This agent is used for treating **non-small-cell lung cancer** in patients who have failed at least one trial of prior chemotherapy, and **advanced pancreatic cancer**.
      (3) **Rash, diarrhea,** and **cough** are common side effects of this oral agent.
5. *Monoclonal antibodies (MABs)*
   a. **Rituximab (Rituxan)**

    (1) Rituximab is a chimeric (human/mouse) **antibody to IgG** that binds to **CD20 antigen on B cells**. This antigen is overexpressed on B cells of non-Hodgkin lymphoma tissues. The net effect of this interaction is cell lysis, possibly secondary to antibody-dependent cytotoxicity or complement cytotoxicity.

    (2) This agent is used for treating relapsed **non-Hodgkin lymphoma** (R-CHOP regimen). It is also used for treating **mantle cell lymphoma.**

    (3) Dermatologic and GI side effects are most common; however, neutropenia has been reported.

  b. Trastuzumab (Herceptin)

    (1) Trastuzumab is a humanized **IgG antibody** against the **epidermal growth factor receptor, HER2/neu**, which is overexpressed in 25%–30% of breast cancers. Expression of this protein is associated with **decreased survival due to more aggressive disease**. The net effect is the **arrest of the cell cycle** via antibody-mediated cytotoxicity.

    (2) This agent is used in treating **HER2/neu-positive metastatic breast cancers** in combination with **paclitaxel**. It is also used after the first-line therapy has failed.

    (3) Diarrhea and hematologic effects are the most common side effects.

  c. Cetuximab (Erbitux)

    (1) Cetuximab is a chimeric human–mouse **IgG antibody to epidermal growth factor receptor (EGFR)**. Its mechanism of action differs from that of **imatinib** in that cetuximab actually **blocks the receptor**. The action of this drug results in **inhibition of cancer cell growth** and **induction of apoptosis. Overexpression** of EGFR in colorectal cancer is associated with **decreased survival** and overall poor prognosis.

    (2) Cetuximab is currently approved for treating **EGFR-expressing metastatic colon cancer** alone or in combination with **irinotecan.**

    (3) The most common effect is rash that may be severe.

  d. Bevacizumab (Avastin)

    (1) Bevacizumab is the first humanized **IgG directed against human vascular endothelial growth factor (VEGF) interaction with its receptors (VEGFR1, VEGFR2)**, which are involved in **angiogenesis,** an important process in cancer proliferation and metastasis.

    (2) This agent is approved for **metastatic colon cancer in combination with 5-FU**.

    (3) Toxicities are mainly dermatologic and GI, but can include proteinuria, hypertension, and congestive heart failure. Reports implicate this agent in rare cases of **bowel perforation.**

VI. STEROID HORMONE AGONISTS AND ANTAGONISTS AND RELATED DRUGS

General properties of hormones and their antagonists are covered in Chapter 10. Their use in malignancy is considered here.

A. Use in neoplasia. The use of these agents in neoplasia is often predicated on the **presence of hormone receptors in target cells** and on the ability of the hormone to stimulate or inhibit cell growth. In the former case, hormonal antagonists are used; in the latter, hormonal agonists.

B. Adrenocorticosteroids (e.g., Prednisone, Hydroxycortisone, Dexamethasone)

  1. Adrenocorticosteroids are **lymphocytic and antimitotic agents**.

  2. Adrenocorticosteroids can be administered orally. They are useful in treating **acute leukemia** in children, **malignant lymphoma**, and both **Hodgkin and non-Hodgkin lymphoma** (CHOP and MOPP regimens).

  3. Adrenocorticosteroids have significant systemic effects, and their long-term use is not recommended.

C. **Mitotane (*o,p'-DDD*) (Lysodren)**
1. Mitotane is an oral agent specific available for the compassionate treatment of **inoperable adrenocortical carcinoma**.
2. Mitotane **inhibits glucocorticoid biosynthesis** and selectively causes atrophy of the tumors within zona reticularis and fasciulata by an unknown mechanism.
3. Nausea, vomiting, lethargy, and dermatitis are common side effects. **CNS depression** is the dose-limiting toxicity.

D. **SERMS: Tamoxifen (Nolvadex), Toremifene (Fareston), Raloxifen (Evista)**
1. The SERMS (**selective estrogen receptor modulators**) are drugs that have estrogen receptor agonist or antagonist properties depending on the target tissue. In the breast, tamoxifen and toremifene, and raloxifen are estrogen antagonists.
2. These agents inhibit estrogen-dependent cellular proliferation and may increase the production of the growth inhibitor TGF-β (transforming growth factor-beta).
3. Tamoxifen and toremifene are used in postmenopausal women with or recovering from **metastatic breast cancer**.
4. Tamoxifen and raloxifen are used as **prophylactic** agents in women at high risk for breast cancer.
5. Moderate nausea, vomiting, and **hot flashes** are the major adverse effects of tamoxifen; **endometrial cancer and thrombosis** are potential adverse effects of long-term therapy.

E. **Antiestrogens: Fulvestrant (Faslodex)** is an estrogen receptor antagonist used to treat **breast cancer**.

F. **Gonadotropin-releasing hormone (GnRH) analogs: Leuprolide (Lupron), triptorelin (Trelstar), goserelin (Zoladex), and histrelin (Vantas)**
1. These agents are peptides that, on long-term administration, **inhibit luteinizing hormone (LH) and follicle-stimulating hormone (FSH) secretion** from the pituitary and reduce the circulating levels of gonadotropins, and consequently estrogen and testosterone. The use of these agents results in **castration** levels of testosterone in men and **postmenopausal levels of estrogen** in women.
2. These agents are effective in treating **prostatic carcinoma**. They are also used for treating **breast and ovarian cancer.**
3. **Initial administration** of these agents, before pituitary-receptor desensitization occurs, may result in **increased LH and FSH release,** with a transitory increase in testosterone and an **exacerbation of disease**. They are often administered with the antiandrogen **flutamide** (Eulexin), **bicalutamide** (Casodex), or **nilutamide** (Nilandron) which **block the translocation of androgen receptors to the nucleus** and thereby prevent testosterone action.
4. *Degarelix (Firmagon)* is a GnRH antagonist that is used to treat advanced prostate cancer. It acts more rapidly than GnRH agonists to reduce gonadotropins and androgen.

G. **Aromatase inhibitors: Anastrozole (Arimidex), Letrozole (Femara), Exemestane (Aromasin), Fulvestrant (Faslodex)**
1. *Anastrozole* and *letrozole* are reversible aromatase inhibitors that have no effect on synthesis of steroids other than estrogens. They are used as an adjunct for **postmenopausal women with ER-positive early breast cancer**, women with breast cancer who have progressed on tamoxifen, and as first-line treatment of ER-positive or ER-unknown **advanced local breast cancer**. An adverse effect of these drugs is **hot flashes and vasomotor symptoms**. Long-term effects include **osteopenia** and **osteoporosis**.
2. *Exemestane* inhibits aromatase irreversibly. This agent is used for treating **postmenopausal women with breast cancer** who have progressed on tamoxifen. Exemestane does not exhibit cross-resistance with other aromatase inhibitors. Its side-profile includes hot flashes and fatigue.

H. **Androgen antagonists: Flutamide (Eulexin), Bicalutamide (Casodex), Nilutamide (nilandron)**
   1. *Flutamide and bicalutamide* are competitive antagonists of the androgen receptor; **nilutamide** is an irreversible inhibitor of the androgen receptor.
   2. These agents are used in combination **with either chemical or surgical castration** for the treatment of prostate cancer.
   3. *Adverse effects* are due to decreased androgen activity and include fatigue, **loss of libido, and impotence.** Other adverse effects are decreased hepatic function and GI disturbances.

VII. ADJUNCT AGENTS

A. **Leucovorin** (folinic acid, [Fusilev]) is a form of folate that is used to **"rescue"** patients from **methotrexate toxicity** (Fig. 12.3) as well as in combination regimens with 5-FU.

B. **Filgrastim (recombinant human G-CSF; Neupogen), pegfilgastim** (Neulasta) are recombinant human granulocyte colony-stimulating hormone (G-CSF) agents that **increase neutrophil production** and are used for prophylaxis and treatment of chemotherapy-induced **neutropenia. Pegfilgastim** is the long acting form. **Sargramostim (GM-CSF; Leukine)** is a recombinant human granulocyte/macrophage colony-stimulating hormone (GM-CSF) used for the same purpose, but more likely to cause myalgia and fever.

C. **Epoetin alfa (Epogen)** and **darbepoetin alfa (Aranesp) stimulate erythroid production and differentiation** and are used to address **anemia** caused by chemotherapy (or renal failure). They are analogs of erythropoietin. **Darepoetin** is the long-acting form.

D. **Allopurinol (Alloprim)** is a purine analog. It **inhibits xanthine oxidase** and is frequently used during chemotherapy to **prevent acute tumor cell lysis** that results in severe hyperuricemia and nephrotoxicity.

E. **Oprelvekin (Neumega)** is a recombinant **interleukin (IL-11)** that is indicated for chemotherapy-induced **thrombocytopenia** as well as for prophylaxis of this potentially dangerous complication.

F. **Amifostine (Ethyol)** is a **cytoprotective agent** that is dephosphorylated to active-free thiol, which then acts as a **scavenger of free radicals**. It is used to **reduce the incidence of neutropenia-related fever and infection** induced by **alkylating agents** and **platinum-containing agents (e.g., cisplatin)**, and to **reduce renal toxicity** associated with platinum-based drug therapy. It is also used to **reduce xerostoma** in patients undergoing irradiation of head and neck regions.

DRUG SUMMARY TABLE

Alkylating Agents
Cyclophosphamide (Cytoxan, generic)
Mechlorethamine (Mustargen)
Ifosfamide (Ifex, generic)
Melphalan (Alkeran)
Chlorambucil (Leukeran)
Busulfan (Myleran)
Carmustine (BiCNU)
Lomustine (CeeNU)
Streptozocin (Zanosar)
Thiotepa (generic)
Dacarbazine (DTIC-Dome, generic)
Mitomycin (Mutamycin, generic)
Temozolomide (Temodar)
Cisplatin (Platinol, generic)
Carboplatin (Paraplatin, generic)
Oxaliplatin (Eloxatin, generic)
Procarbazine (Matulane)
Methotrexate (Trexall, generic)
Pemetrexed (Alimta)
Cytarabine (generic)
5-Fluorouracil (Adrucil, generic)
Floxuridine (generic)
Capecitabine (Xeloda)
Gemcitabine (Gemzar)
6-Mercaptopurine (Purinethol,
   generic)
6-Thioguanine (Tabloid)
Cladribine (Leustatin, generic)
Fludarabine (Fludara, generic)

Natural Products
Vinblastine (generic)
Vincristine (generic)
Vinorelbine (Navelbine, generic)

Paclitaxel (Taxol, generic)
Docetaxel (Taxotere, generic)
Cabazitaxel (Jevtana)
Etoposide (generic)

Antibiotics
Doxorubicin (Adriamycin, generic)
Daunorubicin (Cerubidine, generic)
Idarubicin (Idamycin, generic)
Dactinomycin (Cosmegen, generic)
Epirubicin (Ellence, generic)
Valrubicin (Valstar)
Mitoxantrone (Novantrone, generic)
Mitomycin (Mutamycin, generic)
Bleomycin (Blenoxane, generic)
Topotecan (Hycamtin, generic)
Irinotecan (Camptosar, generic)

Miscellaneous Agents
Hydroxyurea (Hydrea, generic)
L-Asparaginase (Elspar)
Interferon alfa-2b (Intron A)
Interleukin-2 (aldesleukin)
   (Proleukin)
Thalidomide (Thalomid)
Lenalidomide (Revlimid)
Imatinib (Gleevec)
Dasatinib (Sprycel)
Bortezomib (Velcade)
Gefitinib Wessel
Erlotinib (Tarceva)
Sorafenib (Nexavar)
Pazopanib (Votrient)
Nilotib (Tasigna)
Cetuximab (Erbitux)

Panitumumab (Vectibix)
Rituximab (Rituxan)
Trastuzumab (Herceptin)
Bevacizumab (Avastin)

Steroid Hormones and Antagonists
Mitotane (Lysodren)
Megestrol (Megace, generic)
Tamoxifen (Soltamox, generic)
Toremifene (Fareston)
Raloxifen (Evista)
Fulvestrant (Faslodex)
Degarelix (Firmagon)
Leuprolide (Lupron, generic)
Triptorelin (Trelstar, generic)
Goserelin (Zoladex)
Histrelin (Vantas)
Anastrozole (Arimidex, generic)
Letrozole (Femara, generic)
Exemestane (Aromasin, generic)
Fulvestrant (Faslodex)
Flutamide (generic)
Bicalutamide (Casodex, generic)
Nilutamide (Nilandron)

Adjunct Agents
Leucovorin (generic)
Filgrastrim (Neupogen, generic)
Pegfilgrastim (Neulasta)
Sargramostim (Leukine)
Epoetin alfa (Epogen, generic)
Darbepoetin alfa (Aranesp)
Allopurinol (Alloprim, generic)
Oprelvekin (Neumega)
Amifostine (Ethyol, generic)

Review Test

Directions: Each of the numbered items or incomplete statements in this section is followed by answers or by completion of the statement. Select the ONE-lettered answer or completion that is BEST in each case.

1. A second-year medical student finds a few hours a week to work in a cancer research laboratory. Her project involves testing various chemotherapy agents (including adriamycin and etoposide) on colon cancer lines established from patient biopsies. She performs Northern blot analysis on multiply resistant cell lines and is likely to find increased expression of what gene?

(A) *Bcr–Abl*
(B) *EGFR*
(C) *MDR*
(D) *HER2*
(E) *HGPRT*

2. A 25-year-old man presents with recurrent bouts of hypoglycemia with mental status changes that are rapidly reversed by eating. He is not diabetic, and his serum levels of insulin are markedly elevated. His C-peptide levels are also elevated. You begin treating the patient for a presumed insulinoma with which of the following agents?

(A) Cyclophosphamide
(B) Melphalan
(C) Carmustine
(D) Thiotepa
(E) Streptozocin

3. A 73-year-old woman with breast cancer and history of congestive heart failure is placed on a chemotherapy regimen that includes the use of methotrexate (MTX) after her mastectomy. This agent's activity is related to its ability to do what?

(A) Carbamylate intracellular macromolecules
(B) Indirectly inhibit DNA synthesis
(C) Block chromosomal migration and cell differentiation
(D) Complex with DNA to form crosslinks
(E) Inhibit estrogen-dependent tumor growth

4. A 53-year-old man presents with changes in bowel frequency and pencil-thin stools with occasional bright red blood in the stool. A further work-up, including computed tomography (CT) scanning of the chest, abdomen, and pelvis, demonstrates lesions consistent with metastasis in the liver. His therapy will likely include which of the following chemotherapeutic agents?

(A) Carmustine
(B) 5-Fluorouracil
(C) Leuprolide
(D) Temozolamide
(E) Tamoxifen

5. A 53-year-old woman with breast cancer undergoes a breast-conserving lumpectomy and lymph node biopsy. The pathology report returns with mention of cancer cells in two of eight lymph nodes removed. Following radiation therapy, chemotherapy is started that includes the use of paclitaxel. Which side effect is the patient likely to complain of?

(A) Blood in the urine
(B) Easy bruising
(C) Hot flashes
(D) Shortness of breath
(E) Numbness and tingling

6. A 74-year-old man with a 100-pack/year history of smoking is evaluated for hemoptysis. A computed tomography (CT) scan of the chest shows numerous pulmonary nodules. A nodule on the pleural surface is selected for CT-guided biopsy by the interventional radiologist. The biopsy report is small-cell carcinoma of the lung, and chemotherapy containing etoposide is started. This drug works by

(A) Inhibiting topoisomerase II
(B) Inhibiting dihydrofolate reductase
(C) Alkylating double-stranded DNA

(D) Stabilizing microtubules, with resultant mitotic arrest

(E) Causing DNA chain scission and fragmentation

7. A 56-year-old woman with metastatic breast cancer is started on chemotherapy. Her initial treatment will include both cyclophosphamide and doxorubicin. Careful attention is required because of doxorubicin's well-documented toxicity, which is

(A) Hemorrhagic cystitis
(B) Acne
(C) Peripheral neuropathy
(D) Hot flashes
(E) Cardiomyopathy

8. A world-class cyclist was diagnosed with metastatic testicular cancer with lesions in both his lung and brain. He forgoes the standard treatment for his condition because he learns one of the drugs typically used for his condition could ultimately compromise his pulmonary function. Which of the following is included in the standard regimen and is associated with his feared complication?

(A) Cisplatin
(B) Busulfan
(C) Aminoglutethimide
(D) Bleomycin
(E) Cyclophosphamide

9. A 35-year-old otherwise healthy man presents with fullness in the inguinal region with swelling of the ipsilateral leg. A computed tomography (CT) scan demonstrates several confluent enlarged lymph nodes. Biopsy specimens demonstrate malignant $CD20^+$ B cells. A diagnosis of diffuse B-cell lymphoma is made. Which of the following biologics will likely be given to the patient?

(A) Traztuzumab
(B) Rituxaimab
(C) Dactinomycin
(D) l-Asparaginase
(E) Interferon-α

10. A 17-year-old girl sees her physician for swollen lymph nodes in the supraclavicular region. A core biopsy demonstrates Reed–Sternberg cells and fibrotic bands, a finding characteristic of nodular sclerosis Hodgkin disease. Which of the following combined regimens might be used in this patient?

(A) R-CHOP
(B) CMF

(C) FOLFOX
(D) BEP
(E) ABVD

11. A 63-year-old postmenopausal woman is diagnosed with early stage breast cancer, which is initially managed by partial mastectomy and radiation therapy. Her tumor was positive for expression of estrogen receptors. Which agent would you recommend to this patient to prevent relapse?

(A) Leuprolide
(B) Hydroxyurea
(C) Anastrozole
(D) Carboplatin
(E) Goserelin

12. A 56-year-old man complains of fatigue and malaise. On physical examination he has significant splenomegaly. His white blood cell count is dramatically elevated, and the physician suspects leukemia. Chromosomal studies indicate a (9:22) translocation, the Philadelphia chromosome, confirming the diagnosis of chronic myelocytic leukemia (CML). Which of the following might be used in his treatment?

(A) Anastrozole
(B) Rituximab
(C) Imatinib
(D) Gefitinib
(E) Amifostine

13. A 37-year-old man presents with changes in bowel habits for the last several months. He complains of small stool caliber along with occasional blood in his stools. Colonoscopy reveals the diagnosis of colon adenocarcinoma. Further work-up demonstrates that there are metastatic lesions in his liver. The oncologist recommends the use of bevacizumab. This agent

(A) Inhibits cell cycle progression
(B) Induces differentiation of cells
(C) Blocks signaling by vascular EGF
(D) Inhibits angiogenesis
(E) Inhibits HER2/neu signaling

14. A 54-year-old woman complains of headache, nausea, and vomiting. A computed tomography (CT) scan of the head reveals a large mass in the frontal lobe. She underwent surgery to remove the mass, which was shown to be a glioblastoma multiforme (GBM). In addition to receiving radiation, which agent should be given?

(A) Thalidomide
(B) Cisplatin
(C) Thioguanine
(D) Temozolomide
(E) Mercaptopurine

15. A 63-year-old African-American man with a history of prostate cancer had his prostate removed 10 years ago. His prostate-specific antigen levels have begun to rise again, and he complains of back pain, suggesting metastatic disease. A computed tomography (CT) scan demonstrates enlarged para-aortic lymph nodes and osteoblastic lesions of his lumbar spine. Therapy with which agent should be started?

(A) Anastrozole
(B) Leuprolide
(C) Tamoxifen
(D) Mitotane
(E) Prednisone

16. A 56-year-old woman with a significant smoking history was diagnosed with small-cell lung cancer 2 years ago and was successfully treated. Now on follow-up computed tomography (CT) scan, there are several new pulmonary nodules, and the oncologist elects to begin second-line chemotherapy with a DNA topoisomerase I inhibitor. Which of the following is such an agent?

(A) Ciprofloxacin
(B) Etoposide
(C) Vinorelbine
(D) Teniposide
(E) Irinotecan

17. A 42-year-old premenopausal woman recently underwent partial mastectomy and radiation therapy for a small tumor in her breast. There were no lymph nodes involved, and the tumor was estrogen-receptor positive. The oncologist explains that there is a little advantage to adding systemic chemotherapy in such an early-stage cancer but does recommend that the patient take tamoxifen. Which of the following is a concerning side effect of tamoxifen?

(A) Thromboembolism
(B) Bowel perforation
(C) Aplastic anemia
(D) Myelosuppression
(E) Hypotension

Answers and Explanations

1. **The answer is C.** Gene amplification of the multidrug resistance (*MDR1*) gene is found in many tumors and confers resistance to many chemotherapy agents. *MDR1* encodes a transport protein that actively pumps various chemotherapy agents out of the cell. Although *Bcr–Abl, EGFR,* and *HER2* may be overexpressed in tumors, they don't necessarily confer resistance to chemotherapy. *HGPRT* is overexpressed in some tumors, but it only confers resistance to methotrexate.

2. **The answer is E.** Streptozocin is toxic to β cells of the islets of Langerhans in the pancreas and is therefore used in the treatment of insulinomas. Melphalan is a derivative of nitrogen mustard used to treat multiple myeloma, melanoma, and carcinoma of the ovary. Carmustine is a drug used to treat neoplasms of the brain, as it has excellent central nervous system (CNS) penetration. Thiotepa is used in the treatment of bladder cancer.

3. **The answer is B.** Methotrexate inhibits the enzyme dihydrofolate reductase, which ultimately decreases the availability of thymidylate to produce DNA. Nitrosoureas can carbamylate intracellular molecules. Vinca alkaloids such as vinblastine block chromosomal migration and cellular differentiation. Cisplatin works primarily by complexing with DNA to form crosslinks. Agents like tamoxifen inhibit estrogen-dependent tumor growth.

4. **The answer is B.** 5-Fluorouracil is an important agent in cases of metastatic colon cancer and is part of the FOLFOX regimen. Carmustine is used in the treatment of brain tumors, as is temozolomide. Leuprolide is used to treat hormone-sensitive prostate cancer, and tamoxifen is used to treat breast cancer.

5. **The answer is E.** Paclitaxel is often used in the treatment of breast as well as ovarian and lung cancer. Its main toxicities are myelosuppression and peripheral neuropathy that usually manifest as numbness and tingling in the distal extremities. Blood in the urine can indicate hemorrhagic cystitis, a complication of cyclophosphamide use. Easy bruising can result from mechlorethamine use. Hot flashes are a common complaint in patients using tamoxifen. Shortness of breath can result from pulmonary fibrosis secondary to busulfan or bleomycin use.

6. **The answer is A.** Etoposide is used in the treatment of small-cell lung carcinomas as well as testicular tumors. Its mechanism of action is related to its ability to inhibit topoisomerase II. Methotrexate inhibits dihydrofolate reductase. Alkylating agents include mechlorethamine, cyclophosphamide, and ifosfamide. Paclitaxel and docetaxel stabilize microtubules and thereby disrupt mitosis. Bleomycin causes DNA chain scission and fragmentation.

7. **The answer is E.** Doxorubicin is associated with dose-limiting cardiomyopathy. Before using this agent, a thorough cardiac evaluation is required, including an echocardiogram or nuclear medicine scan of the heart. Hemorrhagic cystitis is a complication of cyclophosphamide, prevented by co-administration of MESNA. Acne is a side effect of prednisone and EGFR inhibitors. Peripheral neuropathy is a result of taxanes such as paclitaxel. Hot flashes often accompany tamoxifen use.

8. **The answer is B.** Bleomycin is included in the treatment of metastatic testicular neoplasms and can cause pulmonary fibrosis. Busulfan can also cause pulmonary fibrosis; however, it is not used in the treatment of testicular neoplasms. Cisplatin is highly emetogenic and can cause nephrotoxicity as well as ototoxicity. Aminoglutethimide is an inhibitor of steroid synthesis used in Cushing syndrome as well as in some cases of breast cancer. Cyclophosphamide can cause hemorrhagic cystitis.

9. **The answer is B.** Rituximab is used in conjunction with cyclophosphamide, hydroxydaunomycin (doxorubicin), vincristine, and prednisone (R-CHOP), one of the regimens for non-Hodgkin lymphoma. Traztuzumab is used for HER2$^+$ breast cancer. Dactinomycin is a protein synthesis inhibitor used to treat such pediatric tumors as rhabdomyosarcoma

and Wilms tumor. L-Asparaginase is a recombinant enzyme used to treat leukemias. Lastly, interferon-α can be used to treat hairy cell leukemia.

10. **The answer is E.** ABVD is a treatment regimen used for Hodgkin disease and includes adriamycin, bleomycin, vinblastine, and dacarbazine. R-CHOP is used for treating non-Hodgkin's disease. CMF, or cyclophosphamide, methotrexate, and fluorouracil, is used for breast cancer. FOLFOX, a regimen that uses 5-fluorouracil, oxaliplatin, and leucovorin, is used in the treatment of colon cancer. BEP (bleomycin, etoposide, and platinum [cisplatin]) is used in the management of metastatic testicular neoplasms.

11. **The answer is C.** Anastrozole is an aromatase inhibitor used to inhibit estrogen synthesis in the adrenal gland, a principle source in postmenopausal women. Hydroxyurea is used in the treatment of some leukemias as well as myeloproliferative disorders. Leuprolide and goserelin are GNRH antagonists used to treat prostate cancer. Carboplatin is used in the treatment of ovarian cancers and others.

12. **The answer is C.** Imatinib is an orally active small molecule inhibitor of the oncogenic Bcr–Abl kinase produced as a result of the Philadelphia chromosome, used to treat CML. It also inhibits the c-Kit receptor and can be used in GI stromal tumors (GISTs). Anastrozole is used in the management of breast cancer. Rituximab is an antibody used in the treatment of non-Hodgkin lymphoma. Gefitinib is an orally active small-molecule inhibitor of the EGF receptor used in the treatment of some lung cancers. Amifostine is used as a radio-protectant with or without cisplatin.

13. **The answer is D.** Bevacizumab is a monoclonal antibody against vascular endothelial growth factor (VEGF) interaction with its receptor. Trastuzumab is also a monoclonal antibody, but it inhibits HER2/neu signaling.

14. **The answer is D.** Temozolomide is an orally active alkylating agent related to dacarbazine', which is used along with radiation for the treatment of glioblastoma multiforme and other high-grade astrocytomas. Thalidomide is used in the treatment of multiple myeloma. Thioguanine and mercaptopurine are purine analogs that are used primarily in acute lymphoblastic leukemia. Cisplatin is also often used with radiation in tumors of the lung, head, and neck.

15. **The answer is B.** Leuprolide is used to treat metastatic prostate cancer by decreasing the secretion of luteinizing hormone (LH) and follicle-stimulating hormone (FSH) from the pituitary, leading to decreased testosterone, used by the tumor cells to grow. Anastrozole is used in breast cancer in postmenopausal women to decrease the estrogen levels. Tamoxifen is also used in the treatment of breast cancer to inhibit estrogen-mediated gene transcription. Mitotane is used in the treatment of inoperable adrenocortical carcinomas. Prednisone is used in the treatment of leukemias and lymphomas.

16. **The answer is E.** Irinotecan and topotecan are two antineoplastic agents that inhibit DNA topoisomerase I. Etoposide and teniposide are epipodophyllotoxins that inhibit DNA topoisomerase II. Ciprofloxacin is an antibiotic that inhibits bacterial DNA topoisomerase I. Vinorelbine is a vinca alkaloid that disrupts microtubule assembly.

17. **The answer is A.** Patients with estrogen receptor-positive tumors benefit from tamoxifen adjunct treatment. It, however, carries a risk of thromboembolism as well as the potential to develop endometrial cancer. Bevacizumab has been associated with the risk of bowel perforation. Many traditional chemotherapeutic agents are associated with myelosuppression, and in fact, that is the mechanism for the effects against leukemias. The antibiotic chloramphenicol has been associated with both myelosuppression and aplastic anemia. Many of the therapeutic monoclonal antibodies can cause infusional hypotension.

chapter 13 | Toxicology

I. PRINCIPLES AND TERMINOLOGY

A. Toxicology is concerned with the deleterious effects of physical and chemical agents (including drugs) in humans (Table 13.1).

1. *Occupational toxicology* is concerned with chemicals encountered in the workplace (there are over 100,000 in commercial use). For many of these agents (air pollutants and solvents), the **threshold limit values** (TLVs) are defined in either parts per million (ppm) or milligrams per cubic meter (mg/m^3) (Table 13.2). These limits are either time-weighted averages (TLV-TWA; i.e., concentrations for a workday or workweek); short-term exposure limits (TLV-STEL), which reflect the maximum concentration that should not be exceeded in a 15-minute interval; or ceilings (TLV-C), which are the concentrations to which a worker should never be exposed.

2. *Environmental toxicology* is concerned with substances encountered in food, air, water, and soil; some chemicals that enter the food chain are defined in terms of their **acceptable daily intake (ADI)**, the level at which they are considered safe even if taken daily. **Ecotoxicology** is concerned with the toxic effects of physical and chemical agents on populations and organisms in a defined ecosystem.

B. The dose–response relationship implies that higher doses of a drug or toxicant in an individual can result in a graded response and that higher doses in a population result in a larger percentage of individuals responding to the agent (quantal dose–response). The most commonly used index of toxicity for drugs used therapeutically is the **therapeutic index** (TI), which is defined as the ratio of the dose of drug that produces a toxic effect (TD_{50}) or a lethal effect (LD_{50}) to the dose that produces a therapeutic effect (ED_{50}) in 50% of the population as determined from quantal dose–response curves for toxicity and therapeutic effect.

C. Risk and hazard: Risk is defined as the expected frequency of occurrence of unwanted effects of a physical or chemical agent. The benefits to risks ratios influence the acceptability of compounds. Hazard is defined as the ability of a toxicant to cause harm in a specific setting; it relates to the amount of a physical or chemical agent to which an individual will be exposed.

D. No-observable-effect level (**NOEL**) is defined as the **highest dose of a chemical that does not produce an observable effect in humans**. This value, based on animal studies, is used for chemicals for which a full dose–response curve for toxicity in humans is unknown or unattainable. The ADI of a chemical according to the World Health Organization (WHO) is the "daily intake of a chemical, which during the entire lifetime appears to be without appreciable risk on the basis of all known facts at that time." ADI values are calculated from NOELs and certain other "uncertainty" factors, including estimated differences in human and animal sensitivity to the toxic agent.

t a b l e **13.1**	Acute and Evident Changes in the Poisoned Patient and Possible Causes
Changes	**Causes**
Cardiorespiratory abnormalities	
Hypertension, tachycardia	Amphetamines, cocaine, phencyclidine (PCP), nicotine, antimuscarinic drugs
Hypotension, bradycardia	Opioids, clonidine, β-receptor blocking agents, sedative-hypnotics
Hypotension, tachycardia	Tricyclic antidepressants, phenothiazines, theophylline
Rapid respiration	Sympathomimetics (including amphetamines, salicylates), carbon monoxide, any toxin that produces metabolic acidosis (including alcohol)
Hyperthermia	Sympathomimetics, salicylates, antimuscarinics, most drugs that induce seizures or rigidity
Hypothermia	Alcohol, phenothiazines, sedatives
Central nervous system effects	
Nystagmus, dysarthria, ataxia	Phenytoin, alcohol, sedatives
Rigidity, muscular hypertension	Phencyclidine, haloperidol, sympathomimetics
Seizures	Tricyclic antidepressants, theophylline, isoniazid, phenothiazines
Flaccid coma	Opioids and sedative hypnotics
Hallucinations	LSD, poisonous plants (nightshade, jimsonweed)
Gastrointestinal changes	
Ileus	Antimuscarinics, narcotics, sedatives
Cramping, diarrhea, increased bowel sounds	Organophosphates, arsenic, iron, theophylline, *Amanita phalloides*
Nausea, vomiting	*Amanita phalloides*
Visual disturbances	
Miosis (constriction)	Clonidine, opioids, phenothiazines, cholinesterase inhibitors (including organophosphate insecticides)
Mydriasis (dilation)	Amphetamines, cocaine, LSD, antimuscarinics (including atropine)
Nystagmus	Phenytoin, alcohol, sedatives (including barbiturates), phencyclidine
Ptosis, ophthalmoplegia	Botulism
Skin changes	
Flushed, hot, dry skin	Antimuscarinics (including atropine)
Excessive sweating	Nicotine, sympathomimetics, organophosphates
Cyanosis	Drugs that induce hypoxemia or methemoglobinemia
Icterus	Hepatic damage from acetaminophen or *Amanita phalloides*
Mouth and taste alterations	Caustic substances
Burns	Garlicky breath: arsenic, organophosphates
Odors	Bitter almond breath; cyanide
	Rotten egg odor: hydrogen sulfide
	Pear-like odor: chloral hydrate
	Chemical smell: alcohol, hydrocarbon solvents, paraldehyde, gasoline, ammonia
Green tongue	Vanadium
Metallic taste	Lead, cadmium

E. Duration of Exposure is Used to Classify Toxic Response

1. **Acute exposure** resulting in a toxic reaction represents a single exposure or multiple exposures over 1–2 days.
2. **Chronic exposure** resulting in a toxic reaction represents multiple exposures over longer periods of time.
3. **Delayed toxicity** represents the appearance of a toxic effect after a delayed interval following exposure.

F. Route of exposure can determine the extent of toxicity and outcome (e.g., **anthrax** exposure).

G. Most toxicants to which humans are exposed (e.g., **heavy metals**) cause toxic effects directly, including binding to functional groups on proteins containing O, S, and N atoms. In other

t a b l e **13.2**	Threshold Limit Values for Selected Air Pollutants and Solvents		
		TLV (ppm)	
		TWA	*STEL*
Air Pollutant			
Carbon monoxide		25	–
Nitrogen dioxide		3	5
Ozone		0.05	–
Sulfur dioxide		2	5
Solvent			
Benzene		0.5	2.5
Carbon tetrachloride		5	10
Chloroform		10	–
Toluene		50	–

instances, in a process referred to as **toxication** (or bioactivation), a substance may be converted in the body to a chemical form that is directly toxic or participates in reactions that generate other highly reactive toxic species, such as **superoxide anion (O_2^-)** and **hydroxyl (OH) free radicals** and **hydrogen peroxide (H_2O_2)**, which can cause DNA, protein, and cell membrane damage and loss of function.

H. Endogenous **glutathione** plays a central role in detoxication of these reactive species either directly, or coupled to **superoxide dismutase** and **glutathione peroxidase** (Fig. 13.1). Superoxide dismutase coupled to **catalase** is also involved in detoxication pathways (Fig. 13.1). Endogenous metallothionine offers some limited protection from metal toxicity.

II. AIR POLLUTANTS

A. **General Characteristics**
   1. Air pollutants enter the body primarily through inhalation and are either absorbed into the blood (e.g., gases) or eliminated by the lungs (e.g., particulates). Five major agents account for 98% of known air pollutants (see below). Ozone is also of special concern in certain geographic locations.
   2. Air pollutants are characterized as either **reducing types** (sulfur oxides) or **oxidizing types** (nitrogen oxides, hydrocarbons, and photochemical oxidants).

B. **Carbon Monoxide (CO)**
   1. *Properties and mechanism of action*
      a. Carbon monoxide is a colorless, odorless, nonirritating gas produced from the incomplete combustion of organic matter. It is the **most frequent cause of death from poisoning** (see Table 13.2 for threshold limit values).
      b. Carbon monoxide competes for and **combines with the oxygen-binding site of hemoglobin to form carboxyhemoglobin**, resulting in a functional anemia. The binding affinity of carbon monoxide for hemoglobin is 220 times higher than that of oxygen itself. Carboxyhemoglobin also interferes with the dissociation in tissues of the remaining oxyhemoglobin.
      c. Carbon monoxide also binds to cellular respiratory cytochromes.
      d. CO concentrations of 0.1% (1,000 ppm) in air will result in 50% carboxyhemoglobinemia. Smokers may routinely exceed normal carboxyhemoglobin levels of 1% by up to 10 times.

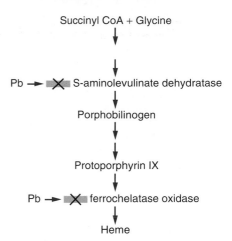

FIGURE 13.1. Inhibition of heme synthesis by lead (Pb).

2. *Poisoning and treatment*
   a. CO intoxication (>15% carboxyhemoglobin) results in **progressive hypoxia**. Symptoms include headache, dizziness, nausea, vomiting, syncope, seizures, and at carboxyhemoglobin concentrations above 40%, a cherry-red appearance and coma.
   b. Chronic low-level exposure may be harmful to the cardiovascular system. Populations at special risk include smokers with ischemic heart disease or anemia, the elderly, and the developing fetus.
   c. **Treatment** includes removal from the source of CO, maintenance of respiration, and administration of oxygen. Hyperbaric oxygen may be required in severe poisoning.

C. Sulfur Dioxide (SO$_2$)
   1. *Properties and mechanism of action*
      a. Sulfur dioxide is a colorless, irritant gas produced by the combustion of sulfur-containing fuels (see Table 13.2 for threshold limit values).
      b. Sulfur dioxide is converted to some extent in the atmosphere to **sulfuric acid** (H$_2$SO$_4$), which has irritant effects similar to those of sulfur dioxide.
   2. *Poisoning and treatment*
      a. At low levels (5 ppm), SO$_2$ has irritant effects on exposed membranes (eyes, mucous membranes, skin, and upper respiratory tract with bronchoconstriction). Asthmatics are more susceptible. **Delayed pulmonary edema** may be observed after severe exposure.
      b. SO$_2$ poisoning is treated by therapeutic interventions that reduce irritation in the respiratory tract.

D. Nitrogen Dioxide (NO$_2$)
   1. *Properties and mechanism of action*
      a. Nitrogen dioxide is an irritant brown gas produced in fires and from decaying silage. It is also produced from a reaction of nitrogen oxide (from auto exhaust) with O$_2$ (see Table 13.2 for threshold limit values).
      b. Nitrogen dioxide causes the degeneration of alveolar type I cells, with rupture of alveolar capillary endothelium.
   2. *Poisoning and treatment*
      a. Acute symptoms include irritation of eyes and nose, coughing, dyspnea, and chest pain.
      b. Severe exposure for 1–2 hours may result in **pulmonary edema** that may subside and then recur more than 2 weeks later. Chronic low-level exposure may also result in pulmonary edema.
      c. NO$_2$ poisoning is treated with therapeutic interventions that reduce pulmonary irritation and cdcma.

E. Ozone (O_3)
   1. *Properties and mechanism of action*
      a. Ozone is an irritating, naturally occurring bluish gas found in high levels in polluted air and around high-voltage equipment (see Table 13.2 for threshold limit values).
      b. Ozone is formed by a complex series of reactions involving NO_2 absorption of ultraviolet light with the generation of free oxygen.
      c. Ozone causes functional pulmonary changes similar to those with NO_2. Toxicity may result from free radical formation.
   2. *Poisoning and treatment*
      a. Ozone irritates mucous membranes and can cause decreased pulmonary compliance, pulmonary edema, and increased sensitivity to bronchoconstrictors. Chronic exposure may cause decreased respiratory reserve, bronchitis, and pulmonary fibrosis.
      b. Treatment is similar to that used in NO_2 poisoning.

F. Hydrocarbons
   1. Hydrocarbons are oxidized by sunlight and by incomplete combustion to short-lived aldehydes such as **formaldehyde** and **acrolein**; aldehydes are also found in, and can be released from, certain construction materials.
   2. Hydrocarbons irritate the mucous membranes of the respiratory tract and eyes, producing a response similar to that seen with SO_2 exposure.

G. Particulates
   1. Inhalation of particulates can lead to **pneumoconiosis**, most commonly caused by **silicates (silicosis)** or **asbestos (asbestosis). Bronchial cancer** and **mesothelioma** are associated with asbestos exposure, particularly in conjunction with cigarette smoking.
   2. Particulates adsorb other toxins, such as polycyclic aromatic hydrocarbons, and deliver them to the respiratory tract.
   3. Particulates also increase susceptibility to pulmonary dysfunction and disease. They may yield fibrotic masses in the lungs that develop over years of exposure.

III. SOLVENTS

A. Aliphatic and Halogenated Aliphatic Hydrocarbons
   1. Aliphatic and halogenated aliphatic hydrocarbons include fuels and industrial solvents such as ***n*-hexane, gasoline, kerosene, carbon tetrachloride, chloroform**, and **tetrachloroethylene** (see Table 13.2 for threshold limit values).
   2. These agents are central nervous system (CNS) depressants and cause neurologic, liver, and kidney damage. Cardiotoxicity is also possible.
   3. *Polyneuropathy* from cytoskeletal disruption predominates with ***n*-hexane** poisoning. **Neural effects**, such as memory loss and peripheral neuropathy, predominate with **chloroform** and **tetrachloroethylene** exposure. **Chloroform** also causes **nephrotoxicity**.
   4. *Hepatotoxicity* (delayed) and **renal toxicity** are common with carbon tetrachloride poisoning. **Carcinogenicity** has been associated with **chloroform, carbon tetrachloride**, and **tetrachloroethylene**. All of these effects may be mediated by free radical interaction with cellular lipids and proteins.
   5. *Chloroform* can sensitize the heart to **arrhythmias**.
   6. Aspiration with **chemical pneumonitis** and **pulmonary edema** is common.
   7. *Treatment* is primarily supportive and is oriented to the organ systems involved.

B. Aromatic Hydrocarbons
   1. *Benzene*: Of this class of solvents, benzene poisoning is the **most common; CNS depression is the major acute effect**. Chronic exposure can result in severe **bone marrow depression**, resulting in aplastic anemia and other blood dyscrasias. Low-level benzene exposure has been linked to leukemia. No specific treatment is available for benzene poisoning.

2. ***Toluene, Xylene*** depress the CNS. They can cause fatigue and ataxia at relatively low levels and loss of consciousness at high levels (10,000 ppm).

C. **Polychlorinated Biphenyls (PCBs)**
   1. PCBs are stable, highly lipophilic agents that, although not used since 1977, still persist in the environment.
   2. Dermatologic disorders are the most common adverse effect. Possible reproductive dysfunction and carcinogenic effects linked to PCBs may be largely due to other contaminating polychlorinated agents such as the **dioxin**, 2,3,7,8-tetrachlorodibenzo-p-dioxin **(TCDD)**.

IV. INSECTICIDES AND HERBICIDES

A. **Organophosphorus Insecticides**
   1. ***Properties and mechanism of action***
      a. Organophosphorus insecticides include **parathion, malathion**, and **diazinon**.
      b. Organophosphorus insecticides have replaced **organochlorine pesticides** (except for a very restricted use in the U.S. of dichlorodiphenyltrichloroethane, i.e., **DDT**), which persist in the environment and have been associated with an increased risk of cancer. Organophosphorus insecticides do not persist in the environment; however, their potential for acute toxicity is higher.
      c. Organophosphorus insecticides are characterized by their ability to **phosphorylate the active esteratic site of acetylcholinesterase (AChE)**. Toxic effects result from acetylcholine (ACh) accumulation (see Chapter 2).
      d. These agents are well absorbed through the skin and via the respiratory and gastrointestinal (GI) tracts.
      e. Some other organophosphate insecticide compounds (e.g., **triorthocresylphosphate**) also phosphorylate a "neuropathy target esterase," which results in **delayed neurotoxicity** with sensory and motor disturbances of the limbs.
   2. ***Treatment of poisoning***
      a. Assisted respiration and decontamination are needed as soon as possible to prevent the irreversible inhibition ("aging") of AChE, which involves strengthening of the phosphorus–enzyme bond.
      b. **Atropine** reverses all muscarinic effects but does not reverse neuromuscular activation or paralysis.
      c. **Pralidoxime** (2-PAM) (Protopam) reactivates AChE, particularly at the neuromuscular junction. It is often used as an adjunct to **atropine** (may reverse some toxic effects); however, it is very effective in **parathion** poisoning.

B. **Carbamate Insecticides**
   1. Carbamate insecticides include, among others, **carbaryl, carbofuran, isolan**, and **pyramat**.
   2. These agents are characterized by their ability to **inhibit AChE by carbamoylation**.
   3. Carbamate insecticides produce toxic effects similar to those of the phosphorus-containing insecticides. Generally, the toxic effects of carbamate compounds are less severe than those of the organophosphorus agents because carbamoylation is rapidly reversible.
   4. Treatment for carbamate poisoning is similar to that used for organophosphate poisoning except that pralidoxime therapy is not an effective antidote because it does not interact with carbamylated acetylcholinesterase.

C. **Botanical Insecticides**
   1. ***Nicotine*** stimulates nicotinic receptors and results in membrane depolarization. Poisoning is characterized by salivation, vomiting, muscle weakness, seizures, and respiratory arrest; it can be treated with anticonvulsants and agents for symptomatic relief (see Chapters 2 and 5).

2. *Pyrethrum*, a common household insecticide, is toxic only at high levels. Allergic manifestations and irritation of the skin and respiratory tract are the most common adverse effects. These are treated symptomatically.

3. *Rotenone* poisoning is rare in humans and generally results in GI disturbances that are treated symptomatically.

D. Herbicides

1. *Glyphosate*, now widely used world-wide, is a relatively safe herbicide that does not persist in the environment. Its major reported adverse effects are irritation of the skin and eyes.

2. *Paraquat*

   a. Paraquat causes acute GI irritation with bloody stools, followed by delayed respiratory distress and the development of **congestive hemorrhagic pulmonary edema**, which is thought to be caused by superoxide radical formation and subsequent cell membrane disruption. Death may ensue several weeks after ingestion.

   b. Treatment consists of prompt gastric lavage; administration of cathartics and adsorbents benefits some victims.

3. *2,4-Dichlorophenoxyacetic acid (2,4-D)* causes neuromuscular paralysis and coma. Long-term toxic effects are rare. 2,4,5-Trichlorophenoxyacetic acid (2,4,5-D-T; "agent orange") is no longer used.

E. Fumigants and Rodenticide: Cyanide

1. Cyanide possesses a high affinity for ferric iron; it **reacts with iron and cytochrome oxidase** in mitochondria to inhibit cellular respiration, thereby blocking oxygen use.

2. It is absorbed from all routes (except alkali salts, which are toxic only when ingested).

3. Poisoning is signaled by bright red venous blood and a characteristic **odor of bitter almonds**.

4. Cyanide causes transient CNS stimulation followed by **hypoxic seizures** and death.

5. Treatment must be immediate with administration of 100% oxygen. **Amyl or sodium nitrite**, which oxidizes hemoglobin and produces methemoglobin, which effectively competes for cyanide ion, can also be administered. **Sodium thiosulfate** can be administered to accelerate the conversion of cyanide to nontoxic thiocyanate by mitochondrial rhodanase (sulfurtransferase). Activated charcoal may also be used. Hydroxocobalamin, which binds with cyanide, is also available as an antidote.

V. HEAVY METAL POISONING AND MANAGEMENT

A. Inorganic Lead Poisoning

1. Historically, paint and gasoline were major sources of lead exposure and still can be found in the environment. Other sources of inorganic lead include "home crafts" such as pottery and jewelry making. Organic lead poisoning is increasingly rare due to phased elimination of tetraethyl and tetramethyl lead (antiknock components in gasoline).

2. Inorganic metallic lead oxides and salts are slowly absorbed through all routes except the skin. Organic lead compounds are also well absorbed across the skin. The GI route is the most common route of exposure in nonindustrial settings (children absorb a higher fraction than adults); the respiratory route is more common for industrial exposure.

3. Inorganic lead binds to hemoglobin in erythrocytes, with the remainder distributing to soft tissues such as the brain and kidney. Through redistribution, it later accumulates in bone, where its elimination half-life is 20–30 years.

4. **CNS effects** (lead encephalopathy) are common after chronic exposure to lead, particularly in children, for whom no threshold level has been established. Early signs of poisoning include vertigo, ataxia, headache, restlessness, and irritability; **wristdrop** is a common sign of **peripheral neuropathy**. Projectile vomiting, delirium, and seizures may occur with the progression of encephalopathy with lead concentrations >100 µg/dL. Mental deterioration with lowered IQ and behavioral abnormalities may be a consequence of childhood exposure.

  5. GI upset, including epigastric distress, is also seen, particularly in adults. Constipation and a metallic taste are early signs of exposure to lead. Intestinal spasm with severe pain (lead colic) may become evident in advanced stages of poisoning. Renal fibrosis may also occur with chronic exposure. Lead also may increase spontaneous abortion. It is associated with altered production of sperm.

B. Inorganic Arsenic
  1. *Properties and mechanism of action*
     a. Inorganic arsenic can be found in coal and metal ores, herbicides, seafood, and drinking water. It is absorbed through the GI tract and lungs.
     b. Trivalent forms (arsenites) of inorganic arsenic are generally more toxic than the pentavalent forms (arsenates). Methylated metabolites may account for their adverse effect.
     c. **Arsenites inhibit sulfhydryl enzymes** (pyruvate dehydrogenase/glycolysis is especially sensitive), resulting in damage to the epithelial lining of the GI and respiratory tracts and damage to tissues of the nervous system, liver, bone marrow, and skin.
     d. Arsenates uncouple mitochondrial oxidative phosphorylation by "substituting" for inorganic phosphate.
     e. Symptoms of acute poisoning include severe nausea, vomiting, abdominal pain, laryngitis, and bronchitis; capillary damage with dehydration and shock may occur. Diarrhea is characterized as "rice-water stools." There is often a garlicky breath odor.
     f. Initial episodes of arsenic poisoning may be fatal; if the individual survives, bone marrow depression, severe neuropathy, and encephalopathy may occur.
     g. Symptoms of chronic poisoning include weight loss due to GI irritation; perforation of the nasal septum; hair loss; sensory neuropathy; depression of bone marrow function; and kidney and liver damage. The skin often appears pale and milky ("milk and roses" complexion) because of anemia and vasodilation. Skin pigmentation, hyperkeratosis of the palms and soles, and white lines over the nails may be observed after prolonged exposure. Inorganic arsenicals have been implicated in cancers of the respiratory system.
     h. **Treatment** is primarily supportive after acute poisoning and involves termination of exposure, emesis, gastric lavage, rehydration, and restoration of electrolyte imbalance. Chelation therapy with **dimercaprol** (BAL) or its analogue, **unithol**, is indicated in severe cases. **Succimer**, another derivative of dimercaprol, may also be used. Treatment of chronic poisoning is supportive, including termination of exposure.
     i. Organic arsenicals are excreted more readily and are less toxic than inorganic forms; poisoning is rare.
  2. **Arsine gas** (AsH_3) poisoning may occur in industrial settings. The effects are **severe hemolysis** and subsequent renal failure; symptoms include jaundice, dark urine, and severe abdominal pain. Treatment includes **transfusion** and **hemodialysis** for renal failure. Chelation therapy is ineffective.

C. Mercury
  1. *Inorganic mercury*
     a. **Properties and mechanism of action**
        (1) Inorganic mercury occurs as a potential hazard primarily because of occupational or industrial exposure. The major source of poisoning is by consumption of contaminated food.
        (2) **Elemental mercury (Hg)** is poorly absorbed by the GI tract but is volatile and can be absorbed by the lungs. Hg itself causes CNS effects; the ionized form, **Hg^{2+}**, accumulates in the kidneys and causes damage in the proximal tubules by combining with **sulfhydryl enzymes**.
        (3) **Mercuric chloride ($HgCl_2$)** is well absorbed by the GI tract and is toxic.
        (4) **Mercurous chloride (HgCl)** is also absorbed by the GI tract but is less toxic than $HgCl_2$.

    b. Acute poisoning and treatment

       (1) Mercury vapor poisoning produces chest pain, shortness of breath, nausea, vomiting, and a metallic taste. Chemical pneumonitis and gingivostomatitis may also occur. Muscle tremor and psychopathology can develop.

       (2) Inorganic mercury salts

         (a) Inorganic mercury salts cause hemorrhagic gastroenteritis producing intense pain and vomiting. Hypovolemic shock may also occur.

         (b) Renal tubular necrosis is the most prevalent and serious systemic toxicity.

    c. Treatment involves removal from exposure, supportive care, and chelation therapy with **dimercaprol, unithol**, or **succimer**. Hemodialysis may be necessary.

    d. Chronic poisoning

       (1) Mercury vapor poisoning may lead to a **fine tremor** of the limbs that may progress to choreiform movements, and **neuropsychiatric symptoms** that may include insomnia, fatigue, anorexia, and memory loss, as well as changes in mood and affect. **Gingivostomatitis** is also common. Erethism (a combination of excessive perspiration and blushing) may also occur. Excessive salivation and gingivitis are often present.

       (2) Inorganic mercury salts. Renal injury predominates. Erythema of extremities **(acrodynia)** is often coupled with anorexia, tachycardia, and GI disturbances.

       (3) For the treatment, unithol or succimer may be helpful. Dimercaprol should be avoided as it will redistribute mercury to the CNS.

  2. *Organic mercurials (methylmercury)*

    a. Organic mercurials are found in seed dressings and fungicides.

    b. Organic mercurials can be absorbed from the GI tract and often distribute to the CNS, where they exert their toxic effects, including paresthesias, ataxia, and hearing impairment. **Visual disturbances** often predominate.

    c. Exposure of the fetus to methylmercury in utero may result in mental retardation and a syndrome resembling cerebral palsy.

    d. Treatment is primarily supportive. Unithol or succimer may be helpful.

D. Iron (see Chapter 7)

E. Metal-chelating Agents

  1. *General properties*

    a. Metal-chelating agents usually contain two or more electronegative groups that form stable coordinate-covalent complexes with cationic metals that can then be excreted from the body. The greater the number of metal–ligand bonds, the more stable the complex and the greater the efficiency of the chelator.

    b. These agents contain functional groups such as –OH, –SH, and –NH, which compete for metal binding with similar groups on cell proteins. Their effects are generally greater when administered soon after exposure.

  2. *Ethylenediamine tetraacetic acid (EDTA)*

    a. EDTA is an efficient chelator of many transition metals. Since it can also chelate body calcium, **EDTA** is administered intramuscularly or by intravenous (IV) infusion as the **disodium salt of calcium**.

    b. EDTA is rapidly excreted by glomerular filtration.

    c. This agent is used primarily in the treatment of **lead poisoning**.

    d. EDTA is nephrotoxic, particularly of renal tubules, at high doses. Maintenance of urine flow and short-term treatment can minimize this effect.

  3. *Dimercaprol (BAL)*

    a. Dimercaprol is an oily, foul-smelling liquid administered intramuscularly as a 10% solution in peanut oil.

    b. Dimercaprol interacts with metals, reactivating or preventing the inactivation of cellular sulfhydryl-containing enzymes. It is most effective if administered immediately following exposure.

    c. This agent is useful in **arsenic, inorganic mercury**, and lead poisoning (with EDTA). It may redistribute arsenic and mercury to the CNS and is, therefore, not recommended for the treatment of chronic poisoning with these agents.

    d. The adverse effects of dimercaprol include tachycardia, hypertension, gastric irritation, and pain at the injection site.

    e. **Succimer** (Chemax) is a derivative of dimercaprol that can be taken orally and is approved for use in children to treat **lead poisoning**. It does not mobilize other essential metals to any appreciable extent. The adverse effects of succimer are generally minor and include nausea, vomiting, and anorexia. A rash indicating hypersensitivity may require the termination of therapy. It is also used to treat **arsenic** and **mercury** poisoning.

    f. **Unithol** (Dimaval) is another analogue of dimercaprol used to treat acute **arsenic** and **inorganic mercury** poisoning. Skin reactions are its most common adverse effect.

4. *Penicillamine (Cuprimine, Depen)*

    a. Penicillamine, a derivative of penicillin, is used primarily to chelate excess copper in individuals with **Wilson's disease**.

    b. Allergic reactions and rare **bone marrow toxicity** and **renal toxicity** are the major adverse effects.

5. *Deferoxamine (Desferal), Desferasirox (Exjade)*

    a. Deferoxamine is a specific **iron-chelating agent** that on parenteral administration binds with ferric ions to form ferrioxamine; it also binds to ferrous ions. Deferoxamine can also remove iron from ferritin and hemosiderin outside bone marrow, but it does not capture iron from hemoglobin, cytochromes, or myoglobin.

    b. Deferoxamine is metabolized by plasma enzymes and is excreted by the kidney, turning urine red.

    c. Rapid IV infusion of deferoxamine may result in hypotensive shock due to the release of histamine. It may also be administered intramuscularly.

    d. Deferoxamine may cause allergic reactions and rare **neurotoxicity** or **renal toxicity**. Deferoxamine therapy is contraindicated in patients with renal disease or renal failure.

    e. **Desferasirox** is an oral iron chelator approved for the treatment of **iron overload.**

VI. DRUG POISONING

A. General Management of the Poisoned Patient (see Table 13.1)
1. Observe vital signs.
2. Obtain history.
3. Perform a toxicologically oriented physical examination.

B. Symptoms
1. More than a million cases of acute poisoning occur each year in the United States, many in children and adolescents.
2. The symptoms of most drug and chemical poisonings are extensions of their pharmacologic properties. The common causes of death include CNS depression with respiratory arrest, seizures, cardiovascular abnormalities with severe hypotension and arrhythmias, cellular hypoxia, and hypothermia.

C. Treatment: Measures to support vital functions, slow drug absorption, and promote excretion are generally sufficient for the treatment. If available, specific antidotes can also be used.

1. *Vital function support*

    a. In the presence of severe CNS depression, it is important to clear the **airway** and maintain adequate **breathing** and **circulation (ABC)**. Comatose patients may die as a result of airway obstruction, respiratory arrest, or aspiration of gastric contents into the tracheobronchial tube.

b. Other important supportive measures include maintaining electrolyte balance and maintaining vascular fluid volume with IV **dextrose infusion (D)**.

2. ***Drug absorption***

   a. Drug absorption may be slowed or prevented by decontamination of the skin. Induction of vomiting with **ipecac syrup** orally is no longer recommended for routine use at home, and is contraindicated in children under 6 years. Its use is also limited in the emergency room in favor of activated charcoal.

   b. Emesis is **contraindicated** if corrosives have been ingested (reflux may perforate the stomach or esophagus), petroleum distillates have been ingested (may induce chemical pneumonia if aspirated), the patient is comatose or delirious and may aspirate gastric contents, or CNS stimulants have been ingested (may induce seizure activity with stimulation of emesis).

     (1) Gastric lavage is performed only when the airway is protected by an endotracheal tube.

     (2) Chemical adsorption with activated charcoal

       (a) Activated charcoal will bind many toxins and drugs, including **salicylates, acetaminophen**, and **antidepressants**.

       (b) This procedure can be used in combination with gastric lavage.

     (3) Laxatives, such as a **polyethylene glycol electrolyte solution** (e.g., GoLYTELY), are used occasionally to speed up the removal of toxins from the GI tract.

3. ***Promotion of elimination*** may be achieved by the following:

   a. Chemically enhancing urinary excretion: Urinary excretion can be enhanced by the administration of agents such as **sodium bicarbonate** which raises the urinary pH and decreases the renal reabsorption of certain organic acids such as aspirin and phenobarbital.

   b. Hemodialysis is an efficient way to remove certain low molecular weight, water-soluble toxins and restore electrolyte balance. **Salicylate, methanol, ethanol, ethylene glycol, paraquat**, and **lithium** poisonings are effectively treated this way; hemoperfusion may enhance the whole-body clearance of some agents **(carbamazepine, phenobarbital, and phenytoin)**. Drugs and poisons with large volumes of distribution are not effectively removed by dialysis.

4. ***Antidotes*** (see respective agents) are available for some poisons and should be used when a specific toxin is identified. Some examples include **naloxone, flumazenil, acetylcysteine, physostigmine, metal chelators** (see above), **atropine, pralidoxime,** and **ethanol**.

▨ DRUG SUMMARY TABLE

Deferasirox (Exjade)	EDTA (ethylenediamine tetraacetic	Pralidoxime (Protopam)
Deferoxamine (Desferal)	acid) (calcium disodium versenate)	Succimer (Chemet)
Dimercaprol (BAL)	Penicillamine (Cuprimine, Depen)	Unithol (Dimaval)

Review Test

Directions: Each of the numbered items or incomplete statements in this section is followed by answers or by completions of the statement. Select the ONE-lettered answer or completion that is BEST in each case.

1. What treatment would be appropriate in a 3-year-old boy with a dramatically elevated blood level of lead?

(A) Pyridoxine
(B) Glucagon
(C) Digibind
(D) Calcium disodium EDTA
(E) Deferoxamine

2. A 56-year-old chronic alcoholic is brought to the emergency room with altered mental status and complains of not being able to see. He reports running out of "whiskey" and ingesting wood alcohol (methanol). His laboratory test results demonstrate a severe anion gap and acute renal failure. Which of the following would be an appropriate therapy?

(A) Hyperbaric oxygen
(B) Fomepizole
(C) Lidocaine
(D) Ethylene glycol
(E) Methylene blue

3. An 18-year-old man is brought to the emergency room by his friends because he "passed out." His friends tell the physician that they were at a party and the patient drank a couple of beers and took several Valium (diazepam). On examination the patient was unresponsive, with decreased respirations (8 per minute). What would be an appropriate treatment?

(A) Flumazenil
(B) Ethyl alcohol
(C) Dextrose
(D) Strychnine
(E) Carbon tetrachloride

4. A 23-year-old known heroin addict is brought to the emergency room for unresponsiveness. On examination he is found to have pin-point pupils and respiratory depression. His fingerstick glucose measurement is normal. What is the most appropriate agent to administer at this point?

(A) Insulin
(B) Naloxone
(C) Dimercaprol
(D) Penicillamine
(E) Atropine

5. A 2-year-old child is brought to the emergency room because he recently ingested numerous "iron pills" his mother was taking for her anemia. The child now has severe abdominal pain, bloody diarrhea, nausea, and vomiting. His serum iron is dramatically elevated. What should be given to treat this toxicity?

(A) Activated charcoal
(B) Mercury vapor
(C) Deferoxamine
(D) Succimer

6. Which of the following is a sensitive indicator of lead toxicity?

(A) Wristdrop
(B) "Rice-water" stools
(C) "Milk and roses" complexion
(D) Odor of bitter almonds

7. Central nervous system (CNS) disturbances and depression are a major toxic effect of

(A) Ionic mercury (Hg^{2+})
(B) Trivalent arsenic
(C) Pentavalent arsenic
(D) Elemental mercury

8. Which of the following toxic agents would pose a systemic problem with dermal exposure?

(A) Inorganic arsenic
(B) Organophosphate insecticides
(C) Inorganic lead
(D) Cadmium

9. Which of the following is the most common result of benzene poisoning?

(A) Central nervous system (CNS) depression
(B) Stimulation of red blood cell production
(C) Delayed hepatotoxicity
(D) Cardiotoxicity

10. Atropine can be used effectively as an antidote to poisoning by which toxic agent?

(A) Parathion
(B) Carbaryl
(C) Methanol
(D) DDT

Answers and Explanations

1. **The answer is D.** Calcium disodium EDTA is a chelator used in the treatment of inorganic lead poisoning. The drug is given intravenously for several days along with dimercaprol. Deferoxamine is used in cases of iron toxicity. Pyridoxine is used in a toxicology setting to reverse seizures due to isoniazid overdose. Digibind is a Fab fragment antibody used in cases of Digoxin toxicity. Glucagon has been used to treat beta-blocker toxicity.

2. **The answer is B.** Fomepizole is an inhibitor of alcohol dehydrogenase, which might otherwise convert methanol to formic acid, which is the true toxin in such cases causing blindness and renal failure. Ethylene glycol (antifreeze) can cause similar toxicity and is also treated with fomepizole. Hyperbaric oxygen is used in the treatment of carbon monoxide poisoning. Lidocaine can be used to help manage arrhythmias in the case of digoxin toxicity. Methylene blue is used in the treatment of methemoglobinemia.

3. **The answer is A.** Flumazenil is a benzodiazepine antagonist used in the management of such overdoses. Ethyl alcohol can be used to treat ingestion of both methanol and ethylene glycol; however, such use often results in ethanol intoxication, and fomepizole is preferred as it does not cause the same effects. Dextrose is an effective treatment for altered mental status due to hypoglycemia in a diabetic patient. Strychnine is a rat poison that can cause seizures when ingested, which are managed by giving diazepam. Carbon tetrachloride is an industrial solvent that can cause fatty liver and kidney damage.

4. **The answer is B.** Given the patient's history and clinical findings, he is likely to be experiencing opioid overdose. The drug of choice in such a scenario is naloxone, an opioid-receptor antagonist. Insulin is used to treat hyperglycemia, which is less likely to cause altered mental status than is hypoglycemia. Dimercaprol is a chelator used in many cases of heavy metal toxicity (i.e., lead). Penicillamine is used in the treatment of copper toxicity, as in Wilson's disease. Atropine is used to treat cholinergic toxicity, which can cause miosis, although an unlikely cause in this clinical presentation.

5. **The answer is C.** Deferoxamine is an iron chelator that is given systemically to bind iron and promote its excretion. Activated charcoal, good for the absorption of numerous toxic ingestions, is ineffective in this case as it does not bind iron. Succimer is an orally available substance related to dimercaprol, and is used for treating lead toxicity. Mercury vapor is toxic and its ingestion is treated with dimercaprol or penicillamine.

6. **The answer is A.** The most common neurologic manifestation of lead poisoning is peripheral neuropathy, a common sign of which is wristdrop. Lead poisoning also affects the hematopoietic system. In children, lead poisoning may be manifested by encephalopathy.

7. **The answer is D.** The central nervous system (CNS) is the major target organ for elemental mercury. Ionic Hg^{2+} predominantly affects the renal system.

8. **The answer is B.** In contrast to the organophosphate insecticides, inorganic forms of arsenic, lead, and cadmium are poorly absorbed through the skin.

9. **The answer is A.** The major acute effect of benzene poisoning is central nervous system (CNS) depression. Chronic exposure may lead to bone marrow depression.

10. **The answer is A.** If administered early in poisoning, atropine reverses the muscarinic cholinoceptor effects of organophosphate insecticides such as parathion, which inhibit acetylcholinesterase (AChE). Pralidoxime (2-PAM) is often used as an adjunct to atropine. Inhibition of AChE by carbamate insecticides such as carbaryl is reversed spontaneously. The toxicity of methanol and chlorophenothane (DDT) is unrelated to acetylcholine action.

Comprehensive Examination

Directions: Each of the numbered items or incomplete statements in this section is followed by answers or by completions of the statement. Select the ONE-lettered answer or completion that is BEST in each case.

1. A 17-year-old male patient was placed on carbamazepine therapy by his neurologist to control newly developed seizures of unknown etiology. The patient was also recently given a macrolide antibiotic by his family physician for a presumed "walking pneumonia." Halfway through his antibiotic course, the patient again developed seizures. What could account for this new seizure activity?

(A) Inhibition of the cytochrome P-450 monooxygenase system
(B) Induction of the cytochrome P-450 monooxygenase system
(C) Impairment of renal excretion of the antiseizure medication
(D) Induction of glucuronyl transferase activity in the liver
(E) Reduction in the amount of nicotinamide adenine dinucleotide phosphate (NADPH)

2. A 21-year-old man sustains multiple blunt traumas after being beaten with a baseball bat by a gang. Aside from his fractures, a serum creatine kinase measurement is dramatically elevated and the trauma team is worried as the myoglobinuria caused by the trauma can cause kidney failure. Although controversial because no randomized trials have been conducted to show efficacy, they immediately begin to administer bicarbonate to alkalinize the urine. How might this serve to decrease myoglobin levels?

(A) Increasing glomerular filtration
(B) Promoting renal tubular secretion
(C) Inhibiting renal tubular reabsorption
(D) Increasing hepatic first-pass metabolism
(E) Inducing the P-450 system

3. Which of the following correctly describes the formula for an intravenous loading dose?

(A) Loading dose = (desired plasma concentration of drug) × (clearance)
(B) Loading dose = (clearance) × (plasma drug concentration)
(C) Loading dose = (0.693) × (volume of distribution)/(clearance)
(D) Loading dose = (amount of drug administered)/(initial plasma concentration)
(E) Loading dose = (desired plasma concentration of the drug) × (volume of distribution)

4. A 32-year-old HIV-positive man follows up with an infectious disease (ID) specialist in the clinic. The results of his recent blood work suggest that the virus has become resistant to multiple nucleoside reverse transcriptase inhibitors. The ID specialist decides to include in the treatment a nonnucleoside inhibitor (nevirapine), which works by binding to a site near the active site on the reverse transcriptase. Nevirapine is an example of what?

(A) Full agonist
(B) Reversible competitive antagonist
(C) Partial agonist
(D) Noncompetitive antagonist
(E) Irreversible competitive antagonist

5. Which of the following drugs is a selective α-adrenergic receptor agonist that is available over the counter?

(A) Epinephrine
(B) Phenylephrine
(C) Isoproterenol
(D) Norepinephrine
(E) Phentolamine

6. Pilocarpine is what type of pharmacologic agent?

(A) Indirect muscarinic agonist
(B) α_2-Adrenergic agonist
(C) Carbonic anhydrase inhibitor
(D) β-Adrenergic antagonist
(E) Direct-acting muscarinic agonist

7. Which of the following is a short-acting acetylcholinesterase inhibitor?

(A) Pyridostigmine
(B) Bethanechol
(C) Edrophonium
(D) Scopolamine
(E) Methantheline

8. Dantrolene

(A) Inhibits calcium release from the sarcoplasmic reticulum
(B) Functions as a $GABA_B$ receptor agonist
(C) Facilitates GABA activity in the central nervous system (CNS)
(D) Reactivates acetylcholinesterase
(E) Competitively inhibits the effects of acetylcholine

9. A 63-year-old man with a history of multiple myocardial infarctions is admitted for shortness of breath. A diagnosis of congestive heart failure is made on clinical grounds, and a cardiologist orders a positive inotropic agent for his heart failure. He is also concerned about maintaining perfusion to the kidneys, so an agent that increases renal blood flow is also desirable. Which of the following agents produces both of these effects?

(A) Epinephrine
(B) Dopamine
(C) Isoproterenol
(D) Terbutaline

10. Clonidine works by

(A) Activating β_1-adrenergic receptors
(B) Activating α_1-adrenergic receptors
(C) Activating β_2-adrenergic receptors
(D) Activating α_2-adrenergic receptors
(E) Blocking β-adrenergic receptors

11. A 23-year-old woman presents with hypertension, anxiety, and palpitations. Her thyroid-stimulating hormone levels are normal, but she has increased levels of urinary catecholamines. She is referred to an endocrine surgeon after a computed tomography (CT) scan shows a unilateral pheochromocytoma. The surgeon should start therapy with which of the following agents prior to removing the lesion?

(A) Dopamine
(B) Phenoxybenzamine
(C) Pancuronium
(D) Pseudoephedrine
(E) Isoproterenol

12. A 45-year-old man with a history remarkable for both asthma and angina now has a kidney stone stuck in his right ureter. The urologist needs to perform cystoscopy, but the anesthesiologist is concerned about using a β-blocker during surgery to control the patient's blood pressure in light of his history of asthma. Ultimately, it is decided to use an ultra-short acting β-blocker and closely monitor both his blood pressure and respiratory status. Which of the following is the best to use in this situation?

(A) Atenolol
(B) Norepinephrine
(C) Albuterol
(D) Pseudoephedrine
(E) Esmolol

13. A neurosurgeon decides to start a patient on a diuretic that works by altering the diffusion of water relative to sodium (an osmotic diuretic) that is helpful in reducing cerebral edema. Which agent did the physician likely prescribe?

(A) Furosemide
(B) Hydrochlorothiazide
(C) Spironolactone
(D) Acetazolamide
(E) Mannitol

14. Which of the following would be useful in treating nocturnal enuresis?

(A) Mannitol
(B) Indomethacin
(C) Furosemide
(D) Vasopressin
(E) Probenecid

15. Vasopressin …

(A) Reduces ADH levels
(B) Increases Na^+ permeability of the collecting duct
(C) Inserts aquaporins into the plasma membrane of collecting duct cells
(D) Increases diffusion of sodium
(E) Reduces production of prostaglandins

16. A 45-year-old male with a 60-pack/year history of smoking presents to his primary care provider with loss of appetite, nausea, vomiting, and muscle weakness. His chest CT reveals enlarged hilar lymph nodes and a suspicious mass in the left hilar region. A presumptive diagnosis of lung cancer is made. Laboratory results reveal low levels of sodium, which in this setting has likely contributed to the syndrome of inappropriate ADH secretion. Which medication might be helpful for this patient's symptoms?

(A) Clofibrate
(B) Conivaptan
(C) Allopurinol
(D) Acetazolamide
(E) Furosemide

17. Which of the following drugs inhibits xanthine oxidase?

(A) Colchicine
(B) Indomethacin
(C) Probenecid
(D) Clofibrate
(E) Allopurinol

18. Which of the following is a common adverse effect of quinidine?

(A) Cinchonism
(B) Lupus-like syndrome
(C) Seizures
(D) Constipation
(E) Pulmonary fibrosis

19. What is the mechanism of action of β-blockers in heart disease?

(A) Prolongation of AV conduction
(B) Activation of the sympathetic system
(C) Promotion of automaticity
(D) Increase in heart rate
(E) Arteriolar vasodilation

20. Which of the following would be useful in the management of arrhythmia due to Wolf-Parkinson-White syndrome?

(A) Digoxin
(B) Lidocaine
(C) Amiodarone
(D) Adenosine
(E) Atropine

21. Which of the following inhibit HMG-CoA reductase?

(A) Nicotinic acid
(B) Rosuvastatin
(C) Ezetimibe
(D) Cholestyramine
(E) Gemfibrozil

22. Which of the following would be a good option to help a patient fall asleep with minimal "hangover"?

(A) Secobarbital
(B) Zolpidem

(C) Chlordiazepoxide
(D) Flumazenil
(E) Buspirone

23. Which of the following is a good choice to treat newly diagnosed generalized anxiety disorder (GAD) in a patient who is a truck driver?

(A) Alprazolam
(B) Triazolam
(C) Buspirone
(D) Trazodone
(E) Thiopental

24. A 57-year-old man with a strong family history of Parkinson's disease sees a neurologist for an evaluation. On examination, the neurologist notes a slight pill-rolling tremor and subtle gait abnormalities. He begins the treatment with levodopa, along with the addition of carbidopa. How does carbidopa work in this setting?

(A) Restores dopamine levels in the substantia nigra
(B) Inhibits monoamine oxidase (MAO)
(C) Inhibits catechol-O-methyltransferase (COMT)
(D) Functions as a dopamine agonist
(E) Inhibits the metabolism of levodopa outside the central nervous system (CNS)

25. The patient in the previous question returns to see his neurologist 3 years later. At this time the patient's symptoms have progressed, and he has now marked bradykinesia and a profound shuffling gait. In an attempt to prevent further deterioration, the neurologist prescribes a catechol-O-methyltransferase (COMT) inhibitor on top of the patient's levodopa and carbidopa. Which agent below is likely to have been added?

(A) Entacapone
(B) Selegiline
(C) Ropinirole
(D) Amantadine
(E) Benztropine

26. Which of the following is a noncompetitive NMDA receptor inhibitor that can be used to treat Alzheimer disease?

(A) Memantine
(B) Donepezil
(C) Tacrine
(D) Tolcapone
(E) Pramipexole

27. A 43-year-old high-profile attorney sees a psychiatrist with expertise in addiction medicine. He explains that he has recently received his third drunk driving citation and fears losing his license to practice unless he stops drinking altogether. He says he "just can't stop" once he starts. He tells the physician that he doesn't have time to attend Alcoholics Anonymous and "wants a pill." The physician explains that there is something that might work if the patient is truly serious. What agent is the physician considering?

(A) Lorazepam
(B) Flumazenil
(C) Naloxone
(D) Disulfiram
(E) Carbamazepine

28. A nonstimulant agent that can be used to treat attention-deficit/hyperactivity disorder (ADHD) is

(A) Methylphenidate
(B) Caffeine
(C) Dextroamphetamine
(D) Atomoxetine
(E) Modafinil

29. Which of the following can be used to treat a 22-year-old with a recent diagnosis of schizophrenia?

(A) Baclofen
(B) Haloperidol
(C) Chloral hydrate
(D) Phenobarbital
(E) Imipramine

30. Soon after drug administration, the patient in the above question begins making odd faces with spastic movements of his neck. Which of the following should be administered to treat these dystonic reactions?

(A) Fluphenazine
(B) Bromocriptine
(C) Dantrolene
(D) Prolactin
(E) Benztropine

31. Which of the following is a potential side effect of clozapine?

(A) Cholestatic jaundice
(B) QT prolongation
(C) Agranulocytosis
(D) Photosensitivity
(E) Galactorrhea

32. Risperidone works primarily through inhibition of receptors for

(A) Dopamine
(B) Serotonin
(C) Histamine
(D) Acetylcholine
(E) Norepinephrine

33. A 7-year-old boy is brought to the neurologist by his mother. She states that the boy's teacher says there are times in class when he stares "into space" and smacks his lips. In the office the boy has one such episode while having an electroencephalogram (EEG), which demonstrates a 3-per-second spike and wave tracing. Which drug is the best for this condition?

(A) Phenytoin
(B) Carbamazepine
(C) Prednisone
(D) Lorazepam
(E) Ethosuximide

34. Compared to valproic acid, carbamazepine, and ethosuximide, which of the following is a unique complication of phenytoin use?

(A) Hepatotoxicity
(B) Gingival hyperplasia
(C) Thrombocytopenia
(D) Aplastic anemia
(E) Stevens-Johnson syndrome

35. Tiagabine works by

(A) Inhibiting GABA uptake by inhibiting the GABA transporter
(B) Increasing GABA by stimulating its release from neurons
(C) Increasing GABA-stimulated chloride channel opening
(D) Prolonging GABA-induced channel opening
(E) Blocking T-type calcium channels

36. Which of the following agents is FDA approved for first line treatment of diabetic neuropathy?

(A) Phenytoin
(B) Carbamazepine
(C) Acetazolamide
(D) Valproic acid
(E) Pregabalin

37. A 5-year-old boy is brought to the emergency room by his parents after they found him with an empty bottle of aspirin. They are not sure how many tablets the boy has consumed. On examination, the child is hyperpneic and lethargic. While an emergency treatment is started, a sample is drawn for an arterial blood determination. What pattern is most likely to be indicated by the arterial blood gas values?

(A) Mixed metabolic alkalosis and respiratory alkalosis
(B) Mixed respiratory alkalosis and metabolic acidosis
(C) Mixed respiratory acidosis and metabolic acidosis
(D) Mixed respiratory acidosis and metabolic alkalosis
(E) Mixed metabolic acidosis and metabolic alkalosis

38. Which of the following is an antineoplastic agent that has been shown to help patients with rheumatoid arthritis?

(A) Valdecoxib
(B) Ketorolac
(C) Methotrexate
(D) Entocort
(E) Auranofin

39. Which of the following is true regarding infliximab?

(A) It is a recombinant antibody to TNF-α
(B) It is a humanized antibody to TNF-α
(C) It is a fusion protein that binds to TNF-α receptor
(D) It is a recombinant protein resembling IL-1
(E) It is a recombinant protein composed of a portion of LFA-3

40. Which of the following is useful in an acute gout attack?

(A) Probenecid
(B) Sulfinpyrazone
(C) Allopurinol
(D) Colchicine
(E) Celecoxib

41. What is the mechanism of action of tacrolimus?

(A) It inhibits transport to the nucleus of the transcription factor NF-AT
(B) It stimulates apoptosis of some lymphoid lineages
(C) It decreases the activity of calcineurin

(D) It inhibits mTOR, which in turn delays the G_1–S transition
(E) It inhibits proliferation of promyelocytes

42. Which of the following is an alkylating agent that may cause hemorrhagic ceptitis and cardiomyopathy?

(A) Azathioprine
(B) Cyclosporine
(C) Tacrolimus
(D) Cyclophosphamide
(E) Basiliximab

43. Your resident asks you what the mechanism of action of tPA is. What is your answer?

(A) It inhibits platelet aggregation
(B) It increases antithrombin activity
(C) It impairs inhibits fibrin polymerization
(D) It blocks GPIIa/IIIb
(E) It activates plasminogen bound to fibrin

44. Which of the following is an antidote for iron overdose?

(A) Protamine
(B) Deferoxamine
(C) Vitamin K
(D) Fresh frozen plasma
(E) Charcoal

45. Which of the following medications would provide the best relief from episodic attacks of Ménière's disease?

(A) Furosemide
(B) Ondansetron
(C) Diazepam
(D) Emetrol
(E) Phentermine

46. A 56-year-old female with severe rheumatoid arthritis returns to see her rheumatologist. She had been referred to a gastroenterologist, who had found multiple gastric ulcers on esophogastroduodenoscopy. She is reluctant to give up the use of NSAIDS and afraid of the potential cardiovascular toxicity of COX-2 inhibitor. At this point, what would be reasonable for the rheumatologist to prescribe?

(A) Omeprazole
(B) Lansoprazole
(C) Nizatidine
(D) Metronidazole
(E) Misoprostol

47. A 29-year-old male who recently immigrated to the United States sees his physician for a burning sensation in his epigastrium. He is referred to a gastroenterologist who performs esophogastroduodenoscopy with biopsy that demonstrate ulcers with the presence of *Helicobacter pylori.* Use of which of the following regimens would provide the most effective and shortest treatment?

(A) Pepto Bismol, clarithromycin, amoxicillin, and omeprazole
(B) Pepto Bismol, metronidazole, tetracycline, and ranitidine
(C) Clarithromycin, metronidazole, and omeprazole
(D) Clathromycin, amoxicillin, and omeprazole
(E) Pepto Bismol, metronidazole, and amoxicillin

48. An 83-year-old male with multiple medical problems develops worsening constipation during his hospitalization for lower extremity cellulitis. The hospitalist decides to start giving a laxative. Which of the following is an appropriate choice and why?

(A) Psyllium, because it is a bulk-forming laxative good for chronic constipation
(B) An osmotic agent, such as senna, which is administered rectally
(C) A stool softener such as lactulose administered rectally
(D) A stool softener such as methyl cellulose that inhibits water reabsorption
(E) A salt-containing osmotic agent such as docusate, useful in preventing constipation

49. A 35-year-old intravenous drug abuser in a methadone maintenance program is admitted to the hospital for a work-up of suspected pulmonary tuberculosis. While in the hospital, he complains of diarrhea and cramping. After stool studies return with a negative result, you decide to begin an antidiarrheal. Which of the following is a good choice for this patient?

(A) Kaolin
(B) Codeine
(C) Diphenoxylate
(D) Loperamide
(E) Propantheline

50. Which of the following would be an appropriate treatment to begin in a patient with Crohn's disease?

(A) Glucocorticoids
(B) Sulfasalazine
(C) Bismuth subsalicylate
(D) Octreotide
(E) Loperamide

51. The above patient returns for follow-up, and she still complains of bloody diarrhea, fever, and weight loss. The gastroenterologist has placed her on a trial of steroids, and yet she still complains of her symptoms. The gastroenterologist could consider using which of the following agents?

(A) Infalyte
(B) Opium tincture
(C) Mesalamine
(D) Infliximab
(E) Diphenoxylate

52. Adverse effects seen with high blood levels of theophylline include

(A) Seizures
(B) Arrhythmias
(C) Nervousness
(D) Nausea and vomiting
(E) All of the above

53. A 62-year-old male alcoholic being treated for non-insulin-dependent diabetes mellitus comes to the emergency department with a 1-hour history of nausea, vomiting, headache, hypotension, and profuse sweating. What is the most likely causative agent?

(A) Clomiphene
(B) Glyburide
(C) Chlorpropamide
(D) Nandrolone
(E) Vasopressin

54. An 81-year-old man with a history of coronary artery disease and a recent diagnosis of hypothyroidism presents to the emergency department with an acute myocardial infarction (MI). What is the most likely causative agent?

(A) Medroxyprogesterone
(B) Levothyroxine
(C) Thiocyanate
(D) Flutamide
(E) Diethylstilbestrol (DES)

55. A 32-year-old woman being treated for an acute exacerbation of lupus erythematosus complains of pain on eating. What is the most likely causative agent?

(A) Oxytocin

(B) Androlone

(C) Vasopressin

(D) Prednisone

(E) Clomiphene

56. It is likely that the acquisition of antibiotic resistance in gram-negative bacilli such as vancomycin is a result of

(A) Spontaneous mutation

(B) Transformation

(C) Transduction

(D) Conjugation

(E) Transposition

57. A 30-year-old patient is undergoing chemotherapy for Hodgkin's disease and develops a fever, prompting an admission by his oncologist. He is found to have a severely decreased white blood cell count, and therapy is started with several antibiotics for febrile neutropenia. Assuming his regimen contains imipenem, which of the following must also be administered?

(A) Probenecid

(B) Clavulanic acid

(C) Sulbactam

(D) Cycloserine

(E) Cilastatin

58. A 17-year-old boy presents with right lower quadrant pain with guarding and rebound. A computed tomography (CT) scan demonstrates appendicitis, and he is taken to the operating room. What would be a good antibiotic to administer prophylactically before the surgery?

(A) Cefazolin

(B) Cefoxitin

(C) Ceftriaxone

(D) Aztreonam

(E) Oxacillin

59. A 23-year-old woman, who is 23 weeks pregnant, develops a bladder infection due to *Pseudomonas* spp. She has a documented allergy to penicillin. What is the best choice of treatment given the patient's history and condition?

(A) Cefoxitin

(B) Aztreonam

(C) Imipenem

(D) Piperacillin

(E) Ciprofloxacin

60. A 37-year-old alcoholic is recovering in the hospital from pneumonia due to *Haemophilus influenzae*. His treatment included the use of intravenous antibiotics. The nurse calls you to evaluate the patient as he returned from a visit from his "buddy" outside. The nurse tells you he smells like alcohol and he is flush, warm, and uncomfortable. You suspect a disulfiram-like reaction. Which antibiotic was he likely to be treated with?

(A) Vancomycin

(B) Bacitracin

(C) Chloramphenicol

(D) Isoniazid

(E) Cefamandole

61. Which of the following can occur in an adult patient treated with chloramphenicol?

(A) Gray baby syndrome

(B) Bone marrow suppression

(C) Disulfiram-like reaction

(D) Nephrotoxicity

(E) Ototoxicity

62. A 32-year-old man complains of a persistent, dry cough for several days with a mild fever and fatigue. The family physician suspects a diagnosis of "walking pneumonia" on clinical grounds, presumably due to *Mycoplasma pneumoniae*. Which of the following groups of antibiotics would be effective?

(A) Penicillins

(B) Cephalosporins

(C) Vancomycin

(D) Chloramphenicol

(E) Macrolides

63. Which of the following is a side effect of clindamycin?

(A) Dizziness

(B) Bruising

(C) Difficulty in hearing

(D) Diarrhea

(E) Tendon pain

64. An 18-year-old African-American army recruit with a history of G-6-PDH deficiency is to be stationed in Somalia. During his tour of duty he develops a cyclic fever, malaise, and weakness. A thin blood smear shows malarial organisms within red blood cells. Which antimalarial is likely to exacerbate the hemolysis, given his enzyme deficiency?

(A) Chloroquine
(B) Pyrimethamine
(C) Doxycycline
(D) Primaquine
(E) Sulfasalazine

65. A 54-year-old diabetic woman was seen in the emergency room 3 weeks ago with complaints of swelling, warmth, and pain in her foot. She was diagnosed with cellulitis and sent home on a 10-day course of an oral first-generation cephalosporin. She returns with severe diarrhea, and *Clostridium difficile* is suspected. What is the initial treatment for this condition?

(A) Clindamycin
(B) Metronidazole
(C) Ciprofloxacin
(D) Neomycin
(E) Silver sulfadiazine

66. A 37-year-old woman recently had a large soft tissue sarcoma surgically resected from her retroperitoneum. She is to receive both radiation and chemotherapy, with cyclophosphamide as part of her chemotherapy. Which agent should be given in conjunction with this drug?

(A) MESNA
(B) Allopurinol
(C) Leucovorin
(D) Cilastatin
(E) MOPP

67. A 54-year-old woman is undergoing an experimental high-dose regimen with adriamycin and cyclophosphamide for breast cancer. As this treatment is particularly myelosuppressive, the oncologist is worried that her white blood cell count will drop dangerously low, making her susceptible to opportunistic infections. In addition to the chemotherapy, what is the oncologist likely to administer to prevent neutropenia?

(A) Epoetin alfa
(B) Filgrastim
(C) Interferon alfa-2b
(D) Oprelvekin
(E) Amifostine

68. Trastuzumab works by

(A) Inhibiting the oncoprotein bcr–abl
(B) Blocking estrogen-mediated gene transcription
(C) Preventing phosphorylation of a receptor tyrosine kinase
(D) Targeting cells for destruction by antibody-mediated cellular cytotoxicity (ADCC)
(E) Reducing circulating levels of tumor necrosis factor (TNF)

69. Which of the following might be considered for the treatment of acute myelocytic anemia (M3 variant)?

(A) Cisplatin
(B) Lomustine
(C) Tretinoin
(D) Fluorouracil
(E) Streptozocin

70. Chromosomal studies in a 56-year-old man indicate a (9:22) translocation, the Philadelphia chromosome, confirming the diagnosis of chronic myelocytic leukemia (CML). Which of the following might be used in his treatment?

(A) Anastrozole
(B) Rituximab
(C) Imatinib
(D) Gefitinib
(E) Amifostine

71. Which agent is most likely to be used to treat hairy cell leukemia?

(A) Interferon alfa-2b
(B) Interleukin-2
(C) All-*trans*-retinoic acid
(D) Rituximab
(E) Daunorubicin

72. A 63-year-old woman develops metastatic colon cancer. The pathologist confirms that a biopsy specimen retrieved from a recent colonoscopy demonstrates that the tumor overexpresses epidermal growth factor receptor (EGFR). The oncologist decides to add a monoclonal antibody to EGFR to her treatment. Which of the following would be added?

(A) Rituximab
(B) Erlotinib
(C) Gefitinib
(D) Cetuximab
(E) Traztuzamab

73. Which of the following should be considered to treat an acetaminophen overdose in a 17-year-old girl?

(A) Trientine
(B) Sorbitol
(C) N-acetylcysteine
(D) Ipecac
(E) Diazepam

74. Organophosphate poisoning is treated with

(A) Pralidoxime
(B) Parathion
(C) Amyl nitrate
(D) Bethanechol
(E) Nicotine

75. What should be given to correct coagulopathy due to an overdose of warfarin in a 73-year-old man?

(A) Aminocaproic acid
(B) Vitamin K
(C) Heparin
(D) Vitamin D
(E) Oprelveldn

76. A 60-year-old male patient has had pain from chronic gout for more than 20 years. Until recently, he has been managed successfully with allopurinol but he has recently suffered a series of debilitating attacks. Which of the following would be a reasonable next approach in treating his gout?

(A) Febuxostat
(B) Pegloticase
(C) Indomethacin
(D) Furosemide
(E) Celocoxib

77. The antihypertensive action of which of the following drugs is due, in part, to diminished degradation of bradykinin?

(A) Enalapril
(B) Losartan

(C) Aliskiren
(D) Fludrocortisone
(E) Furosemide

78. A prediabetic female 52-year-old patient with COPD, hypertension, and 2+ proteinurea is being treated with losartan. She complains that she has had a rash and a mild itching since she started losartan. Which of the following drugs would inhibit RAAS and be most suitable for this patient?

(A) Captopril
(B) Enalapril
(C) Aliskirin
(D) Epleronone
(E) Spironolactone

79. A male patient with HTN is being treated with a thiazide and a potassium sparing diuretic. His blood pressure is well controlled with this combination but he complains of tenderness fatty deposits in his pectoral area. Which of the following is the most likely to be causing this adverse effect?

(A) Indapamide
(B) Spironolactone
(C) Amiloride
(D) Chlorthalidone
(E) Hydrocholorothiazide

80. Since the patient in the previous question was treated successfully in terms of his blood pressure, you elect to keep the same overall pharmacologic strategy. Which of the following would allow you to do this?

(A) Aliskirin
(B) Epleronone
(C) Amiloride
(D) Enalapril
(E) Metazolone

Answers and Explanations

1. **The answer is B.** Both carbamazepine and macrolide antibiotics are known inducers of the cytochrome P-450 system. Thus, it is likely that the original therapeutic levels of antiseizure medicine were decreased to nontherapeutic levels when the metabolism of the drug was increased with the addition of the antibiotic. Some common drugs that inhibit P-450 include cimetidine, chloramphenicol, and disulfiram. Impaired renal excretion results in increased, not decreased, levels of drugs. The induction of glucuronyl transferase is a possible drug interaction, although less likely in this case. The P-450 system requires nicotinamide adenine dinucleotide phosphate (NADPH); therefore, a deficiency would result in decreased, not increased, activity by the system.

2. **The answer is C.** Alterations in urinary pH alters renal reabsorption of substances. In this case, alkalinization traps filtered myoglobin in the urine so that it cannot be reabsorbed, which leads to decreased levels in the serum. The other mechanisms such as increasing glomerular filtration and promoting tubular secretion are other potential ways to alter plasma drug/metabolite levels. Myoglobin is not hepatically metabolized; therefore, hepatic or P-450 metabolism would not alter myoglobin levels.

3. **The answer is E.** Loading dose = (desired plasma concentration of the drug) × (volume of distribution). Once the loading dose is given, the formula for the maintenance dose = (desired plasma concentration of drug) × (clearance). The elimination rate = (clearance) × (plasma drug concentration). The half-life of a drug = (amount of drug administered)/(initial plasma concentration). And lastly, the volume of distribution = (amount of drug administered)/(initial plasma concentration).

4. **The answer is D.** By definition, drugs that do not bind to the active site, such as nonnucleotide reverse transcriptase inhibitors, are noncompetitive antagonists. They function by causing changes in the active site so that it cannot bind its native substrate. Agonists are drugs that elicit the same activity as the endogenous substrate, whereas partial agonists only induce some of the activities of the endogenous substrate. Competitive inhibitors, like nucleoside reverse transcriptase inhibitors, can be either reversible or irreversible.

5. **The answer is B.** Phenylephrine is a selective α_1-adrenoreceptor agonist that causes nasal vasoconstriction, which results in decreased nasal secretion. Epinephrine is the most potent of the adrenergic receptor agonists, followed by norepinephrine. Isoproterenol is the weakest antagonist. But the previous three agents also bind β-adrenergic receptors and are not available over the counter. Phentolamine is just the opposite, an α_1-adrenergic antagonist.

6. **The answer is E.** Pilocarpine is a direct-acting muscarinic agonist used in the management of acute narrow-angle glaucoma, often with an indirect-acting muscarinic agonist like physostigmine. Carbonic anhydrase inhibitors (e.g., acetazolamide), β-adrenoreceptor agonists, and even α_2-adrenoreceptor agonists can be used in the treatment of glaucoma.

7. **The answer is C.** In myasthenia gravis, autoantibodies develop to nicotinic acetylcholine receptors, causing impaired neuromuscular dysfunction, which results in muscular fatigue. This fatigue can be treated with acetylcholinesterase inhibitors. Edrophonium is the shortest-acting agent in this class and used to diagnosis this disorder, with such weakness immediately corrected with its use. Pyridostigmine is a longer acting agent used in the treatment of the disease. Bethanecol is a direct-acting muscarinic cholinergic agonist, whereas both scopolamine and methantheline are both muscarinic-receptor antagonists.

8. **The answer is A.** Dantrolene is used in the treatment of malignant hyperthermia and works by inhibiting the release of calcium from the sarcoplasmic reticulum. Baclofen, an

antispasmatic used in the treatment of multiple sclerosis, inhibits synaptic transmission as a GABA$_B$-receptor agonist. Benzodiazepines function to facilitate GABA activity in the central nervous system (CNS) and spinal cord. Pralidoxime (2-PAM) reactivates acetylcholinesterase. Nondepolarizing neuromuscular junction blockers such as atracurium competitively inhibit the effects of acetylcholine.

9. **The answer is B.** Dopamine is useful in the management of congestive heart failure, as it has both positive inotropic effects on the heart and preserves blood flow to the kidneys. Epinephrine and isoproterenol increase cardiac contractility while decreasing peripheral resistance. Albuterol is a β_1 agonist used in the management of asthma, and terbutaline is another β-2 agonist used to suppress labor, in the event of threatened labor of a premature fetus.

10. **The answer is D.** Clonidine activates prejunctional α_2-adrenergic receptors in the central nervous system (CNS) to reduce sympathetic tone, thereby decreasing blood pressure. Activation of α_1-adrenergic receptors increases blood pressure, which is useful for the treatment of hypotension. β_1-Adrenoreceptor agonists are used primarily for increasing heart rate and contractility. β_2-Adrenergic agonists are used to dilate airways in the management of asthma. β-Adrenoreceptor antagonists are used in the treatment of angina and hypertension.

11. **The answer is B.** An α-adrenoreceptor antagonist such as phenoxybenzamine is indicated for the treatment of pheochromocytomas in the preoperative state as well as if the tumor is inoperable. β-Blockers, such as isoproterenol, are then used systemically, following effective α-blockade, to prevent the cardiac effects of excessive catecholamines. Pseudoephedrine is an α-adrenoreceptor antagonist available over the counter to relieve nasal discharge. There is no role for adrenergic receptor agonists such as dopamine or for that matter nondepolarizing muscle relaxants such as pancuronium.

12. **The answer is E.** Esmolol is an ultra-short acting β_1 antagonist that is relatively specific for the heart; however, the short half-life of this drug should allow the anesthesiologist to fine tune the delivery and readily reverse the effects should there be problems with respiration. Atenolol is a much longer acting agent that would not provide such control. Norepinephrine would actually adversely affect the patient's angina, as it is stimulatory to the heart. Albuterol is a β agonist used in the treatment of asthma. Pseudoephedrine is an over-the-counter α agonist used in cold formula preparations.

13. **The answer is E.** Mannitol is an osmotic diuretic frequently used in the management of cerebral edema caused by various insults. This agent works by altering the diffusion of water relative to sodium by "binding" the water, with a resultant reduction of sodium reabsorption. Furosemide and hydrochlorothiazide act by directly altering reabsorption of sodium in various parts of the nephron (choices A and B). Spironolactone (choice C) antagonizes mineralocorticoid receptor. Acetazolamide inhibits carbonic anhydrase (choice D).

14. **The answer is D.** Vasopressin can be tried in cases of recalcitrant nocturnal enuresis. Mannitol is most commonly used in the management of cerebral edema (choice A). Indomethacin can occasionally be used as an antidiuretic agent in diabetic patients (choice B). Furosemide is used in congestive heart failure (choice C). Probenecid is used in the treatment of gout (choice E).

15. **The answer is C.** Vasopressin causes specific water channels termed aquaporins II to be inserted into the plasma membrane of the luminal surface of the medullary collecting ducts. This directly affects permeability of the collecting duct (choice B). Under the conditions of dehydration, as is the case with this patient, the ADH levels increase (choice A). Choice D represents the mechanism of action of osmotic diuretics. Production of prostaglandins is reduced with the use of agents such as indomethacin (choice E).

16. **The answer is B.** Conivaptan is a non-peptide ADH antagonist and as such is useful in the treatment of SIADH, which is commonly seen in patients with lung cancer. Clofibrate (choice A) increases the release of ADH centrally. Allopurinol, acetazolamide, and furosemide do not affect actions of ADH to an appreciable degree (choices C, D, and E).

17. **The answer is E.** Allopurinol is a xanthine oxidase inhibitor and is most commonly used in the treatment of gout. It is not used for acute attacks, rather for the prevention of recurrent episodes. Colchicine (choice A) may be used for an acute episode, as well as in long-term therapy; however, it has a high incidence of side effects. Indomethacin (choice B) is useful for symptomatic treatment of gout. Probenecid (choice C) is also useful for prophylaxis of gout; however, it is not a xanthine oxidase inhibitor. This agent increases the secretion of uric acid. Clofibrate (choice D) is used in the treatment of hypercholesterolemia.

18. **The answer is A.** Cinchonism, or ringing in the ears and dizziness, is common after quinidine use. Lupus-like syndrome (B) can be observed after the use of procainamide. Seizures may occur with the use of lidocaine (C). Diarrhea can occur with the use of quinidine, not constipation (D). Pulmonary fibrosis is a long-term complication of using amiodarone (E).

19. **The answer is A.** β-Blockers prolong AV conduction. They reduce sympathetic stimulation (B). These agents depress automaticity (C). β-Blockers decrease heart rate (D), and can cause arteriolar vasoconstriction (E).

20. **The answer is D.** Adenosine, a class V antiarrhythmic, is used for the treatment of paroxysmal supraventricular tachycardias, including those of Wolf-Parkinson-White syndrome. Digoxin (A) and amiodarone (C) can be used for the management of atrial fibrillation. Lidocaine is used in the treatment of many arrhythmias (B). Atropine is used for bradyarrhythmias.

21. **The answer is B.** Rosuvastatin is an HMG–CoA reductase inhibitor. Nicotinic acid (A) inhibits the process of esterification of fatty acids, thereby reducing plasma triglyceride levels. Ezetimibe (C) reduces cholesterol absorption. Cholestyramine can bind bile acids and prevents their enterohepatic circulation (D). Gemfibrozil (E) reduces hepatic synthesis of cholesterol.

22. **The answer is B.** Zolpidem has actions similar to those of benzodiazepines, although it is structurally unrelated. It is used as a hypnotic and anxiolytic with minimal abuse potential. Barbiturates such as secobarbital are rarely used because of their lethality on overdose. Chlordiazepoxide is a long-acting benzodiazepine, whereas most hypnotics are short-acting benzodiazepines. Flumazenil is a benzodiazepine receptor antagonist that will not reverse the effects of zolpidem. Buspirone is not used as a hypnotic and has little sedative effect.

23. **The answer is C.** Buspirone is a partial serotonin 5-HT$_{1A}$-receptor agonist that has efficacy comparable to that of benzodiazepines for the treatment of anxiety, but is significantly less sedating. Alprazolam is an intermediate-acting benzodiazepine used in the treatment of generalized anxiety disorder (GAD) but still has some sedation, which would be undesirable in this situation. Triazolam is a short-acting benzodiazepine, and trazodone is a heterocyclic antidepressant, both used to induce sleep. Thiopental is a barbiturate sometimes used to induce anesthesia.

24. **The answer is E.** Carbidopa, unlike levodopa, does not penetrate the central nervous system (CNS); it does inhibit levodopa's metabolism in the gi tract, allowing lower doses of levodopa and decreased side effects. Levodopa is a precursor to dopamine and can help restore levels of dopamine in the substantia nigra. Monoamine oxidase inhibitors should be used with caution along with levodopa, as this can lead to a hypertensive crisis. Bromocriptine is a dopamine agonist used in the treatment of Parkinson's disease.

Catechol-*O*-methyltransferase (COMT) inhibitors are yet another class of agents used in the treatment of Parkinson's disease.

25. **The answer is A.** Levodopa is metabolized, in part by catechol-*O*-methyltransferase (COMT); therefore, an inhibitor such as entacapone is an adjunct treatment for patients on levodopa. It does however increase the side effects including diarrhea, postural hypotension, nausea, and hallucinations. Selegiline is a monoamine oxidase inhibitor (MAOI) used in the treatment of Parkinson's disease. Ropinirole is a nonergot dopamine agonist used in early Parkinson's disease that may decrease the need for levodopa in later stages of the disease. Amantadine has an effect on the rigidity of the disease as well as the bradykinesia, although it has no effect on the tremor. Benztropine is muscarinic cholinoceptor antagonist used as an adjunct drug in Parkinson disease.

26. **The answer is A.** Memantine is an NMDA-receptor inhibitor that is well tolerated and, although controversial, has been shown in some studies to slow the rate of cognitive decline in Alzheimer patients. Donepezil and tacrine are acetylcholinesterase inhibitors that have been shown, like memantine, to have similar controversial activities. Tolcapone is a catechol-*O*-methyltransferase (COMT) inhibitor rarely used in Parkinson disease because of the possibility of hepatic necrosis. Pramipexole is used as a dopamine receptor agonist in the management of Parkinson disease.

27. **The answer is D.** Disulfiram is an inhibitor of aldehyde dehydrogenase, which blocks the breakdown of acetaldehyde to acetate during the metabolism of alcohol. The buildup of acetaldehyde results in flushing, tachycardia, hypertension, and nausea to invoke a conditioned response to avoid alcohol ingestion, including that found in over-the-counter medications and in some foods. Lorazepam is useful in the prevention of seizures as a result of alcohol withdrawal, whereas carbamazepine is used should they develop. Flumazenil is used for benzodiazepine overdose and naloxone for opioid overdose.

28. **The answer is D.** Atomoxetine is a nonstimulant drug used in the management of attention-deficit/hyperactivity disorder (ADHD) that works by inhibiting norepinephrine reuptake. The stimulate agents used for the treatment of ADHD include methylphenidate and dextroamphetamine and work by inhibiting dopamine reuptake. Caffeine is a stimulant in many beverages, which may have some role in the management of some headaches. Modafinil is a newer agent used in the treatment of narcolepsy.

29. **The answer is B.** Haloperidol is an antipsychotic agent used in acute psychotic attacks and for the treatment of schizophrenia. It is a dopamine-receptor antagonist that acts predominately at the dopamine D_2 receptor. Baclofen is a $GABA_B$ receptor antagonist that is used in the treatment of spinal cord injuries. Choral hydrate is a hypnotic agent that works similarly to ethanol. Phenobarbital is a barbiturate used in the treatment of seizures and as an anesthetic. Imipramine is a tricyclic antidepressant and is not used in schizophrenia.

30. **The answer is E.** Acute dystonias are a complication of antipsychotics that work primarily through dopamine D_2 receptors and therefore have a high incidence of extrapyramidal effects. Haloperidol and agents such as fluphenazine are the most likely offenders. Such reactions are best managed with an anticholinergic agent such as benztropine. Another complication of haloperidol is the neuroleptic malignant syndrome, which is treated with a dopamine agonist receptor and dantrolene. Hyperprolactinemia with galactorrhea is common with agents that block dopamine's actions, as dopamine normally represses prolactin release.

31. **The answer is C.** Agranulocytosis occurs more frequently with clozapine than with other agents, requiring routine blood tests. It is the only agent that improves the negative symptoms of schizophrenia. Cholestatic jaundice and photosensitivity are common with chlorpromazine. Galactorrhea is a side effect of older high-potency agents that block dopamine. QT prolongation is a complication of agents such as thioridazine and ziprasidone.

32. **The answer is B.** The unique affinities of various antipsychotics result in their unique activities and their unique side effects. Risperidone is an atypical antipsychotic that works by blocking the 5-HT$_{2A}$ serotonin receptor. The older high-potency antipsychotics inhibit dopamine receptors. Agents such as clozapine inhibit histamine receptors. Atropine is an antagonist at cholinergic receptors.

33. **The answer is E.** Ethosuximide is the drug of choice for absence seizures in children. Valproic acid has more side effects and therefore is a second-line drug. Prednisone is used in infantile seizures. Phenytoin and carbamazepine can be used in partial seizures or in tonic-clonic seizures. Lorazepam is often used in the treatment of status epilepticus.

34. **The answer is B.** Gingival hyperplasia is a unique side effect of phenytoin, which can be partially avoided by meticulous oral hygiene. Several anticonvulsants can cause hepatotoxicity, including valproic acid. Aplastic anemia is a rare, but a potential complication of carbamazepine, ethosuximide. Valproic acid is also associated with thrombocytopenia. Ethosuximide has been associated with a severe form of erythema multiforme, the Steven-Johnson syndrome.

35. **The answer is A.** Tiagabine is an anticonvulsant used in conjunction with drugs such as phenytoin. Its mechanism is related to its ability to inhibit GABA transport into the cell, thereby decreasing GABA uptake. Gabapentin works by stimulating the release of GABA from neurons. Benzodiazepines function to increase GABA-stimulated chloride channel opening, whereas barbiturates prolong GABA-induced chloride channel opening. Ethosuximide works by blocking T-type calcium channels.

36. **The answer is E.** Many antiseizure drugs find applications for other diseases. Pregabalin is approved for the treatment of diabetic nephropathy, an unfortunate consequence in this patient's presentation. Phenytoin is also used for the treatment of arrhythmias. Carbamazepine is used in the management of trigeminal neuralgia. It is occasionally used as a third-line agent to treat diabetic nephropathy. Acetazolamide, sometimes used as a treatment for absence seizure control, is used in the treatment of glaucoma. Valproic acid can be used in the prophylaxis of migraine headaches.

37. **The answer is B.** Salicylate toxicity initially increases the medullary response to carbon dioxide, with resulting hyperventilation and respiratory alkalosis. Increase in lactic acid and ketone body formation results in a metabolic acidosis. All other choices are incorrect in this particular setting. The treatment includes correction of acid–base disturbances, replacement of electrolytes and fluids, cooling, alkalinization of urine, and forced diuresis.

38. **The answer is C.** From the presented list, only methotrexate is known to be an antineoplastic agent. This medication has been used successfully in rheumatoid arthritis and other rheumatologic conditions. Valdecoxib (A) is a COX-2 inhibitor that has been recently removed from the market. Ketorolac (B) is a powerful analgesic used for multiple autoimmune conditions. Entocort (D) is a glucocorticoid that can be used in some arthritides. Auranofin (E) is a gold compound that is rarely used anymore.

39. **The answer is A.** Infliximab is a recombinant antibody to TNF-α; it has been successfully used in the treatment of Crohn's disease, rheumatoid arthritis, and some other autoimmune conditions. Choice B represents Humira, an agent also used for rheumatoid arthritis. Choice C is Etanercept, a subcutaneous agent approved for the treatment of rheumatoid arthritis. Choice D represents anakinra, an IL-1 blocker also used for rheumatoid arthritis. Choice E is alefacept, an agent used for psoriasis.

40. **The answer is D.** Colchicine is often used to treat an acute gouty attack. Probenecid (A) and sulfinpyrazone (B) reduce urate levels by preventing reabsorption of uric acid. These agents are used for chronic gout. Allopurinol (C) is a xanthine oxidase inhibitor; it is also used for the treatment of chronic gout. Celecoxib is a COX-2 inhibitor.

41. **The answer is C.** Tacrolimus decreases the activity of calcineurin, which leads to a decrease in nuclear NF-AT and the transcription of T-cell-specific lymphokines and early T-cell activation. Choice A refers to mechanism of action of cyclosporine. Choice B refers to glucocorticoids. Choice D represents the mechanism of action of sirolimus. Choice E refers to azathioprine.

42. **The answer is D.** Cyclophosphamide has been successfully used for the treatment of lupus nephritis; however, it does carry significant morbidity associated with its use. Azathioprine works by suppressing T-cell activity (A). Cyclosporine inhibits T-helper cell activation (B). Tacrolimus inhibits transcription of T-cell-specific lymphokines (C). Baciliximab is a monoclonal antibody against CD-25 used to reduce the incidence and severity of renal transplant rejection.

43. **The answer is E.** As the name suggests, tPA activates plasminogen bound to plasmin, thereby acting as a thrombolytic. Choice A refers to clopidogrel and ticlopidine. Choice B refers to heparin and its analogues. Choice C refers to dextran. Finally, choice D refers to abciximab.

44. **The answer is B.** Deferoxamine is an iron-chelating agent and as such can be given in cases of iron supplement overdose. Protamine (A) is an antidote for heparin. Vitamin K (C) and fresh frozen plasma (D) are given for coumarin reversal. Charcoal is an agent sometimes used for gastric lavage.

45. **The answer is C.** Diazepam and lorazepam are very effective in treating the vertigo associated with Ménière's disease. Loop diuretics, such as furosemide, can precipitate vertigo secondary to volume depletion and resultant orthostatic hypotension. Ondansetron is a powerful antiemetic. Emetrol is an over-the-counter (OTC) antiemetic for infants. Phentermine is an amphetamine derivative that has been used for weight loss.

46. **The answer is E.** Misoprostol is approved for use in patients taking NSAIDS, both to decrease acid production and to increase bicarbonate and mucous production. Both omeprazole and lansoprazole are proton inhibitors that would not increase the protective mucous and bicarbonate. Nizatidine is an H_2-blocker that would also do nothing to increase the production of protective prostaglandins. Metronidazole is an antibiotic used to treat *Helicobacter pylori.*

47. **The answer is A.** Pepto Bismol, clarithromycin and amoxicillin, and omeprazole can be used for 7 days to eradicate *Helicobacter pylori* associated with peptic ulcer disease (metronidazole and tetracycline are additional choices for antibiotics). Choice E (Pepto Bismol, metronidazole, and amoxicillin) was the original triple therapy. The use of a proton pump inhibitor is usually preferred to an H_2-blocker, as in Choice B. Regimens containing clarithromycin are used for cases of resistance to metronidazole.

48. **The answer is A.** Psyllium and methyl cellulose are bulk-forming agents good for chronic constipation. The osmotic agent lactulose is given orally. Stool softeners such as docusate are useful in preventing constipation. Salt-containing osmotic agents such as magnesium sulfate are good for acute evacuation of the bowels. Senna is an irritant agent that stimulates intestinal motility.

49. **The answer is D.** Loperamide would be a good choice in this patient as it effectively controls diarrhea. Both codeine and diphenoxylate are opioids with abuse potential, especially in patients with abusive histories. Diphenoxylate is available in combination with atropine to reduce the potential for abuse. Anticholinergics such as propantheline prevent cramping but have little effect on diarrhea. Kaolin is good for absorbing toxins from the intestines.

50. **The answer is A.** Glucocorticoids are used in the management of moderate cases of Crohn's disease. 5-Amino salicylic acid (5-ASA) compounds such as sulfasalazine are used in mild cases of ulcerative colitis. Octreotide is used for diarrhea secondary to increased

release of gastrointestinal hormones. Bismuth subsalicylate and loperamide can be used in the treatment of uncomplicated diarrhea.

51. **The answer is D.** Infliximab is an anti-TNFα monoclonal antibody approved for the treatment of refractory Crohn's disease when mesalamine or steroids fail. Infalyte is an oral rehydration solution used in cases of childhood diarrhea. Opium tincture and diphenoxylate are opioid preparations for uncomplicated diarrhea.

52. **The answer is E.** Theophylline is associated with all of the reactions listed. They usually occur at elevated blood levels, generally accepted as greater than 20 µg/dL. However, adverse drug reactions may occur at any blood level.

53. **The answer is C.** A disulfiram-like reaction may be seen in noninsulin-dependent diabetics treated with chlorpropamide, an oral hypoglycemic, when used in combination with alcohol.

54. **The answer is B.** Elderly patients with subclinical hypothyroidism are at risk for arrhythmias, angina, or myocardial infarction (MI) if they have underlying cardiovascular disease when they begin treatment with thyroid hormones such as levothyroxine. These potential adverse effects occur because of increased cardiovascular work load as well as the direct effect of thyroid hormone on the heart.

55. **The answer is D.** Prednisone, a steroid commonly used to treat exacerbations of lupus erythematosus, can cause peptic ulcer disease due to the inhibition of the prostaglandins that normally protect the mucosa.

56. **The answer is D.** Conjugation is the principal mechanism for the acquisition of antibiotic resistance among enterobacteria and involves the transfer of resistance transfer factors on plasmids through sex pili. The other mechanisms for gene transfer, including random mutation, transformation, transduction, and transposition are not as common among these organisms.

57. **The answer is E.** Cilastatin must be given with imipenem. It is an inhibitor of renal dehydropeptidase, which normally would degrade imipenem. Probenecid increases penicillin concentrations by blocking their excretion by the kidney. Both clavulanic acid and sulbactam are penicillinase inhibitors used to increase the spectrum against penicillinase-producing species. Cycloserine is a second-line agent for gram-negative organisms and tuberculosis.

58. **The answer is A.** Cefazolin, a first-generation cephalosporin, is often used for surgical prophylaxis because it has activity against most gram-positive and some gram-negative organisms. Second-generation agents (cefoxitin) and third-generation agents (ceftriaxone) are not used because they have less gram-positive coverage. Aztreonam lacks activity against anaerobes and gram-positive organisms. Oxacillin is primarily active against staphylococci.

59. **The answer is B.** Aztreonam is active against *Pseudomonas* spp., appears to be safe during pregnancy, and does not show cross-hypersensitivity with penicillins. Piperacillin, cefoxitin, and imipenem all have some overlap in penicillin-allergic patients. Although ciprofloxacin is good in nonpregnant patients, it is absolutely contraindicated in pregnancy.

60. **The answer is E.** Cefamandole, a cephalosporin, is known to precipitate a disulfiram-like reaction. Bacitracin is not used intravenously, only topically. Chloramphenicol is associated with bone marrow suppression. Vancomycin can be associated with flush on infusion. Isoniazid is an antituberculoid antibiotic.

61. **The answer is B.** Bone marrow suppression results in pancytopenia in treated patients, which in rare cases can lead to aplastic anemia. Gray baby syndrome is associated with chloramphenicol use in infants. Disulfiram-like reactions can occur with some cephalosporins. Aminoglycosides and vancomycin can result in nephrotoxicity and ototoxicity.

62. **The answer is E.** Macrolides such as azithromycin or clarithromycin are the agents of choice for the treatment of mycoplasmal diseases. As mycoplasmas have no cell wall, drugs such as penicillins, cephalosporins, or vancomycin are ineffective. Chloramphenicol is relatively toxic and reserved for select infections.

63. **The answer is D.** Diarrhea due to pseudomembranous colitis with *Clostridium difficile* overgrowth is common with many broad-spectrum antibiotics, especially clindamycin. Bruising can occur with some cephalosporins. Dizziness is common with tetracyclines, such as minocycline. Ototoxicity can result in hearing loss with vancomycin and aminoglycosides. Tendon pain is possible due to the cartilage toxicity associated with fluoroquinolones.

64. **The answer is D.** Primaquine is associated with intravascular hemolysis or methemoglobinuria in G-6-PDH deficiency patients, as it causes oxidative damage to hemoglobin. Chloroquine and pyrimethamine do not cause hemolysis, although they are often used with sulfa drugs, which can cause hemolysis in such patients. Chloroquine rarely causes hemolysis, and doxycycline is not known to cause problems in G-6-PDH deficiency.

65. **The answer is B.** Metronidazole is the preferred treatment for *Clostridium difficile* colitis, which probably resulted from the patient's use of a broad-spectrum antibiotic for her initial infection. Vancomycin is considered in the treatment of *Clostridium difficile* colitis in refractory cases. The use of Clindamycin is often associated with *Clostridium difficile* colitis. Ciprofloxacin can be used for the treatment of diverticulitis, but not colitis. Neomycin is used to sterilize the bowel, which is not the goal in this case. Silver sulfadiazine is used to treat skin infections in burn patients.

66. **The answer is A.** MESNA is often given with cyclophosphamide and ifosfamide to help detoxify metabolic products that can cause hemorrhagic cystitis. Allopurinol is given with chemotherapy agents such as busulfan to reduce renal precipitation of urate. Leucovorin is given to rescue patients in the case of methotrexate toxicity. Cilastatin is an inhibitor of imipenem degradation. MOPP is a multidrug regimen (mechlorethamine, Oncovin (vincristine), procarbazine, and prednisone) used in the treatment of Hodgkin's disease.

67. **The answer is B.** Filgrastim is a recombinant form of granulocyte colony-stimulating factor (G-CSF) given to prevent chemotherapy-induced neutropenia. Epoetin alfa is commonly used to prevent anemia while on chemotherapy. Oprelvekin is an agent used to help treat chemotherapy-induced thrombocytopenia. Interferon alfa-2b is used in the management of specific leukemias and lymphomas. Amifostine is given to patients receiving radiation to the head and neck to preserve salivary function.

68. **The answer is C.** Trastuzumab is an antibody to the extracellular domain of the receptor tyrosine kinase HER2/neu. In some breast cancers, HER2/neu is expressed in high levels leading to auto-phosphorylation in the absence of ligand binding. Trastuzumab blocks such signaling. Imatinib is used in treating chronic myelogenous leukemia and inhibits bcr–abl. Tamoxifen functions by inhibiting estrogen-mediated gene transcription. Rituximab targets CD20$^+$ cells in B-cell lymphomas for ADCC. Thalidomide works in part by inhibiting TNF production.

69. **The answer is C.** Tretinoin is all-*trans*-retinoic acid and produces remission by inducing differentiation in the M3 variant of acute myelogenous leukemia (AML), characterized by aberrant expression of a retinoic receptor-α gene. Cisplatin is often used in the treatment of cancers of the lung, head, and neck. Lomustine has good central nervous system (CNS) penetration and is used in treating brain tumors. Fluorouracil is also used in treating multiple tumors including those of the breast and colon. Lastly, streptozocin is used in the treatment of insulinomas.

70. **The answer is C.** Imatinib is an orally active small molecule inhibitor of the oncogenic bcr–abl kinase produced as a result of the Philadelphia chromosome, used to treat chronic myelogenous leukemia. It also inhibits the c-Kit receptor and can be used in treating gastrointestinal stromal tumors (GISTS). Anastrozole is used in the management of breast cancer. Rituximab is an antibody used in the treatment of non-Hodgkin lymphoma. Gefitinib is an orally active small molecule inhibitor of the EGF receptor, used in the treatment of some lung cancer. Amifostine is used as a radio-protectant, with or without cisplatin.

71. **The answer is A.** Interferon alfa-2b is used for the treatment of hairy cell leukemia, chronic myeloid leukemia, Kaposi sarcoma, and lymphomas. Interleukin-2 is used in the treatment of metastatic renal cell carcinoma. All-*trans*-retinoic acid is used to induce remission in M3 acute myelogenous leukemia (AML). Although sometimes used to treat hairy cell leukemia, rituximab is used primarily to treat CD20$^+$ non-Hodgkin lymphoma. Daunorubicin is an antibiotic-type compound used in the treatment of some leukemias and lymphomas.

72. **The answer is D.** Cetuximab inhibits the EGF receptor by binding to the extracellular domain of the receptor. Other EGFR signaling inhibitors include erlotinib and gefinitib, although both of these molecules are orally active and penetrate the cell to perturb EGFR signaling from within the cell. Rituximab and Traztuzamab are both antibodies as well, but are used in the treatment of non-Hodgkin lymphoma and breast cancer, respectively.

73. **The answer is C.** N-acetylcysteine is used in the case of acetaminophen toxicity. It provides sulfhydryl groups for the regeneration of glutathione stores in the body. Trientine is a copper-chelating agent sometimes used in Wilson's disease. Sorbitol is used as a cathartic to help remove toxins from the gastrointestinal tract. Ipecac has been used to induce emesis in cases of toxic ingestions. Diazepam can be used to prevent seizures when strychnine is ingested.

74. **The answer is A.** Pralidoxime reactivates acetylcholinesterase to reverse the effects of exposure to organophosphates, of which parathion is actually an example. Amyl nitrate can be used in cases of ingestion of the cytochrome oxidase inhibitor cyanide. Bethanechol is a direct-acting muscarinic cholinoceptor agonist used to treat urinary retention and overdose and can result in symptoms similar to organophosphate poisoning. Nicotine is sometimes found in insecticides and can cause vomiting, weakness, seizures, and respiratory arrest.

75. **The answer is B.** Warfarin is an orally active inhibitor of vitamin K-dependent carboxylation of various clotting factors. In the event of supratherapeutic doses of warfarin, the anticoagulation can be reversed by giving vitamin K. Heparin is an intravenous preparation that is also an anticoagulation agent. Aminocaproic acid inhibits plasminogen activation and is used in the treatment of hemophilia. Vitamin D is used in cases of its deficiency or in the treatment of osteoporosis. Oprelvekin is a recombinant form of interleukin-11 that stimulates platelet production and does not affect the clotting factors.

76. **The answer is B.** Pegloticase is a recombinant uricase, an enzyme mutated and nonfunctional in humans. Uricase metabolizes uric acid to water-soluble allantoin. Pegloticase is approved for cases of refractory gout. It is highly effective but must be administered by infusion and is expensive.

77. **The answer is A.** Inhibition of ACE reduces the formation of the active metabolite AgII, but also reduces the proteolytic breakdown of the potent vasodilator. This contributes significantly to the antihypertensive action of ACE inhibitors. The remaining drugs to not alter bradykinin metabolism.

78. **The answer is C.** Inhibition of RAAS has been shown to slow the progression of kidney damage in Type 2 diabetes. Since the patient has COPD, ACE inhibitors would be contra-indicated because of the potential to worsen cough. She has demonstrated a sensitivity to an ARB; she is likely to have a sensitivity to other ARBs. Aliskerin is a small-molecule inhibitor of renin.

79. **The answer is B.** Spironolactone blocks androgen and glucocorticoid receptors as well as mineralocorticoid receptors. This can cause proliferation and tenderness of mammary tissue.

80. **The answer is B.** Epleronone is a much more specific mineralocorticoid receptor antago-nist than sprinolactone and is not associated with gynocomastia. Amiloride is another potassium-sparing diuretic but acts to block renal ENa channels.

Index

Note: Page numbers in *italics* denote figures; those followed by "t" denote boxes; Q denotes questions; E denotes explanations

A